STAND
UP
STRAIGHT!

STAND UP STRAIGHT!

A History of Posture

SANDER L. GILMAN

REAKTION BOOKS

To Marina V. E. Gilman,

who taught me to stand up straight!

Published by Reaktion Books Ltd
Unit 32, Waterside
44–48 Wharf Road
London N1 7UX, UK
www.reaktionbooks.co.uk

First published 2018
Copyright © Sander L. Gilman 2018

Printed and bound in Great Britain by Bell & Bain, Glasgow

A catalogue record for this book is available from the British Library

ISBN 978 1 78023 924 8

Contents

Preface

POSTURE IS, as we shall see, a contentious as well as a contradictory concept in Western culture. To write its history in any
comprehensive way means being encyclopaedic rather than critical.
The chapters in this book reflect the ambiguity of posture in a number
of cultural and disciplinary realms. As will become obvious, these blend
into one another in odd and often surprising ways over time. Who would
have thought, for example, that the aesthetics of eighteenth century art
was shaped both by ideas of dance education and by medical intervention? Who would have imagined that arguments for and against slavery
both relied on theories of posture?

Each chapter is thus anecdotal rather than exhaustive. Each story
I tell relies on some existing critical work. Yet the totality of thinking
about posture as a structuring element in how we define the human
as an ethical, moral and functioning being has to date been lacking.
The moment we look at the military or at fashion or at pathology or
at aesthetics as independent disciplines, posture seems to become a
limited and rather pedestrian notion. This point has been made to me
often when I have recounted (often at too great a length) to my trapped
listeners my obsession with the ubiquity of posture. Following my presentation at medical humanities rounds at a major medical school, I
overheard one of my listeners comment: 'Who would have imagined
posture was that interesting?' Well, it is, and I hope this book leads to
further queries about its ubiquity and meanings.

By linking all these categories (and many others not directly examined in this book), the use of posture can start to be understood in
the often subtle appeals of its moral, ethical and critical implications.

Stand Up Straight! is a directive to moral action as well as to a phys-ical reaction. Posture comes to be a limiting case for the human. My work on the subject emerged from my work on stereotyping and our anxiety about who we are and whom we can become as humans. It is one more building block in a history of perception. But it is also, and this is perhaps more important, a measure of how much and perhaps how easily we integrate such perceptions of what it means to be human into our bodies and minds. We become the ideal of what we believe we must become, and avoid that which we believe is deleterious to our sense of self. We stand and sit and move not only because of sets of muscles and ligaments and bodily systems that allow us to do so, with real and present limitations, but because of what we believe and what the implications of such beliefs are.

As with many of my earlier works, I rely on a wide range of tex-tual and visual sources for my evidence. Michael Lynch states that 'visibility in science', in the form of data displays, 'constitute[s] the material form of scientific phenomena'.[1] It is certainly the case that scientific data, as we have long known, are made visible within sci-ence through charts and statistical representations. Yet other forms of representations have had (and still have) a role in scientific argument – from photographs to films. As are charts, graphs and data patterns of all sorts, they are often closely related to representations as cultural phenomena. Indeed, the idea that visual data has special significance only as scientific evidence belies its visual presence in all forms in the worlds of advertising, fine art and, indeed, caricature. Visual evidence inhabits a place where general, aesthetic and scientific meanings over-lap, often with unforeseen consequences. *Studying* posture in culture means *seeing* posture.

Stand Up Straight! is the first attempt to provide a sketch (and it is no more than that) of what I hope will be an engaging way of seeing cultural history as a formative aspect across multiple disciplines. These are all disciplines created to explain aspects of human nature using pos-ture as a litmus test. They thus receive their substance from world views that emphasize specialist knowledge but which simultaneously reflect cultural presuppositions. Cutting across disciplines in the way I have in this volume may highlight some connections otherwise not seen and provide links between the various levels of the meaning of posture.

Introduction:
Posture Beyond the Workplace

AT THE CLOSE OF 2015 the health columnist of the *New York Times*, Jane Brody, wrote that she had received a letter from 'a distraught wife [who] begged me to write about the importance of good posture. "My husband sits for many hours a day slouched over his computer," she said. "I've told him repeatedly this is bad for his body – he should sit up straight – but he pays no attention to me. He reads you every week. Maybe he'll listen to you."'¹ Brody's reply began: 'Slouching is bad. It's bad not only for your physical health, but also for your emotional and social well-being.' For her, good posture is good health, and good health demands good posture. Brody doesn't say so, but she views our bodies as ill-fitted for the modern world. Our work habits, our technology, even our vulnerability to crime are all affected by our posture. Indeed, how we think is affected, since 'slouching can also reduce lung capacity by as much as 30 percent, reducing the amount of oxygen that reaches body tissues, including the brain.' The bottom line of this fascination with posture is that we are *Homo economicus*, workers whose posture bears on our ability to function as economic entities.

Posture so defined has long been part of our world of economic productivity. As early as the nineteenth century, 'brain' workers were seen to suffer from 'diverse effects of fatigue' – 'the carriage is enervated; their posture is weighted down.' All feared 'that the energy of mind and body was dissipating under the strain of modernity'.² Today this theme continues in odd ways. The craze for standing desks that exploded among the American intelligentsia in the early twenty-first century (mimicking the desk of Charles Dickens's Bob Cratchit, minus

9

the stool) equates good posture with productivity. Ebenezer Scrooge would have applauded this, since the desks in his counting house assured that he could observe his workers at all times. Indeed, over and over again in the literature on standing desks the idea is put forth that good posture, defined by some authority, determines our physical and mental health and these in turn define our role, for good or ill, in society. As two writers noted in the title of their volume, 'sitting is the new smoking.'[3] Another asked, 'Can chairs kill us?', which was quickly answered in the positive: 'They are out to get us, to harm us, to kill us.'[4] Our bodies, it is claimed, did not evolve to sit but to stand, and standing is our healthier and more natural state. But it is the natural state in which to work. So much so that this association has become the stuff of satire:

> I can tell by looking at your little warped potato body – now don't get offended, that's just how it looks from up here – that you sit all day while working at *your* desk. Don't tell me – probably in a chair? I figured. I used to be like you! Sitting at home, sitting on the train to work, sitting at work, sitting sitting sitting. A quick aside – did you know that sitting in a chair all day will literally cause your body to reject your spine? I *know*.[5]

Such views linking posture, health and sitting are certainly not an invention of the twenty-first century. The standing desk came to be thought of as a cure for specific diseases of 'literary and sedentary persons', as we read in the notes to the English translation of Samuel-Auguste Tissot's thesis *De valetudine litteratorum* (On the Health of Men of

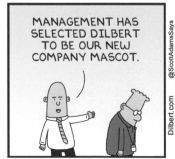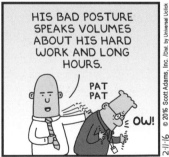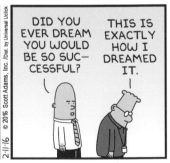

Scott Adams, *Dilbert*, 11 February 2016. Adams's cartoon strip, *Dilbert*, is devoted to the foibles of the contemporary office. One week was devoted to the question of the impact of work on posture.

Letters), originally published in Latin in 1766 and then translated by him into French.[6] Tissot, who is best known for his obsessive interest in the ills resulting from masturbation, turned his eye towards the fragile bodies of scholars and the pathological result of their occupation because he saw a marked increase in such cases in his practice. Three years after the publication of his Latin text, an annotator observed that such occupational diseases of the intelligentsia could be 'palliated, or lessened, by walking at intervals, while a studious person thinks, which does not always retard thought; and by reading and writing, sometimes, in a standing posture, at a desk, which may be raised to different and commodious heights, by a screw, round which it turns'.[7] The physician and medical popularizer Thomas Beddoes urged his middle-class readers 'who are entering on the vocation of trade to endeavour as much as possible to write in an erect posture, and on desks sufficiently high to reach above the pit of the stomach'.[8] Stand well and you will work better! Such mechanistic views of posture, sitting and health always have their moral reading. Work posture, if competently chosen, defines the healthy human.

The moral underpinnings of posture are manifold. The seventh-century English monk the Venerable Bede notes in his interpretation of the Gospel of Luke that standing while reading is appropriate because

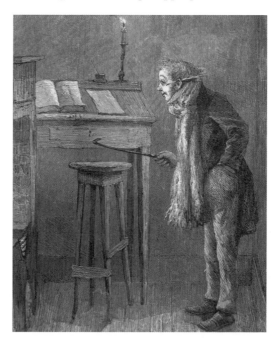

Sol Eytinge, Jr, *In the Tank*, 1869, wood engraving. The hardworking, exploited Bob Cratchit tries to keep warm in Scrooge's counting house.

it is the posture of one who is working, and sitting afterwards is the posture of one resting or passing judgment.[9] Jesus, he notes, stood as he passed his book (the Christian Church) to his disciples before entering the Kingdom of God in preparation for the final judgment. Upright posture makes good Christians. The Enlightenment transforms this view into a moral imperative to preserve one's good health. The Edinburgh-trained physician John Armstrong in *The Art of Preserving Health* (1745), his second blank-verse treatise on health topics, continues to link good health with reading aloud while standing (as did the Venerable Bede) as the means to avoid illness:

> While reading pleases, but no longer, read;
> And read aloud, resounding Homer's strain,
> And wield the thunder of Demosthenes.
> The chest so exercis'd improves its strength;
> And quick vibrations thro' the bowels drive
> The restless blood, which in unactive days
> Would loiter else thro' unelastic tubes.
> Deem it not trifling while I recommend
> What posture suits: to stand and sit by turns,
> As nature prompts, is best. But o'er your leaves
> To lean for ever, cramps the vital parts,
> And robs the fine machinery of its play.[10]

Stand up and read aloud and your health will be preserved; sit and you are condemned to ill health and an unproductive life.

Such popular health works of the Enlightenment continued the notion of the illnesses of employment and the role that poor posture played in them. The fascination of illness and employment came to be a trope of public health concerns with Bernardo Ramazzini's *De morbis artificum diatriba* (The Disease of Workers) in 1713, which appeared in English almost immediately, in 1715. Illnesses, such as rickets, the tailor's disease, took on the qualities ascribed to such occupational illnesses. In one of the most popular Enlightenment volumes on public health (it ran to 22 editions within the first decades), the Edinburgh-trained physician William Buchan observed that 'Many of those who follow sedentary employments are constantly in a bending posture, as shoemakers, taylors, cutlers, etc. Such a situation is extremely hurtful. A bending posture obstructs all the vital motion, and of course must ruin health.'¹¹ The remedy is clear: you must work standing up, or at least sitting with good posture: 'the sedentary artificers are often hurt by their bending postures. They ought therefore to stand or sit erect as the nature of their employment will permit.'[12] Work in such menial occupations leads to postural deficits.

All these comments about work and posture, bad or good, seem to have their starting point in Socrates' complaint in Xenophon's *Oeconomicus* that there are occupations that are

> scorned and, naturally enough, held in low regard in our states. For they spoil the bodies of the workmen and the foremen, forcing them to sit still and stay indoors, and in some cases to spend the whole day by the fire. As their bodies become wom-anish their souls lose strength too. Moreover, these so-called banausic occupations leave no spare time for attention to one's friends and city, so that those who follow them are reputed bad at dealing with friends and bad defenders of their country.[13]

How successful you are in the world is reflected in your posture, and thus your posture is a measure of your value to the world. Indeed, as Socrates continues to argue, such craftsmen not only have bad posture but are poorer citizens of the state, since they have a very different *investment* in it than do the farmers, who are more closely bound to it by the land they till.[14]

To date, this Socratic dialogue, Xenophon's sole surviving attempt to write on economic theory, has functioned critically to examine the power relationships between men and women, mirroring how Greek masculinity controls emotions (according to Michel Foucault in his *History of Sexuality*) or, according to Leo Strauss in his book-length study, as an ironic comment on Greek public virtues.[15] If we think of Xenophon's attempt to root his argument about power and moral value in our posture and its public meanings, it is clear that this dialogue is about all these. This, as we shall see, underpins all our ruminations in this book, encapsulating the seemingly natural link between bodies, emotions and virtues that haunts the idea of posture. We are how we stand or sit or move in every dimension of our interaction with our material world.

To return to our point of departure: a year or so after Jane Brody wrote her advocation of good posture in the workplace, a small commentary appeared in the local section of the *New York Times*. A new denizen of the city, having moved recently from southern California, was suddenly confronted by the thought of wintry weather as he descended in the lift on his way to work:

> Feeling sorry for myself as I contemplated the blast of cold that the January weather would require me to step into, I was slumping a little bit. Suddenly, the only other passenger in the cramped conveyance, an older woman with steel-gray hair and even steelier eyes whom I didn't know, poked me firmly in the ribs through my topcoat with two sharp fingers. 'Lift your head up!' she commanded, harshly but unmistakably for my own good. Well, I lifted it. And what a palpable difference that small adjustment made – not just at that moment but for the rest of the day and beyond.[16]

Can we imagine that the woman was Jane Brody or perhaps her avatar? Just to make sure that we truly 'stand up straight' and face the day, our shivering author could have invested a mere $129.95 in the 'Upright Pro', a 'medically-backed wearable device to improve posture', connected to your iPhone by Bluetooth, to 'train your body to sit upright.'[17] Such a device will, it implies, allow you to be a better and happier cog in the machinery of the modern world, without your nosy neighbour's prodding.

ONE

Posture in the World
of Movement

E VEN THE BEST SCHOLARS have had difficulty dealing with the
complexity of defining posture. The classical scholar Matthew B.
Roller of Johns Hopkins University, in an extraordinary study of
posture in the dining practices of the classical world, defines posture as
'maintaining the body as a whole in a relatively motionless, stable state
for an indefinite period', and contrasts it with gesture 'as nonverbal communicative techniques'. Gesture, for him, is 'a continuous and temporally
restricted movement of a bodily appendage'.[1] Yet do we really gesture
with our feet? Nor can we limit posture to the static world that Roller
finds in classical dining. Rather, posture is a fluid concept that moves
regularly between 'statics' (the position of the body at rest), 'mechanics'
(how the body moves) and 'gait' (how the body moves in space and
time). (Perhaps we can think of gait as gesturing with our feet.[2])

Yet there are moments, as Roller states, when we think of posture
as the image of bodies somehow frozen in space. We see the soldier
standing upright or the corseted body (whether for reason of therapy
or fashion) as rigid. Yet such bodies are always moving imperceptibly,
always self-correcting because of our vestibular system (the inner ear)
and our constant correction of our place in space through proprioscep-
tion, the unconscious interplay among our muscles, tendons and
joints. One anatomical feature seems also to be that two different types
of muscle always govern posture (in the sense of voluntary stiffened or
rigid body position) and 'unimpeded movement', the movement of the
limbs and the torso in action.[3] All these stimuli are integrated in the
brain to provide information about how we relate to the world about
us, even when we attempt to stand upright. Thus we never stop moving,

even when we seem to be fixed and frozen in space. That is why the command 'Stand up straight!' makes us correct and correct again. It is vital to understand that 'normal' posture, an ideal concept created by social norms and disciplines, can also be disrupted by neurological changes in the central and peripheral postural control system, such as errors in context-dependent prediction of the movement, 'leakage' of postural memory, sensory conflict or fault in the receptor system.[4] The bard of such neurological errors of posture is, of course, Oliver Sacks, whose own confrontation with mobility issues and impaired posture *after* recuperating from a leg injury led him to read Henry Head's work on body maps, which we will discuss in our conclusion, as well as to evoke Purdon Martin's groundbreaking work on the pathologies of proprioception. What Sacks discovered was that as a patient he had been 'prostrate, recumbent: doubly so – physically, through weakness and inability to stand; morally, through passivity, the posture of a *patient* – a man reduced, and dependent on his doctor'.[5] After his injury heals he realizes that this postural disability has been heightened rather than healed as he now feels that his wounded leg seemed no longer to be part of his body. 'I was astonished at the profundity of the effect it had: a sort of paralysis and alienation of the leg, reducing it to an "object" which seemed unrelated to me; an abyss of bizarre, and even terrifying effects.'[6] As Sacks observes, while we have self-correcting posture, it too can provide us with false clues about how we stand or move. Yet all such nuances of posture are subsumed to our understanding and internalization of our posture. This internalization is not necessarily understood by the claims of those who define what posture is to be in any given circumstance.

Such postural awareness is also part of our bodily communications system. Just as gestural language requires us to learn specific motor skills in order to communicate, so does posture. It becomes part of kinesics, 'the conscious or unconscious psychomuscularly-based body *movements* and intervening or resulting positions . . . that . . . possess intended or unintended communicative value'.[7] Each culture and time evolves such systems, and they are limited only by the very nature of the body's structure. These systems are imported and exported from culture to culture, nation to nation, historical moment to historical moment, based on their cultural value. Thus we will examine how some patterns of posture that are to be found in the classical world reappear, with their authenticity vouched for by their very antiquity, in the early modern period. These modern reinterpretations, like the rereading of Western notions of posture in revolutionary China, evoke such sources for their emotive power and embed them in the reading of posture in their own world. We shall see how various systems of bodily communication cross millennia when they are needed, as well as crossing what seem to be impervious social barriers. Thus concepts of gender and race employ ideas of posture that are common to both but have radically different implications. These cultural nuances have psychological as well as epistemological significance.

Our Postural Disciplines

Such social activities as 'sport', 'dance' or 'drill' represent the cultural organization of all aspects of posture, even if any given activity seems to stress one or more of our senses of how we hold our bodies. These activities shape and reshape our sense of self. Each has a vocabulary of posture that may or may not rest on meanings intrinsic to other ways of shaping our bodies. The army recruit on the first day of training responds to the command 'Stand up STRAIGHT!' very differently from the child first learning to play the piano to the request that they 'Sit up straight.'

If we are uncomfortable in our bodies, or are told that our bodies could be improved, our sense of our body may come under the aegis of the health sciences. When we think about bodily health in terms of posture, we think of postural correction, whether through exercise or through implements such as corsets or corrective shoes. All such approaches demand a sense of what correct or normal posture is and why pathological or different posture must be corrected, whether by the drill sergeant or the physician. This may be accomplished 'by ridicule . . . , verbal scolding, or by physical punishment where deviation from the postural norms verges on lese majesty or deliberate indignity to a superior'. While Western postural codes have 'perhaps relaxed . . . since the nineteenth century, certain areas of it preserve archaic postural etiquettes backed up by formidable sanctions, as in the military drill regulations'.[8] As we shall see, there are many other arenas where postural norms are enforced by discipline.

The boundary between the two poles of the healthy and the unhealthy, the correct and the incorrect, seems absolute when we

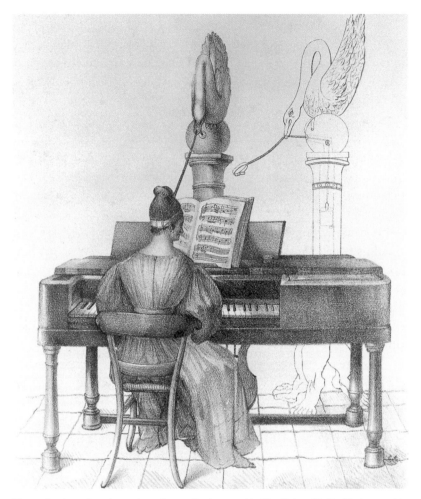

Illustration from the atlas to the orthopaedist Jacques Mathieu Delpech's *De l'Orthomorphie, par rapport a L'espèce humaine* (Orthomorphism; or, An Account of Human Space; Paris, 1828). Correct musical posture is an inherent quality demanded of the musician in training. Here a swan restraint is used to correct the head position of a pianist.

imagine posture in such social categories, but we are constantly correcting and altering these absolute boundaries for a wide range of reasons. Once we imagine posture as something constant, as having meaning, as communicating who we are to ourselves and to others, we see that posture shows how body and mind are truly inseparable.

Posture is simultaneously of the mind and of the body. That is, it is one of the clearest proofs of the absence of any mind-body dichotomy. The way our body imagines itself in the world is the product of our sense of posture and of the cultural meanings attached to that sense. Our personal sense of our body, the way we unconsciously move or remain static in space, is a psychological phenomenon tied to our culture but also to our bodies. If we sense our selves as out of sync with our internal map of our body, we become disorientated; if it remains untested, it becomes our 'norm'. But the testing of our body may, as we shall see, come from many directions. These can often be contradictory even though they overlap. Posture comes into play when we are moving and when we are standing seemingly still; it defines how we march and how we dance and how we walk. Posture is also the absence of movement, as in when we stand or sit. While we can begin with examining 'statics' – posture as a fixed position of the body – this concept of posture is also affected by the rules by which one should sit, stand and present oneself in social situations in order to become healthy or beautiful or functional. These rules are generated by the disciplines of the body that exist and overlap in our social world. They define what it means to be 'human' and then how, over time, we have transformed the merely human into a 'modern', civilized citizen.

Posture can thus be used to separate 'primitive' from 'advanced' peoples, the 'ugly' from the 'beautiful', and the 'ill' from the 'healthy'. Indeed, an entire medical sub-speciality developed during the nineteenth century in which gymnastics defined and reinvigorated the body through 'postural correction'. This sub-speciality morphed into a wide range of alternative and complementary ways of changing, correcting, improving or modifying our posture, from steel braces to Western yoga, from chiropractic to Pilates. (Joseph Pilates (1883–1967), whose system undergirded the postural tradition that now bears his name, was convinced that poor posture and the related speed of modern life inevitably lead to bad health.) In this world of alternative therapy for posture, as well as in the world of allopathic (mainstream) medicine, the fascination with the mechanics of posture, including the many meanings that come to be associated with the spine, plays an ever greater role. Posture becomes anatomical just as much as it becomes psychological. Even scientific presentations of posture in the twenty-first century treat posture in such terms:

Individuals with poor posture look less well and are more likely to have a poor self-image, and self-confidence. It has also been demonstrated that certain posture defects predispose the individual to . . . injuries.[9]

Poor posture is claimed to define our relationship to the external world, and it shapes our sense of self.

All these claims and methods that concern defining and modifying the ill and the healthy were and are also parallel to and often part of a Western attempt to use posture (and the means of altering it) as the litmus test for the modern body of the perfect or healthy or responsible citizen. There is a national politics of posture that imagines the perfect body of an ideal citizen. Such ideas of bodily reform bring together the earlier debates about how to reform the body in education and medicine, in popular culture and in organized and structured activities. But, most importantly, ideas about posture become habituated in our very sense of our own bodies. While this present book is divided into the various self-defined disciplines of posture, from theology to disability studies, its central theme is that the boundaries between such ways of defining our body are often arbitrary and capricious. Posture links (and divides) the disciplines that we use to define our body, and that linkage is central to our tale. We think about posture as we think about ourselves in the world, but such thought processes quickly become habituated and we forget, if we ever knew, that we are constantly learning appropriate postures for appropriate activities.

The Language of Posture

Posture is comprised of discourses that, on the one hand, clearly define in any given setting the rules of posture and yet, on the other, incorporate into our understanding of such rules a wide and often contradictory sense of what we are and what we are doing at any time and in any setting. But our vocabulary to describe posture is just as entangled, for 'the body is not mute, but it is inarticulate; it does not use speech, yet begets it.'[10] The language we use (and will use in this study) to describe posture is also ambiguous, even though it seems quite straightforward.

Take the complex anglophone understanding of the very word 'posture', for instance. The *Oxford English Dictionary* defines posture in many ways that are inherently intertwined. The root of the word is the French *posture* – meaning the position of the body – documented from 1588 in Middle French and then in 1580 as *posteure* in a figurative use, which in turn has its origin in the classical Latin *positura*. As in French, its first meaning is as

> the relative disposition of the various parts of something; *esp.*
> the position and carriage of the limbs or the body as a whole,
> often as indicating a particular quality, feeling, etc.; an attitude,
> a pose. Hence, more generally: the manner in which a person
> bears himself or herself; natural carriage or deportment.

It is the phrase 'natural carriage or deportment' that captures the core problem of the term. The way one 'naturally' appears is the way one acts in a social setting. Sir Philip Sidney's *The Countesse of Pembrokes Arcadia* (1586) is listed by the OED as the first usage: 'In another table was Atalanta; the posture of whose lims was so liuelie expressed, that if the eyes were the only iudges, . . . one would haue sworne the very picture had runne.' A generation later, in 1616, William Shakespeare uses the word freely in *Antony and Cleopatra*, as in Act v, Scene 2, when Cleopatra comments on what would happen to her if she were transported as war booty to Rome, where her relationship with Antony would become the stuff of Roman comedy:

> . . . saucy lictors
> Will catch at us, like strumpets; and scald rhymers
> Ballad us out o' tune: the quick comedians
> Extemporally will stage us, and present
> Our Alexandrian revels; Antony
> Shall be brought drunken forth, and I shall see
> Some squeaking Cleopatra boy my greatness
> I' the posture of a whore.

Here the double meaning of posture, which certainly affects English speakers, is evident.[11] Cleopatra's posture would be mimicked by boy actors: both the recumbent state of the prostitute, according to Shakespeare, and the very attitude of mind that makes her a prostitute in the eyes of the Romans.[12] Her double use of posture reflects on her and Antony's military defeat and thus also plays on the other meaning of posture at the time, the sort of pun that Shakespeare truly loved. For posture also comes to mean military bearing, how one holds oneself in the regimented world of soldiers' bodies.

Indeed, the complexity of the concept of posture generates a slew of synonyms: carriage, bearing, deportment, pose, stance and mien, among many others. Each has multiple and often contradictory meanings, some of them very particular to a specific discipline of posture (as in the golfer's or boxer's stance) and some laden with moral qualities, as in Falstaff's clearly ironic self-description as having 'a most noble carriage' in *Henry IV* (Part 1, II.iv). Once posture is evoked, even when the word goes unmentioned, the entanglements of our language for posture are present. So we can also speak of carriage as a form of moral posture, as our 'political stance' toward any public issue or, as Luciana says to Antipholus of Syracuse in Shakespeare's *Comedy of Errors* (III. ii. 14), where he as a new husband is told to dissemble to his spouse, at least act as if he is moral, 'teach sin the carriage of a holy saint.' The way we hold ourselves, the way we move in the world, reveals who we are, but exactly what it reveals is never quite clear.

If, as Terry Eagleton observed, the sayable must be demarcated from the unsayable, 'certain normative regulations' must emerge to bring order, value and interest to cultural discourse.[13] The bourgeois public sphere, he points out, is a realm that is 'unable to withstand . . . the inruption into it of . . . interests in palpable conflict with its own "universal" rational norms'.[14] Thus we have romances of upright posture when the norms of posture come to be equated with the norms of morality.

In Leviticus 21:18–20, those whose bodily imperfections make it impossible for them to serve the Lord in the Temple include, according to the King James translation, 'a blind man, or a lame, or he that hath a flat nose, or any thing superfluous, or a man that is brokenfooted, or brokenhanded, or crookbackt, or a dwarf, or that hath a blemish in his eye, or be scurvy, or scabbed, or hath his stones broken'. For the readers of this version (and most subsequent translations) the blind, the halt, the lame and the hunchback, with his (and they are all men) crooked posture, may not serve.[15] Indeed, their imperfections result in their uncleanliness in much the same way that certain animals could never be sacrificed because of their imperfections. Posture reveals the inner nature of the human. And it is immutable. The hunchback (גִבֵּן) becomes one of the categories that, when evoked explicitly, provides a moral lesson to the reader about the relationship between the body and the spirit.[16]

The 'hunchback', the person with kyphosis – excessive curvature of the spine (remember, the 'normal' thoracic lumbar has a slight curvature) – comes to be the icon of postural excess. The malevolent hunchback whose body reflects his character shapes Richard III's image – at least in Shakespeare's accounts of Richard Crookback (the name of Ben Jonson's lost play of 1602).[17] Shakespeare's Richard, murderer of children, bemoans his fate to have 'an envious mountain on my back,/ Where sits deformity to mock my body' (*Henry VI*, Part 3, III. iii.ii).

But the early modern hunchback can be comical as well as purposelessly nasty, as in the ubiquitous figure of Pulcinella from the Neapolitan *commedia dell'arte* in the seventeenth century. He morphs into Mr Punch, the mean-spirited hunchback in the Punch and Judy shows that plagued Victorian beachfront holidaymakers, besting all social conventions. Each shows his malign character writ large in his hideous posture. And each is fascinating exactly because of this link. A four-year-old child, evacuated from the Blitz in 1939, suddenly finds himself in rural North Yorkshire, among a group of children

> taken to see a Punch and Judy show and, although a bit shocked and frightened, we were fascinated and totally absorbed at the same time. The actions of the hook-nosed, long-chinned, hunchbacked Mr Punch were dreadful.[18]

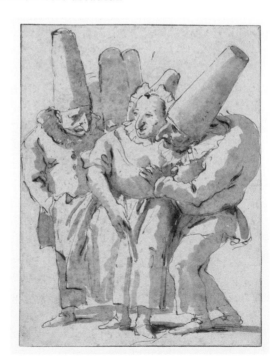

Giovanni Battista Tiepolo, *Punchinellos Approaching a Woman*, late 1730s, pen and brown ink and brush with brown wash over black chalk.

But he more than any other captured the children's attention: would that we could be like him, disrespecting all authority!

In the nineteenth century such postural differences come to be a touchstone of the impossibility of change. Thus the hunchback's mis-shapen posture is echoed in Søren Kierkegaard's odd comment in 1848 on the promises that new governments make to change everything for the better: 'and so a new ministry comes along . . . and in general makes a round-shouldered watchman and a bow-legged journeyman smith into the equal human being. In many ways the age is reminiscent of that of Socrates . . . but there will be nothing left to remind us of Socrates.'[19] Except, we might add, given Kierkegaard's sudden sense of Athens in his own age, the immutable ugliness of Socrates, as unchangeable as the body of the 'round-shouldered watchman'. We need, of course, to recall that Kierkegaard's own round-shouldered or hunchbacked appearance (the Danish term was *skudtrygget*), perhaps the result of a childhood accident exacerbated by spinal tuberculosis, often made him the butt of his contemporaries.[20]

Yet there are counter-readings. In George Eliot's *Adam Bede* (1859), as one commentator notes, the title character 'is characterized by an honesty that is conveyed, for example, by his upright and naturally dignified posture: "he looked neither awkward nor embarrassed, but stood in his usual firm upright attitude . . . in that rough dignity which is peculiar to intelligent, honest, well-built workmen."'[21] While this is often, as we shall see, a reflection of a fascination with mobile physiognomy, as with the Victorians, it comes to be a truism from the early modern period to the present. The historian of sexuality George Mosse notes that 'men of the Enlightenment pass rather easily from an analysis of bodily structures to judgments about character. The Roman slogan "a healthy mind in a healthy body", eventually inscribed on many a school gymnasium throughout Europe, sums up this linkage.'[22] Your external bodily position defines your moral attitude.

Certainly the greatest nineteenth-century novel on the topic, Victor Hugo's *Hunchback of Notre Dame* (1831), is the story of a figure with deformed posture working against type. It is the tale of Quasimodo, the deaf and half-blind bell-ringer of the cathedral, whose love for the gypsy dancer Esmeralda transfigures him. The novel concludes in the sepulchre of the Montfaucon, the cemetery where the hanged body of Esmeralda was interred:

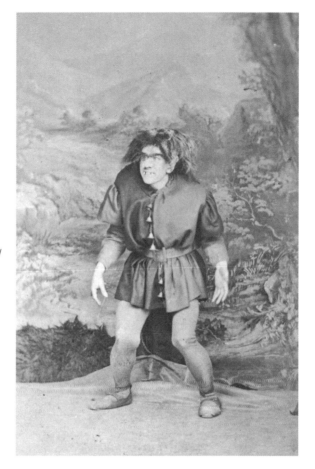

Johnny Clarke as Quasimodo in *Esmeralda* at the Strand Theatre, 1861, sepia photograph on paper. An index of how posture is read in the Victorian public sphere can be seen in how actors portrayed characters defined by such postural variations. This is a *carte-de-visite*. The scene is described as 'While to this picture so extremely frightful, / This round back forms a back-round most delightful.'

they found among all those hideous carcasses two skeletons, one of which held the other in its embrace. One of these skeletons . . . was that of a woman . . . The other, which held this one in a close embrace, was the skeleton of a man. It was noticed that his spinal column was crooked, his head seated on his shoulder blades, and that one leg was shorter than the other. Moreover, there was no fracture of the vertebrae at the nape of the neck, and it was evident that he had not been hanged. Hence, the man to whom it had belonged had come thither and had died there. When they tried to detach the skeleton, which he held in his embrace, he fell to dust.[23]

True even after death, the deformed hero is transfigured. His remains literally vanish, not only into dust, but into a mythopoeic realm of postural transformation. Yet his image continues on the stage, in film, in ballet and indeed even in video games to shape our image of the ability to transcend the limitations of posture. Such an image of posture as moral force continues in Verdi's *Rigoletto* (1851), based on Hugo's *Le Roi s'amuse* (1832), and in Dalton Trumbo's anti-war film *Johnny Got His Gun* (1971), based on his novel from 1938. (It does in German, too: *aufrecht* and its positive cognates, such as *aufrichtig*, cover much the same moral semantic fields as 'upright'.) These are variations on what Jenny Morris has called a 'supercrip', a person with a disability who lives out the popular representation of disability as adversity to be overcome.[24] Posture makes us moral, we fantasize, until we meet a Quasimodo, whose moral force draws our own posture into question.

There is another side, perhaps a necessary counterweight, to the moral sense of uprightness, and that is the notion that posture is itself merely pretence. (This is the same semantic field as *unaufrecht* in German, with the senses of being pertinacious, sanctimonious, feigned and hypocritical.) As early as Charles Dickens's *Pickwick Papers* (1836), such phrases as 'ingenious posturing' define such superficiality.[25] The poet Philip Larkin, writing in 1956, speaks of poetry as 'plain language, absence of posturings, sense of proportion, humour'.[26] Kingsley Amis simply calls it being a 'prancing, posturing phoney'.[27] Is being upright real or is it merely humbug, the false morality and body posture of Uriah Heep (to remain with Charles Dickens)? This question deals with more than metaphors of a moral or immoral body; it is the core of our understanding of the body and character as twinned in a

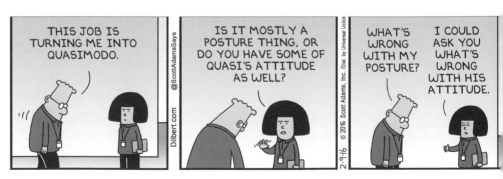

Scott Adams, *Dilbert*, 9 February 2016. Posture in the modern office, in Adams's cartoon strip *Dilbert*, turns the office worker into a modern Quasimodo. Dilbert's body and character are linked in ways that provide an ironic comment on the exploitation of the office worker.

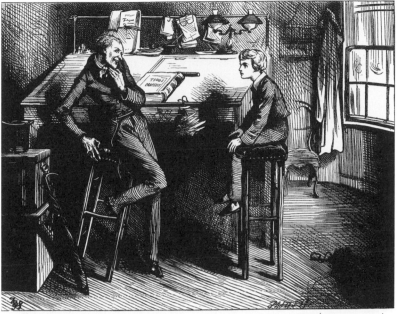

"OH, THANK YOU, MASTER COPPERFIELD," SAID URIAH HEEP, "FOR THAT REMARK! IT IS SO TRUE! UMBLE AS I AM, I KNOW IT IS SO TRUE! OH, THANK YOU, MASTER COPPERFIELD!"

Fred Barnard, *'Oh, thank you, Master Copperfield', said Uriah Heep, 'for that remark! It is so true! Umble as I am, I know it is so true! Oh, thank you, Master Copperfield!'* From Charles Dickens, *David Copperfield*, household edn (London, 1871–9).

Cartesian sense but also confronting real bodies and their moral choices. Intertwined with the notion of how we hold ourselves, how we move in the world, is whether such a visible body reflects any sense of the moral uprightness of the individual. This is rooted in Western traditions of both philosophical and theological understanding of posture.

TWO

Postures of the Mind: Theology and Philosophy Explain Human Posture

O RIGINS ARE ALWAYS FRAUGHT with meaning. The explanation of how we as human beings arose or evolved is perhaps the origin tale that is most contested. In preaching about the origins of man, St Augustine asked, 'Where do the people themselves come from, to be amazed? Where were they? Where have they come out from? Where does the body get its shape from, and the variety of its limbs and organs? And its attractive posture and deportment? From what beginnings, what mean and insignificant origins?'[1] He asked not only where we come from but how we acquire our 'attractive appearance' as human beings, our upright posture, which is the shadow of our character, our 'deportment'.

The very notion of what in the ancient world defines the human being in contrast to all other living things is simple: upright posture. The human being is defined across all aspects of classical thought as 'standing on two feet support[ing] a straight spine'.[2] Indeed, Aristotle defines a human as 'the only being that stands upright':[3]

> In man more than in any other animal the upper posture and the lower parts of the body are determined in accordance with what is naturally upper and lower: in other words, upper and lower in man correspond with upper and lower in the universe itself . . . Of course, in all animals the head is up above with regard to the creature's own body; but, as I have said, man is the only animal which, when fully developed, has the head up above in the sense in which 'up' is applied to the universe.[4]

Upright posture is defined as bipedalism, and being erect moves man towards the gods. Aristotle also notes that erect carriage provides the now front-facing human head with a *prosōpon* (πρόσωπον, a face or mask) with its concomitant ability to speak rationally. The human, he continues, is 'the only animal that stands upright, is the only one that looks straight before him . . . or sends forth his voice straight before him'.[5] Human rationality is proven by speech, which propels upright posture, contradicting Anaxagoras, who had argued that having hands, a sign of upright posture, is what made the human being

> the most intelligent of the animals; but surely the reasonable point of view is that it is because he is the most intelligent animal that he has got hands [or, we might add, upright posture]. Hands are an instrument; and Nature, like a sensible human being, always assigns an organ to the animal that can use it (as it is more in keeping to give flutes to a man who is already a flute-player than to provide a man who possesses flutes with the skill to play them).[6]

The human alone has upright posture because the human alone can employ it. Upright posture defines what is in the end a human and human alone.

How erect posture is read differs from commentator to commentator. Best known of the ancient commentators is Plato, who, according to legend, is claimed to have seen the human as bipedal and featherless. For Plato this featherless, bipedal being strives for the infinite and for knowledge, as in the *Timaeus*, 'so that grasping with these and supported thereon it was enabled to travel through all places, bearing aloft the chamber of our most divine and holy part'.[7] *Anthropos* (ανθρωπος), the word for man, means the animal that looks upwards and considers the gods. Ancient views of anthropogenesis all seem to centre on upright posture as the defining attribute.

Although bipedalism seems to us an obvious way of seeing human beings, it was Plato who used upright posture to move the rational mind as far from the centre of the appetite and the organ of generation as possible:

> we declare that God has given to each of us, as his daemon, that kind of soul which is housed in the top of our body and which

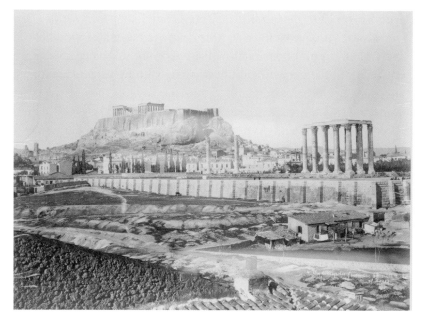

The Parthenon, Athens, far view from southeast, 1925.

raises us – seeing that we are not an earthly but a heavenly plant – up from earth towards our kindred in the heaven.[8]

The head, for Plato, is the 'acropolis' of the body, its highest point both literally and metaphorically. In the *Laws*, he reverses the image, comparing the virtues of the leaders of the upright body as 'we are comparing the State itself to the skull.' The youthful cadre of leaders are those

> who are selected as the most intelligent and nimble in every part of their souls, are set, as it were, like the eyes, in the top of the head, and survey the State all round; and as they watch, they pass on their perceptions to the organs of memory – that is, they report to the elder wardens all that goes on in the State.[9]

The state is to the upright body as the body is to the city-state.

Plato's upright body at its best must also possess wisdom and nobility, *agathos kai sophos* (ἀγαθὸς καὶ σοφὸς), which he abstracts in the *Meno* from the older Greek notion of *kalos kagathos* (καλός καγαθός), beauty and goodness.[10] This older concept describes military posture, in the sense both of the soldier's body and of his loyalty to the state. This is 'the chivalrous ideal of the complete human personality, harmonious in mind and body, foursquare in battle and speech, song and action.'[11] In his reformulation, Plato stressed that such goodness is not visible in the upright body. Even an ugly body (such as Socrates is purported to have had) can be *agathos kai sophos*. Indeed, there is a moment that Xenophon records in the *Apology* when this is exemplified in terms of posture. It is after Socrates has been condemned to death and is about to walk out of the room to drink the hemlock: he states that he had only 'taught the youths of Athens, without charge, every good thing that I could. With that he departed, blithe of eyes, posture, and step, as was fully consonant with the words he had just spoken.'[12] *Agathos kai sophos* is a quality of the soul. (This is very different from the concept of *sophrosyne*, temperance, which Plato discusses in the *Charmides*. That has to do with the balance between the competing forces of the body, not their harmonization.) These Platonic concepts become elided in the course of the early modern period, somehow becoming identical with Juvenal's demand some five hundred years later in the *Satires* (10.356) of the good citizen-soldier having '*mens sana in corpore sano*' (a sound mind in a sound body) and his imperative '*fortem posce animum mortis terrore carentem*' (ask for a heart that is courageous, with no fear of death).[13] For Juvenal's ideal body 'prefers the troubles and grueling Labours of Hercules to the sex and feasts and downy cushions of Sardanapallus', who, according to the Greek historian Diodorus of Sicily, wore female attire and lived a life of slothful luxury. 'Real' men don't slouch on silken divans. The straight/gay dichotomy has deep roots that are reflected in the Roman notions of acceptable and poor posture. Thus upright posture comes to be part not only of why we stand up straight but of the moral force that we have when we stand up straight. The body again reflects the inner nature of the good citizen. Upright posture correctly calibrated allows instant recognition of the inner worth of the individual.

Xenophon, in the *Memorabilia* (1.4.11), builds on the notion of the head as the body's acropolis and takes a more functional view, arguing that

> In the first place, man is the only living creature that they have caused to stand upright; and the upright position gives him a wider range of vision in front and a better view of everything above and exposes him to less injury.[14]

Yet you will remember that Xenophon in the *Oeconomicus* also sees in the healthy body of the farmer a better citizen than the craftsman at his loom or the smith at his forge. For the Greeks, the meaning associated with standing upright is part of a rhetoric of military defence, since the very idea of the acropolis is always understood as a space that is both defensible and defines the new city-state as a national space. The human thus stands upright as metaphor for the human condition, seeking the divine but also defending the citizens of the city-state. (Slaves, even Greek slaves, do not stand up straight.)

To describe humans as 'featherless', as in Plato's definition, sounds odder to modern ears than does the functional association of bipedalism and intelligence, but Plato sees the absence of bodily covering as a move away from the base towards the human, for he is quite aware that the other bipedal animal is the bird. Greek thought gives the bird a middle role between the human and the gods, since birds are connected to the gods through their use in divination. Plato's definition of man as featherless and bipedal is attributed to him by Sextus Empiricus and, most importantly, by Diogenes Laertius in his account of that much more famous Diogenes, Diogenes of Sinope.[15] (Plato really does seem to define man, at least obliquely, as a featherless biped in *The Statesman*.[16]) Responding to Plato's contorted definition of man, Diogenes of Sinope, known as the Cynic, notoriously plucked a (bipedal) chicken and took it to Plato's Academy, declaring, 'Here is Plato's man.'[17]

Diogenes was odd: uniquely calling himself a 'cosmopolitan', a citizen of the world as well as of the city, he avoided all worldliness, lived in a huge barrel in the marketplace, and searched during daylight hours with a lit lantern for an honest man. As a forerunner of the Stoics, Diogenes' ridicule of Plato was as much a critique of his understanding that such a classification of bipedalism as a sign of the divine was too reductive to be compelling. The followers of Plato responded to his mockery by revising Plato's definition of a human being as a featherless biped, expanding it to include 'with straight nails'. While perhaps convincing, even this pointed to the hidden equation between the human and the divine, or at least, to put it in terms that Diogenes might have found more compelling, the *search* for the divine through the human potential to be upright. For the ancient world, there was no question of the primacy of bipedal, upright man. As late as the Renaissance, the Christian humanist Erasmus in his *Ecclesiastes, sive de*

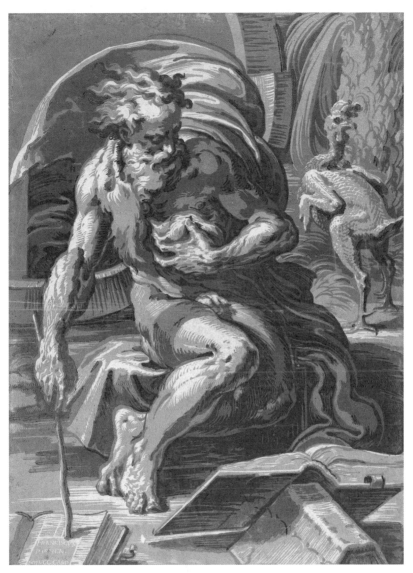

Ugo da Carpi, after Girolamo Francesco Maria Mazzola Parmigianino, *Diogenes and the Chicken*, *c.* 1527, chiaroscuro wood engraving. According to legend, Diogenes the Cynic lived in a barrel and famously represented man as a plucked chicken in ridicule of Plato's description of man as a featherless biped. Jars were depicted in ancient reliefs and sculptures, but in this image Diogenes' home has become a barrel. It has been suggested that the source of this change might be an Italian translation from 1480 of *Lives of the Philosophers*, which used the word *botte* (cask), reflecting the then current practice of storing wine in casks rather than jars.

ratione concionandi (Ecclesiastes: On the Art of Preaching; 1535) continued Platonically to define humans as rational, 'featherless and bipedal' beings.[18] The tension here between absolute definitions of posture, such as the Platonic one, and their antithesis, Diogenes' chicken, sets the pattern for all subsequent debates about posture, even though over time the latter seems to have won the day.

Indeed, our notorious chicken reappears in contemporary debates about 'the boundary of the class for humans' in the philosophy of science, as a grotesque example.[19] Bertrand Russell dissected the implications of this notion for symbolic logic in the early twentieth century when he noted, '"Socrates is a featherless biped" is different from "Socrates is human", in that the latter set of classifications is all-encompassing; the former clearly not.[20] By the twentieth century only such ironic evocations are possible. Russell implies that no one in his world would even imagine this as a possible definition of the human.

Indeed, in his satire of contemporary life *The Isles of the Penguins* (1908), Anatole France has the Venerable St Maël – his short-sighted wandering saint, cast up on a distant island – baptize a flock of upright penguins, having confused them for humans: 'Now what he had taken for men of small stature but of grave bearing were penguins whom the spring had gathered together, and who were ranged in couples on the natural steps of the rock, erect in the majesty of their large, white bellies.'[21] The debate that follows in heaven among the saints over whether the baptism of upright penguins is valid is resolved by the heavenly hosts recognizing the baptism. Thus begins the account of Penguinia, a society composed of penguins more or less transformed into upright, bipedal human beings, which mirrors in all its qualities, including its emphasis on female posture and gait, the world of *fin de siècle* Paris that France inhabited. As one penguin comments about female gait and posture, evoking the penguin's 'pigeon-toed' stance,

> Professor Haddock asserts . . . in a learned article in the 'Anthropological Review', 'a woman attracts a civilized man in proportion as her feet make an angle with the ground. If this angle is as much as thirty-five degrees, the attraction becomes acute. For the position of the feet upon the ground determines the whole carriage of the body.'[22]

The early twentieth-century satiric leap from bipedal chickens to upright penguins is not that great. Yet posture, bipedalism, remains clearly a defining quality of the human. The debate about being upright, with its moral, aesthetic and physiological implications, has abandoned the upright chicken and other bipedal avians for other, more powerful analogies.

Posture as a Sign of the Divine

As the artists, writers and thinkers of the Renaissance adapted classical images of upright posture, they also incorporated classical ideas that upright posture was a comment on the inherently superior, if not divine, nature of man. In the *Metamorphoses* (1.84–6), Ovid observed: 'And, though all other animals are prone, and fix their gaze upon the earth, he gave to man an uplifted face and bade him stand erect and turn his eyes to heaven.'[23] By the high Middle Ages, such pagan definitions had merged with a tradition of interpretations of the biblical account of the creation of Adam. For the Jews, Adam's upright posture was a sign of being superior to the animals created by God, even after the expulsion from Paradise.[24] Yet such a posture is never directly evoked in the Bible in the account of Adam's creation: 'And the LORD God formed man *of* the dust of the ground, and breathed into his nostrils the breath of life; and man became a living soul' (Genesis 2:7). While missing in the work of acculturated Jewish thinkers, such as Philo writing for a Greek reading audience in his various accounts of the Creation in Genesis, it does appear within the early Rabbinic tradition in the Hellenized Middle East.[25]

Bereshit Rabbah, the third-century AD collection of commentaries from Christian Palestine on Genesis, clearly reflects a Jewish reading of the classical explanation of upright posture. Hellenizing culture permeated the cultural and indeed the religious life of Jews and provided an explanation of upright posture. Adam is created, according to the rabbinic commentators, 'with four attributes of the higher beings [that is, angels] . . . : he stands upright, like the ministering angels; he speaks, like the ministering angels; he understands, like the ministering angels; and he sees, like the ministering angels.' But Adam is clearly mortal, having been also given four of the attributes of the lower animals: 'he eats and drinks, like an animal; procreates, like an animal; excretes, like an animal; and dies, like an animal.' What is striking is that uprightness is seen as an attribute of the divine, a rereading of the Greek tradition in a world in which Adam must be suspended between the divine and the material, for, as the commentaries note:

> The Holy One, blessed be He, said: 'If I create him of the celestial elements he will live [forever] and not die, and if I create him of the terrestrial elements, he will die and not live [in a future life]. Therefore I will create him of the upper and of the lower elements: if he sins he will die; while if he does not sin, he will live.'[26]

The mortality of Adam is a sign of his lower nature; his upright posture links him to the angelic sphere.

The merging of the classical and religious view of standing straight becomes the standard explanation of what makes the human being human. One of the greatest of the medieval exegetes, Isidore of Seville, commented that the very word for man, the Latin noun 'homo', reflects man's creation 'de humo terrae', just as the Greek noun anthropos reflects man's upright stature and elevated gaze in contemplation of God.[27] Here, of course, Plato's idea becomes Isidore's Christian deity. But it is even more so, since upright posture is connected by Gregory of Nyssa with that most human of activities, speech: upright posture has freed man's hands to communicate with his fellows, for the 'form of the human body agrees with the rationality of the mind'. He evokes the Platonic image of human beings as 'capable of thought and knowledge, a share of animal life, an upright bearing, risibility, broadness of nail' as the 'signs of human nature'.[28] As has been observed recently on the nature of such debates in redefining not only the exterior of man's body but the very nature of his soul, 'the human body consequently has a role in the drama of salvation, and in its ability to reveal spiritual realities, such as the necessity of the soul to realize its spiritual "uprightness".'[29]

Certainly the best-known image of human 'uprightness' in the Renaissance is to be found on the central panel in the ceiling of the Sistine Chapel, painted between 1508 and 1512, The Creation of Adam. Reproduced and parodied in innumerable images, Michelangelo's supine Adam, painted in 1511, shows the finger of God about to give Adam a soul and thus present mankind with upright posture. This is the only image from Michelangelo's project for which a red-chalk sketch exists.

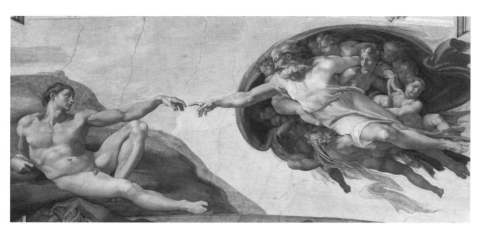

Michelangelo, *The Creation of Adam*, 1511, fresco.

Other Renaissance images exist of Adam in a recumbent posture – Jacopo della Quercia's *Creation of Adam* on the Porta Magna of San Petronio in Bologna, and the languid figure of Adam done by Lorenzo Ghiberti on the doors of the Baptistery in Florence, the *Porta del Paradiso*, for example – but it is Michelangelo's image that sticks in the Western imagination. As the Victorian aesthete Walter Pater noted, Adam is without human strength at that moment, and 'a touch of the finger-tips will suffice' to transform his soul.[30] Thus, as another commentator noted, 'the Life Force passes from God to Man.'[31]

But what is unnoticed is that the recumbent posture of the fully formed Adam is not upright. Michelangelo's understanding of anatomy was 'supported by a classical and Christian tradition of human dignity through erect posture. Michelangelo knew more than the position of bones: he knew the function and purpose of legs. They had a divinely conferred dignity.'[32] Supine, such legs were less than fully human; they were without the soul that dignifies mankind. Upright posture in a Christian world that has rediscovered classical images of the body points now towards a divine posture, as St Cyprian stated in 'To Demetrian': 'God made you erect, and although the other animals are prone and are depressed with posture bent toward earth, you have an exalted stature and a countenance raised upwards toward heaven and the Lord. Look there, direct your eyes there, seek God on high.'[33] Christianity sees upright posture through the eyes of the Greeks, but mankind now becomes much more than a plucked chicken. Thus Adam is redeemed, for 'no medieval thinker could avoid stressing the fact that man, on account of Adam's fall, had lost much of his natural dignity'. This is indeed in 'many ways a pessimistic view of man and his state is typical of medieval thought'.[34] Yet the Renaissance reverses this, positing Adam's upright posture as the one quality that survived the expulsion from the Garden of Eden.

The question of Adam's posture leaves us with ever more complications, however. Do we not have a replication in Adam's posture of the ambiguity of Michelangelo's *David* (1504)? The question about David's posture is whether we are seeing him the instant before he moves to raise his sling or, as earlier representation had him, having thrown the stone and waiting for it to strike Goliath. His stance – body twisted, shoulders at an angle to the hips – is one that lends the figure animation, with its weight resting on one leg in the classical *contrapposto* position so indebted to the work of such classical sculptors as Polykleitos. Donatello's *David* (*c.* 1440) stands in almost the same position over Goliath's decapitated head. In which direction is Michelangelo's David about to move? On the Sistine ceiling, is God about to touch Adam or has he already done so? Is Adam truly recumbent, or is his posture already at that instant moving from the recumbent to the upright state? That ambiguity, so typical of Michelangelo, is mirrored in the figures surrounding his bearded God. Who is it that is nestled in God's arm as he gestures towards Adam? Is it wisdom (*Sapentia*), the quality God is giving (or has given) to Adam?[35] Is it the Virgin Mary present at the creation of man, as Adam's skull is present at the Crucifixion?[36] Is it Eve, who will soon enough be part of the tale? Is it even a female figure at all? The debate about the meaning of this figure has been as intense as that surrounding Adam's posture. Some have seen her as central to the image, because 'her influence radiates to all cardinal points: upward as she grasps the paternal yoke that weighs on her shoulder; sideward to fix upon Adam; rightward, engaging the child; and . . . downward by way of a fatal loincloth. Daughter, bride-designate, mother, she buds here as all woman – while posture and charm convey the venereal attributes of beauty, candor, fecundity.'[37] The posture of both Adam and Eve defines them, but the underlying ambiguity makes it impossible to decide among the various readings of it. Yet it is their posture that we are forced to read and interpret.

The claim that it is divinely created posture that defines the human being continues to the beginning of the Enlightenment, when the theologian-philosopher Johann Gottfried Herder, in his *Ideas for the Philosophy of the History of Humanity* (1784–91), defines posture first and foremost as central to the 'organic difference between man and beast'. Yet, unlike the classical tradition, he discusses this before he discusses human reasoning:

> The form of man is upright: in this he is singular upon the earth . . . to the human species alone is this position natural and constant. . . All the muscles acting in this position are adapted to it. The calf of the leg is enlarged: the pelvis is drawn backward: the hips are spread outwards from each other: the spine is less curved: the breast is widened: the shoulders have clavicles: the hands have fingers endued with the sense of feeling: to crown the structure the receding head is exalted on the muscles of the neck: man is . . . a creature looking far above and around him.[38]

Such ideas of the uniqueness of upright human anatomy reflect contemporary debates about military posture, with the military plumb line running from the top of the head to the feet marking the body of the soldier more and more defining ideal human posture.

In his account of the primacy of posture, Herder also makes a series of distinctions that, while seemingly biblical in their origin, begin to place posture as a major factor in delineating a hierarchy of human beings. Genesis 1:20–25 gives an account of the creation of the hierarchy of beasts, from those who fly to those who 'creepeth upon the earth'. Adam's creation is the penultimate stage: 'Let us make man in our image, after our likeness: and let them have dominion over the fish of the sea, and over the fowl of the air, and over the cattle, and over all the earth, and over every creeping thing that creepeth upon the earth.' Eve, almost an afterthought – 'in the image of God created he him; male and female created he them' – is then made from Adam's rib. Herder's quasi-theological account of posture then provides its own contrast in a hierarchy of creation, 'for though the bear has equally broad foot, and stands erect when he fights: though the ape and the pygmy sometimes walk or run in an erect posture: still to the human species alone is this position natural and constant.'[39] Herder is one of the Enlightenment figures who, although opposed to slavery as well as to the Kantian notion of the innate mental inferiority of the black, saw the pygmy as an intermediate stage between the lower orders of creation and the fully human, and thus not possessing quite human posture.[40] Human posture, like human reason, is an inherent and unchanging quality that defines the human.

Herder does not downplay the role of reason in determining what is human. In his definition of rationality he stresses above all speech, which one might expect; but the noble posture comes first (with appropriate citations about the anatomical differences among animals to the anthropological literature of his time, such as Thomas Camper and his son-in-law Theodor Soemmering, as well as Johann Friedrich Blumenbach).[41] In 1795 Blumenbach argued that human beings are naturally upright and bipedal, countering Carl Linnaeus' view from the 1750s that the human was primarily a quadruped with 'four feet, on two of which he locomotes and the other two of which he uses for prehensile purposes'.[42]

Being upright defined being human in all its anatomical specificity, from the shape of the pelvis to the structure of the hands and feet. But Herder is, in the final analysis, a theologian. Upright posture is a sign of the very nature of Creation, crowned by an upright being whom God tells to 'stand up straight':

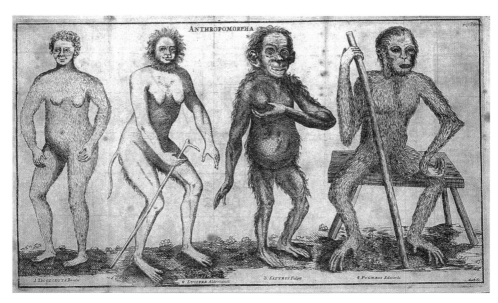

Carl Linnaeus, 'Four "Humanoid" Figures from Linnaeus's *Amoenitates academicae* (Academic Delights, 10 vols, 1749–90)', 1763. These were published in Carl Linnaeus's name, and edited by him (vols I–VII) and J.C.D. Schreber (vols VIII–X). The four 'humanoid' figures are from the volume of 1763: (left to right) Troglodyta Bontu, Lucifer Aldrovandi, Satyrus Tulpii and Pygmaeus Edwardi, from the thesis *Anthropomorpha* by Christianus Emmanuel Hoppius, 1760, published in vol. VI of *Amoenitates academicae* (Stockholm, 1763).

When our creative parent had fulfilled her labours, and exhausted all the forms, that were possible on our Earth, she paused, and surveyed her works . . . With maternal affection she stretched forth her hand to the last creature of her art, and said: 'stand up on the earth! Left to thyself, thou hadst been a beast, like unto other beasts: but through my especial aid and love, *walk erect,* and be of beasts the god.' . . . with wonder shall we perceive, what new organism of powers commenced in the erect position of mankind, and how by it alone man was made a *man*.[43]

Herder's scientific sentiment bridges the gap between Plato's notion of upright posture signifying the seeking of the rational and John Milton's understanding that man's erect posture, created by the hand of God, preceded man's own intelligence.

Such a view can be found in the early modern period among both Christian and Jewish thinkers. In *Paradise Lost* (1667), Milton had illustrated the creation of the first man as a sentient creature through God's gift of upright posture:

> a creature, who, not prone
> And brute as other creatures, but endued
> With sanctity of reason might erect
> His stature, and upright with front serene
> Govern the rest, self knowing; and from thence
> Magnanimous to correspond with Heaven,
> But grateful to acknowledge whence his good
> Descends, thither with heart, and voice, and eyes
> Directed in devotion to adore
> And worship God Supreme, who made him
> Of all his works. (7.506–15)

Here, Milton echoes Job 22:26: 'For then shalt thou have thy delight in the Almighty, and shalt lift up thy face unto God.' Creation is the moment when the human being is able to stand upright in a moral as well as a physical sense.[44] This is reflected in the gender difference 'in the birth scenes of Adam and Eve in *Paradise Lost*, where Eve gazes downward at "herself" in the pool of water while Adam looks upward toward his "creator" in the sky'.[45]

Milton further encodes upright posture as a means of signifying the successful struggle between the divine and the demonic in *Paradise Regained* (1671). As one recent critic observes, the Tempter atop the temple spire says, "'To stand upright / will ask thee skill" (4.551–2), indicating by his understatement that the feat of standing on the spire is physically impossible. If the hero stands, he will reveal his supernatural identity.' For the Tempter says, 'Now show thy progeny; if not to stand, / Cast thyself down (4.554–5)'. Whatever action the hero takes follows Satan's lead.

> The dilemma appears to be an infallible temptation; it invites the despairing conclusion that life in this world necessarily defeats faith. The Son, however, does not betray the smallest tremor of anxiety. He confidently strikes back with a verse from Deuteronomy 5:16: "Also it is written, / Tempt not the Lord thy God, he said and stood" (4.560–61). The reply is a denunciation of Satan's perverse application of Scripture, but it is also the most spectacular of all the hero's verbal gestures of self-denial. Once again he refers the Satanic challenge to higher authority, and climactically identifies himself (to those who are doctrinally informed) as a hero fighting with the Sword of the Spirit.[46]

The heroic posture mirrors God's own image, in which the human is cast, in opposition to the forces of evil that only mimic being morally and physically upright. To stand, in both the physical and the metaphysical sense, defines the divine.

A century before Milton, Judah Loew ben Bezalel (1512–1609), known as the Maharal – the fabled Rabbi of Prague, who is reputed to have created the Golem, the Jewish precursor of Frankenstein's monster – defined upright posture as the essential quality of the human. In his classic commentary on the Torah, *Tiferet Israel* (The Adornment of Israel), he describes the creation of Adam:

> In the fifth [hour] he stood on his feet . . . this thing, which is standing on its feet, is to be found only in the human being . . . the human being walks upright, as he is the king of the lower beings, and it is appropriate for a king to walk in upright posture. And among the lower beings there is nothing like the human being, and therefore all the animals are walking bent

downward, like the slave, who is beneath his king, and only the human being is upright. And there are more miraculous things in his form, that is his upright posture, and all is hinted at in what they said (*Mishna Avot* chapter 3, Mishnah 4), 'Pleasant is the human-being who is created in the image of God,' and it is explained in the book *Derekh Hayim*. The general principle is, that walking upright is what is special to human-beings and makes him superior to animals.[47]

In Jewish Prague, the Golem, the monster shaped from inanimate clay and transformed into a protector of the Jews by having the word of God placed in his mouth, is the baseline for that which is not human. For Rabbi Loew, the human being is created in the divine image through standing up straight like the angels. The Golem in his animate state only approximates the human in his quasi-uprightness – a simulacrum of being upright. Once the word of God is removed from his mouth, his momentary human appearance vanishes and he returns to the clay from which he was made.[48] Being upright is a quality of the human and their relationship to the divine. In Jewish texts dealing with the correct manner of prayer, standing upright is addressed primarily in the context of devotion, for example the correct posture for standing when discussing the human's imitation of angels during the recital of the *Kedusha*, the third section of the *Amidah*, the daily prayers. They (the prayers) begin with the evocation of the angels: 'Holy, Holy, Holy, The Lord of Hosts, The entire world is filled with His Glory' (Isaiah 6:3). It is not directly about 'facing' God, but about resembling the divine through standing upright, and jumping a little upwards. As with the image of the Golem, upright prayer shows the momentary transmutation of the base into the divine, of the human into a form that approaches God.

In the Enlightenment, for Herder, standing upright and erect are not only divine gifts but scientific attributes. However, there is always the possibility of a flaw, a flaw emphasized by Milton in his vision of the Fall. One of Herder's sources is the Italian physician Pietro Moscati (1736–1824), who in 1771, comparing the essential differences of the human and animals, came to the conclusion that upright posture disposed heart, circulation and the intestines to many defects and diseases.[49] Upright posture provides the human with a connection to the Divine, but also to the worm within. Indeed, Moscati imagines that the human being could function much better as a quadruped. Herder's image of feral children, a classical topos of the Enlightenment, had them functioning quite well on all fours. But of course they were bereft of both language and civilization. To be fully human, in spite of the pitfalls, one had to walk upright.

Posture Defines What We Can Become

Immanuel Kant reacted against such a notion of the divine perfection of human posture and the theology that it implied. For him, Herder's views are merely romantic psychologizing rather than an empirical statement about the nature of humans and their future. The human being is not perfect, but, following on from his understanding of what Enlightenment means, must have the potential to alter and change, 'to use [one's own mind] without guidance of another. *Sapere aude*.'[50] Dare to know! And central to that act is to know oneself.

For the human 'is himself an animal', as Kant observed in his *Idea for a Universal History with a Cosmopolitan Purpose* (1784). There he characterized the human, even in the role of the ruler, as 'crooked wood'. Contemporary humans were 'stunted, crooked and twisted' and could attain a 'beautiful, straight stature', but only as a goal after long years of effort. This is Kant's Platonic rereading of the demand for *mens sana in corpore sano*:

> The highest supreme authority, however, ought to be just in itself and yet a human being. This problem is therefore the most difficult of all; indeed its perfect solution is even impossible; out of such crooked wood as the human being is made, nothing entirely straight can be fabricated.[51]

It is human striving that can move towards but perhaps never completely attain 'straightness' and therefore perfection. Kant stresses transformation, not stasis. Yet his image is that of the carpenter, confronted with a piece of wood so misshapen that nothing ever truly plumb can be made of it ('aus so krummem Holze, als woraus der Mensch gemacht ist, kann nichts ganz Gerades gezimmert werde'[52]). No matter how extraordinary the effort, such wood can never become true. Nature, he continues, evoking our image of the garden – if only obliquely – allows us only to approximate such an ideal. Then, in one of his extraordinary footnotes, Kant presents a counterfactual, noting that he cannot imagine how this could be on other planets. But on this earth the role of the human being is extraordinarily malleable (*künstlich*), 'if we discharge well this commission of nature, then we can well flatter ourselves that among our neighbors in the cosmic edifice we may assert no mean rank. With us it is otherwise; only the species can hope for this.'[53] Individuals, even the body of the soldier, can approximate only this, but the totality of human experience over infinite time can bring evidence for it.

A new state – one founded on reason, but on reason acquired through self-knowledge – is the forest in which such 'crooked wood' evolves:

> Yet in such a precinct as civic union is, these same inclinations have afterward their best effect, just as trees in a forest, precisely because each of them seeks to take air and sun from the other, are constrained to look for them above themselves, and thereby achieve a beautiful straight growth; whereas those in freedom and separated from one another, that put forth branches as they like, grow stunted, crooked, and awry. All culture and art that adorn humanity, and the most beautiful social order, are the fruits of unsociability, through which it is necessitated by itself to discipline itself, and so by an art extorted from it, to develop completely the germs of nature.[54]

All value comes from striving to establish oneself within society. One should note here that the ambiguity of 'crooked' and 'upright' as moral terms is also present in Kant's German. For *krumm* also has the moral implication of the antithesis of *gerade* or *aufrecht*, crooked as opposed to just or upright. All these terms can be used to describe posture. This vision of human development and mal-development is at the core of Kant's notion of posture, both in the moral and the political sense. It is no wonder that the metaphor of 'crooked wood' resurfaces in his theodicy essay 'Religion within the Boundaries of Mere Reason' (1791), referring to the creation of religious practice within the limits of the human. All institutions that we create are limited by our own fallibility and fragility.

Isaiah Berlin calls Kant's claim the bedrock upon which human fallibility is grounded in spite of its seeming simplicity, 'And for that reason no perfect solution is, not merely in practice, but in principle possible in human affairs, and any determined attempt to produce it is likely to lead to suffering, disillusionment and failure.'[55] An awareness of imperfection and a striving to overcome it are what make human beings human, even or perhaps especially those with imperfect posture: 'In his ethical writings, too, Kant stressed the virtual impossibility of moral perfection for man. Only when the will was informed by reason alone was human action moral, when the "heteronomous" impulses of the feelings were completely suppressed.'[56]

Enlightenment Prussia saw natural imperfections as problems to be overcome. With 'Dutch engineering bolstered by Prussian military strength', Prussian kings began massive projects to drain swamps and make wildernesses arable.[57] As David Blackbourn notes, 'The well-tempered state was one in which the prince had access to computations, tabulations, and classifications on everything under the sun, including tracts of "useless" land that might, one day, produce a field of corn or support a herd of Frisians.'[58] Or, indeed, through the introduction in the age of Kant of scientific forestry, with its emphasis on producing valuable 'straight timber'. Indeed, Germany produced an entire generation of scientific foresters, who spread across Europe.[59]

Such activities become so inherent to enlightened self-awareness that Goethe places them at the centre of his critique of modernity in *Faust II*, where Faust undertakes the draining of vast swamps, the foul pools, with a vast ditch. A hut mars his view of this new, perfect world, and his casual word encourages Mephistopheles to destroy the idyllic lives of Philemon and Baucis, the aged pair who live there at one with nature. Faust's goal is to create a paradise of green fields and productive humans; he accomplishes only the destruction of those ideal lives. Prussia's draining of the wetlands around Berlin and the systematic planting of straight trees there was meant to maximize the state's income as well as to improve the land. Kant's

> metaphor points to the idea of a parallel development in human society – from *normalbaum* to *normalmensch* [sic], who optimally develops his or her predispositions in the unsocial sociability of civil society. The metaphor supports a social thesis . . . to which foresters might have added after their many failed attempts to maximize sustained yield that trees are too crooked as well.[60]

Kant's image of the 'crooked wood' is a direct answer to Herder's claim about the primacy of upright posture in defining human nature. But Kant's contemporaries saw that there were certainly other forests with other wood that could never become straight. In Goethe's reading of the metaphor of the forest in his essay on the Decalogue, 'Two Important, Yet Unasked Biblical Questions' (1773), he calls the Jews 'a wild, unfruitful stock, which stood in a circle of wild unfruitful trees'.[61] This exception would play a part in the idea of the Jew in 'race science' over the next two hundred years. Kant's forest, too, contained trees that needed to be pruned or eliminated.

Kant had attacked the centrality of erect posture as the defining feature of the human in his review of the first volume of Herder's *Ideas* in 1785.[62] In it, he summarized Herder's account of upward posture as the core to the creation of the sentient human:

> It was not because he was destined to be rational that man was endowed with erect posture which allows him to make rational use of his limbs; on the contrary, he acquired reason as a result of his erect posture, as the natural effect of that same constitution which he required in order to walk upright.[63]

Herder's grounding of reason in physiology rather than abstract concepts was for Kant an aberration, since he demanded as part of his understanding of human development the ability for radical change. Herder is suspicious of such radical claims of human malleability. Rather, he doubts any transcendence of inherent (for him God-given) human nature undertaken purely by human rationality. To acquire the state where the categorical imperative becomes universal demands such transcendence. But the idea that the human being, rooted in this single act of acquiring upright posture, comes to be fully human in all its faculties – moral, aesthetic and rational – was even odder to him. For it assumed the absence of any true development over time, only the possibility of moral decay and postural collapse.

Later, in his *Conjectural Beginning of Human History* (1786), Kant avoids any discussion of posture and has the human being created by God acquiring reason by moving past the initial stages of instinct driven by pure human need. Kant begins his tale in a garden – his version of the Garden of Eden – its climate temperate, a place where man has passed his initial brutish state and has acquired mobility and language.[64] 'I shall consider the human being only after it has made substantial progress in honing it [sic] skills in using its naturally given powers . . . The first human being was thus able to stand and walk. It was able to speak.'[65] It is Adam's disobedience to God that allows him to free himself from the 'womb of nature' and become rational. What 'restless reason' supplies is a sense of need beyond the moment, the capacity

> to develop the abilities within him, [that] will not allow him
> to return to the state of brutishness and naiveté from which it
> had taken him. It urges him to put himself, despite his hating
> it, patiently through the toils of life and to pursue all the glitter
> and baubles that he despises and even to forget death itself,
> which terrifies him, for all the trifles, the loss of which he fears
> even more.[66]

Human beings are thus rooted in the present, but being aware of the future means that they are always anticipating change. They are not born upright, praising God, but only struggle through their reason towards moral perfection.

Herder picks up the thread of Kant's arboreal argument against him in 1785 in further instalments of the *Ideas for the Philosophy of the History of Humanity*, where he claims that,

> [as] far as it may be, no tree is permitted to deprive another of
> air, so as to render it a stunted dwarf, or force it to become a
> crooked cripple, that it may breathe with more freedom. Each
> has its place allotted it, that it may ascend from its root by its
> own impulse, and raise its flourishing head.[67]

Nature is rooted not in struggle and self-assertion but in the equal ability of all to avoid becoming a 'stunted' tree. All humans begin in the perfection of God's creation. Yet it is the Kantian idea of 'crooked wood' that becomes a leitmotif for the orthopaedists as well as educational theorists of the time. Not divine perfection, not the reliance on priests or physicians, but rigorous self-improvement creates good posture. And this is not merely a metaphor for posture.

As early as 1771, in 'On the Essential Corporeal Difference between the Structure of Animals and Human Beings', Kant reviewed Moscati's claim that upright posture had serious biological costs, such as harm to both mother and child in pregnancy, heart disease and problems with the circulatory system and metabolism.[68] Animals have a natural posture, which is walking on all fours. Kant 'claimed that it confirmed the intervention of reason in the natural order, manifesting its power and its autonomy in the case of man'.[69] We are destined, he said, to be social animals, at the very cost of these infirmities of posture, and thus we learn to walk upright. Our posture is very much in our own hands to shape or not.[70] Here Kant echoes Jean-Jacques Rousseau's understanding of the cultural determinants of posture. Kant's own appearance is, of course, the stuff for the physiognomists of the age, such as Johann Kaspar Lavater. As has been observed concerning Kant's debate with Herder about the centrality of upright posture,

> his fantasy [is] of having made his misshaped [sic], unattractive body beautiful and straight through rigorous self-denial. In his imagination, Kant had become moral, righteous, and in this sense beautiful by suppressing his inclinations and instincts. Herder's concept of man broke the spell; Kant was not naturally upright; his asceticism had failed.[71]

But one wonders whether, when Kant imagined the 'crooked wood' of the philosopher's body, his mind's eye caught not on his own tiny, round-shouldered image, but on the hunchbacked portraits of Moses Mendelssohn, the equally tiny Jewish philosopher, who in 1763 won a prize awarded by the Berlin Academy for a paper on the mathematical proof for metaphysics. Kant, who came second, was confronted at almost every turn during the age by Mendelssohn's misshapen visage, in engravings by artists such as Daniel Chodowiecki and a silhouette in Lavater's *Fragments*.[72] Mendelssohn, according to Lavater, is as ugly as Aesop, but brilliant nevertheless. Yet Jews, Kant notes – even his correspondent Mendelssohn – represent a specific subtype of 'crooked wood'. For the Jews are a people frozen in an archaic past, having a statutory religion, who do not and cannot strive for self-improvement as do Christians, whose religion is a moral faith; they are truly 'crooked wood' that cannot develop.[73]

For Kant, human self-improvement leads to the overcoming of our inherently crooked posture. The Romantics, such as Johann Gottlieb Fichte in his *Foundations of Natural Right in Accordance with the Principles of the Wissenschaftslehre* (published in two volumes, in 1796 and

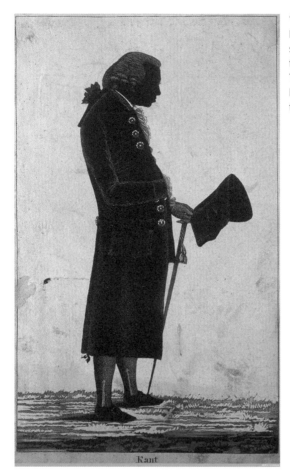

'Immanuel Kant on His Daily Walk', aquatint silhouette in black ink from life by Johann Theodor Puttrich, 1793. Kant's own posture was that of 'crooked wood'.

Kant

1797), built on Kant and Herder in equal proportion. Fichte saw the upright body with its erect posture as freeing the arms and hands from functional tasks and creating a face that is turned upwards, with its eyes towards God and its mouth able to praise the transcendental:

> The cultivated human being is characterized most distinctly by a spiritual eye and a mouth that reflects the heart's inner-most stirrings . . . for the human, the eye, in and of itself, is not simply a dead, passive mirror, like the surface of still water, or an artificially produced mirror, or the eye of an animal. It is a powerful organ that self-actively circumscribes, outlines, and reproduces spatial shapes. It self-actively sketches out the figure that is to emerge from raw marble or that is to be projected upon a canvas before the chisel or paint brush is set in

motion; it self-actively creates an image for a freely constructed mental concept.[74]

Herder's notion that upright posture allows mankind to develop language is extrapolated here, as upright posture permits the mouth to move from purely biological functions to that of language production:

> The mouth, which nature designed for the lowest and most selfish of functions – that of nourishment – becomes, through the human's self-cultivation, the expression of all social sentiments, just as it is the organ of communication. As the individual, or – since we are talking about fixed parts of the species – as the race becomes more animal-like and more self-seeking, the mouth protrudes more; as the race becomes more noble, the mouth recedes beneath the arch of the thinking forehead.[75]

Fichte's rereading of Herder's (and earlier Aristotle's) image of the human face as the mirror of the human soul made possible only by erect carriage is established through the understanding that the human is also Kant's 'crooked wood'. The human demands refashioning through self-awareness and is not simply Aristotle's physical manifestation of the highest good:

> All of this, the whole expressive face, is nothing as we emerge from the hands of nature; it is a soft mass of confluent tissues within which one can detect, at most, only what is yet to become of it once one imposes on it an idea of one's own development; – and it is precisely because of this incompleteness that the human being is capable of such formability.
>
> All of these things . . . are what compels everyone with a human countenance to recognize and respect the human shape everywhere – regardless of whether that shape is merely intimated and must still be transferred (albeit with necessity) to the body that intimates it, or whether that shape already exists at a certain level of completion. The human shape is necessarily sacred to the human being.[76]

This is the material body encompassing the notion of rational freedom, since the human body does not follow a predetermined path but is able to choose. Thus the body, to echo Kant, can always adapt to new tasks, even those that had never before been imagined.

Posture and the Idea of the Beautiful (or its Opposite)

Kant's successor in the chair of philosophy at Königsberg in 1833, the dyed-in-the-wool conservative Hegelian Johann Karl Friedrich Rosenkranz (1805–1879), argued precisely the opposite in his *Aesthetik des Hässlichen* (Aesthetics of Ugliness; 1853), namely that ugliness – the antithesis of beauty – resides in the totality of the essence of human existence on a scale that runs from the beautiful and intelligent to the 'cretin who is yet even uglier than the Black, as they add to the unbalance of the body the stupidity of intelligence and the weakness of the spirit':

> The ugly does not reside in the essence of human beings. Rather, since rationality and freedom define the human being, so too is it clear that being human is defined by the symmetry of the body, the differences in hands and feet, in the human being's upright posture. [If] a human being is, like the Bushman or like the cretin, naturally ugly, such distortions of the body represent their local and relatively inherited lack of freedom. Disease is usually the source of ugliness when it distorts the skeleton, the bones and the muscles, as for example in syphilitic osteomyelitis or gangrenous destruction of the skeleton. It causes ugliness when it colours the skin, as in jaundice, or covers the skin in ulcers as in scarlet fever, the plague and certain forms of syphilis.[77]

Rosenkranz then moves easily from the aesthetic to the moral, seeing in ugliness the 'origin of evil and the ugliness transmitted through evil to the external manifestation of human beings. Evil is not transcendent essence beyond the freedom of human beings.'[78] It is the immutability of the body and its reflection of evil in its ugliness (whether in race, disability or disease) that are defined by the lack of beautiful and therefore good posture. This is reflected in his theories of education, as we shall see later.

The theological argument espoused by Herder and countered by Kant is not uncontested before the age of evolutionary theory. Before

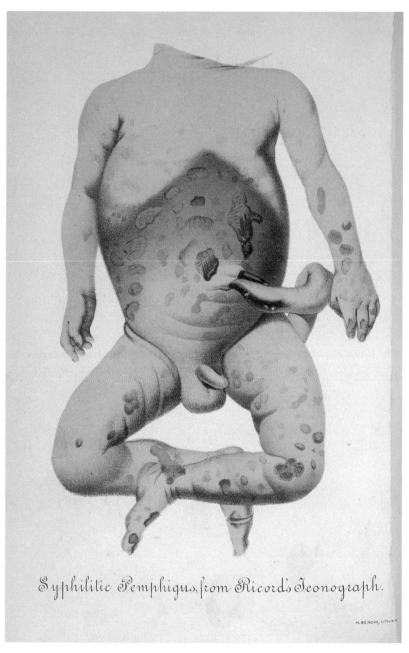

Syphilitic Pemphigus, from Ricord's Iconograph

Syphilitic Pemphigus, from Ricord's Iconograph. The deformed body of a syphilitic infant forms the frontispiece of P. Diday, *A Treatise on Syphilis in New-born Children and Infants at the Breast* (New York, 1883).

the beginning of the American Civil War, the physician and writer Oliver Wendell Holmes, Sr, produced his most widely read novel, *Elsie Venner* (1859 in the *Atlantic Monthly*; published as a book in 1861). It is an account that looks at the problem of degeneration through the lens of science. A snake bites a pregnant woman, and her offspring, the title character, has attributes both human and reptilian. For Holmes, as for his contemporary Nathaniel Hawthorne in the short story 'The Minister's Black Veil' (1837), as well as 'Rappaccini's Daughter' (1844) and then, most explicitly, the romance *The Marble Faun* (1860), the dilemma is one of 'original sin', which Holmes casts (as does Kant) as a question of moral choice rooted in a rational mind. Unlike his contemporaries Ralph Waldo Emerson and Walt Whitman, who 'were trying their best to convert medical facts into inspirational poetry, Holmes was converting a literary form into a vehicle for a case history'.[79] In this case study, Venner's original sin, her supposed reptilian ancestry, is drawn into question by the minister, the Reverend Doctor Chauncy Honeywood, who preaches a sermon on

> the book of Genesis at the eighteenth chapter and read that remarkable argument of Abraham's with his Maker in which he boldly appeals to first principles. He took as his text, 'Shall not the Judge of all the earth do right?' and began to write his sermon, afterwards so famous, 'On the Obligations of an Infinite Creator to a Finite Creature'.[80]

Honeywood skirts a series of heresies in his argument, according to Holmes, 'for which men had been burned so often'. His rejection of original sin and the very idea of disability as proof of the sins of the mother are cast aside:

> He did not believe in the responsibility of idiots. He did not believe a new-born infant was morally answerable for other people's acts. He thought a man with a crooked spine would never be called to account for not walking erect. He thought if the crook was in his brain, instead of his back, he could not fairly be blamed for any consequence of this natural defect, whatever lawyers or divines might call it . . . supposing that the Creator allows a person to be born with an hereditary or ingrafted organic tendency, and then puts this person into the

hands of teachers incompetent or positively bad, is not what is called sin or transgression of the law necessarily involved in the premises?

Kant's 'crooked wood', the moral legacy of all humans, is but one variation on the range of human posture. Poor posture, like poor education, demands of us all the ability still to see the moral law under which we live. Holmes evokes poor posture as a disability of the body, not a predisposition of the soul.

For nineteenth-century thinkers, reading Kant on posture came to define the spark of life itself. On 16 January 1839 Emerson lectured on the very definition of life to a large audience at Boston's Masonic Temple. He stressed that

> the soul pauses not. In its world is incessant movement. Genius has no retrospect. Virtue has no memory. And that is the law for man. Live without interval: if you rest on your oars, if you stop, you fall. He only is wise who thinks now; who reproduces all his experience for the present exigency; as a man stands on his feet only by a perpetual play and adjustment of the muscles. A dead body or a statue cannot be set up in the upright posture without support. You must live even to stand.[81]

Life itself is defined by human posture. Once life is extinguished, posture is no longer possible.

The theological notion of posture as the animating force for the human, echoed by Emerson, never really vanishes, as can be seen in the aesthetics of the nineteenth century. For Georg Wilhelm Friedrich Hegel, posture is at the core of the aesthetic impulse. Here he differs from Kant, whom he often engages in his work. In his lectures on aesthetics from the 1820s, Hegel develops a theory of posture as one of the keys to understanding being not only as self-determining reason (following Kant) but as rationally organized matter. The human being is the rational product of the reason embodied in nature. And that, for Hegel, is to no small degree keyed to 'man's upright posture':

> The animal body runs parallel with the ground, jaws and eye pursue the same direction as the spine, and the animal cannot of itself independently annul this relation of itself to gravity.

The opposite is the case with man, because the eye, looking straight outwards, has its natural direction always at right angles to the line of gravity and the body. Like the animals, man can go on all fours and little children do so in fact; but as soon as consciousness begins to awaken, man tears himself loose from being tied to the ground like an animal, and stands erect by himself. This standing is an act of will, for, if we give up willing to stand, our body collapses and falls to the ground. For this very reason the erect position has in it an expression of the spirit, because this rising from the ground is always connected with the will and therefore with the spirit and its inner life; after all it is common parlance to say that a man 'stands on his own feet' when he does not make his moods, views, purposes, and aims depend on someone else.[82]

Thus upright posture defines the very ability to act. The moment we cease to wish to act, our posture collapses and we revert to the primitive, to the childlike. This is a simple restatement of the complex theological notion that standing upright makes the pre-Edenic human into a volitional being, able to judge right from wrong. But Hegel continues to argue that upright posture alone is not sufficient to define the aesthetic impulse in man. Seeing the world from an upright position does not yet define the beautiful:

But the erect position is not yet beautiful as such; it becomes so only when it acquires freedom of form. For if in fact a man simply stands up straight, letting his hands hang down glued to the body quite symmetrically and not separated from it, while the legs remain tightly closed together, this gives a disagreeable impression of stiffness, even if at first sight we see no compulsion in it. This stiffness here is an abstract, almost architectural, regularity in which the limbs persist in the same position relatively to one another, and furthermore there is not visible here any determination by the spirit from within; for arms, legs, chest, trunk – all the members – remain and hang precisely as they had grown in the man at birth, without having been brought into a different relation by the spirit and its will and feeling. (The same is true about sitting.) Conversely, crouching and squatting are not to be found on the soil of freedom because they indicate something subordinate, dependent, and slavish. The free position, on the other hand, avoids abstract regularity and angularity and brings the position of the limbs into lines approaching the form of the organic; it also makes spiritual determinants shine through, so that the states and passions of the inner life are recognizable from the posture.

Here, Hegel makes a clear distinction between the static and dynamic human, but also between the free human and the crouching slave. The static human may be the embodiment of archaic Greek sculpture, but it stands in sharp contrast to the individual who is able to accentuate their own sensuous self-containment.

For Hegel it is classical Greek sculpture (Praxiteles) but also, un-surprisingly, Michelangelo's works that embody this ideal. This is an aspect of the historical roots of the 'master–slave' dialectic, for Hegel the clearest distinction between the spirit of man, now loosed from the confines of the posture of the repressive societies such as ancient Egypt, with its static and rigid aesthetic form. Separate from the squat-ting position of the slave is the image of upright posture as the core of modern man.[83] Hegel's image is that of the black slave, the slave in revolt on Santo Domingo. At that moment in history, the human being acquires its true aesthetic quality as a dynamic figure with a rich and pure beauty writ large on its body in opposition to that of the slave. The posture of the master is defined by the posture of the slave. We can see Alexandre Kojève's reading of Hegel's master–slave dialectic as demanding the internalization of the idea of the slave in the slave's psyche as well as body, for

> there is no instinct that forces the Slave to work for the Master. If he does it, it is from fear of the Master. But this fear is not the same as the fear he experienced at the moment of the Fight: the danger is no longer immediate; the Slave only knows that the Master can kill him; he does not see him in a murderous posture. In other words, the Slave who works for the Master represses his instincts in relation to an idea, a concept. And that is precisely what makes his activity a specifically human activity, a Work, an *Arbeit*.[84]

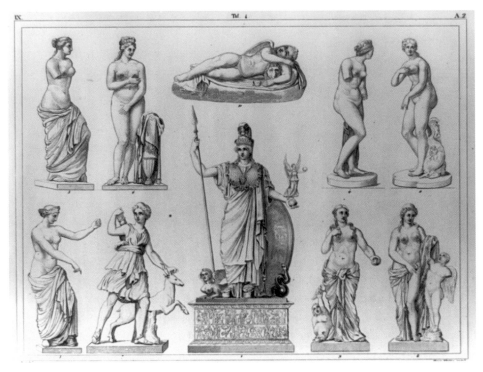

Henry Winkles, 'Greek and Roman Sculpture, Including Phidias' Statue of Pallas in the Parthenon, Several of Venus, Diana the Huntress, and Others'. From J. G. Heck, *Iconographic Encyclopedia of Science, Literature, and Art* (New York, 1851), vol. II. Much of Hegel's awareness of classical art came from the many reproductions of such art both as casts (in the new Berlin university) and in the form of plates from illustrated volumes.

But it is also the case that without such a posture the internalization of the slave's role is illegible.

Perhaps we should remark here on the obvious. The difference between the body in classical sculpture and the real, living body is profound. Oscar Wilde observed this most cogently in his 'Decay of Lying' (1891). His interlocutor asks,

> Do you think that Greek art ever tells us what the Greek people were like? Do you believe that the Athenian women were like the stately dignified figures of the Parthenon frieze, or like the marvellous goddesses who sat in the triangular pediments of the same building? If you judge from the art, they certainly were so. But read an authority, like Aristophanes for instance. You will find that the Athenian ladies laced tightly, wore high-heeled shoes, dyed their hair

yellow, painted and rouged their faces, and were exactly like any silly fashionable or fallen creature of our own day. The fact is that we look back on the ages entirely through the medium of art, and art, very fortunately, has never once told us the truth.[85]

This was also true of their posture. With regard to the postural science of the time, confusion reigned. As late as 1925, an editorial in *The Lancet* claimed that

> It is well known to sculptors and students of ancient art that the male Greek figure, as represented in such statues and reliefs as have come down to us, differs considerably from the best models of modern times. The difference would seem to consist of a greater sharpness of the lumbo-sacral angle . . . We have no means of knowing whether the sculptures were true to nature or not, but at least they show that the ideal of manly beauty in the time of Pheidias differed from that of the orthopaedic surgeon of today.[86]

Or indeed, as the American postural reformer Joel E. Goldthwait notes in 1915, in what came to be a standard American text of the time on posture and health:

> The difference in the anatomic types is also recognized consciously or unconsciously, in art, and nothing can be more perfectly normal than the early (not always the late) Greek figures, or Michael Angelo's 'David', or William Hunt's 'Bathers'. The type which Rubens almost always depicts is the heavy, full-blooded herbivorous type, while the slender, carnivorous type is the one depicted by Botticelli and Fra Angelico, or by Puvis de Chavannes of the modern school.[87]

Actually, it is the sculptures of the Greeks and not their bodies that provide an alternative visual account of human posture. It is clear that when such sculptures are viewed 'from sideways and behind, the body becomes impossible'. Thus in one, 'the spinal column makes a pronounced "S" curve, descending by an unbroken groove into the cleft of the buttocks. The effect is one of symmetry, as if bisecting the

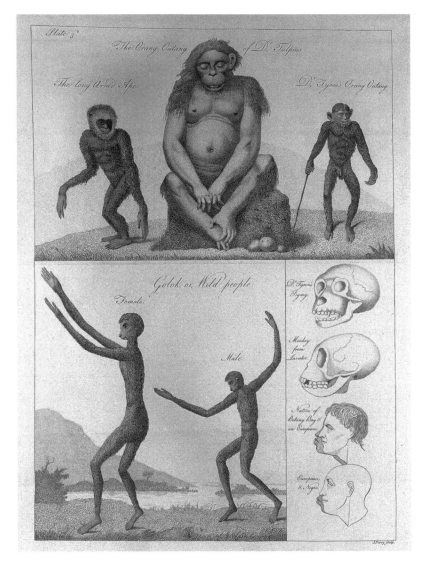

The Orang Outang of Dr Tulpius and Other Apes. An engraving illustrating the orang-utan of Dr Tulpius; the long-armed ape; Dr Tyson's orang-utan; Golok or wild people and various skulls. From Charles White, *An Account of the Regular Gradation in Man and in Different Animals and Vegetables; and from the Former to the Latter* (London, 1799).

body horizontally and vertically; but this is not how the human body is actually designed.'[88]

The elision between aestheticized bodies and actual bodies is a commonplace after Johann Joachim Winckelmann's Enlightenment aesthetics of 'noble simplicity and calm grandeur', embodied in the posture of the *Apollo Belvedere*. For him, that figure combined *arête gymnastike* (physical virtue) with *arête mousike* (spiritual virtue). The emphasis that neoclassical aesthetics placed on the sculptural representation of the body centred on the notion of plasticity and posture. Suzanne L. Marchand maintains that 'Herder, Kant, and Lessing, like Winckelmann, preferred sculpture to other visual arts, especially sculpture that depicted the human body. Winckelmann's exaltation of the human form may have originated . . . in his early training in theology (after all, God created man in his image).'[89] And made him upright, according to thinkers such as Herder. Yet it is the masculinity of the smooth, white body of the *Apollo Belvedere* that defines perfect posture. This projected a specific sense of masculinity; 'for Winckelmann himself, the steeling of the muscles through physical exercise was an integral part of the sculpture's beauty; it signified virility while posture and expression projected harmony.'[90] Indeed, the use of classical sculpture as a model of the ideal posture is one that echoes well into the twentieth century.

In his *Philosophy of Mind* (1830), Hegel stresses that the 'upright posture, has been by will made a habit – a position taken without adjustment and without consciousness – which continues to be an affair of his [the human's] persistent will.'[91] For it is the human will that defines posture, not the deity. Yet being human is defined by posture:

> Man's absolute gesture is his erect posture; he alone is able to do this, whereas even the orang-outang can stand upright only with the aid of a stick. Man does not hold himself erect naturally but stands upright by the energy of his will; and although his erect posture, after it has become a habit, requires no further effort of will, yet it must always remain pervaded by our will if we are not momentarily to collapse.[92]

The ultimate collapse, as Emerson later noted, is the collapse into death. For Hegel it is the collapse into the primitive, into the state of 'slavishness'. This posture is analogous to the contemporary reading of the slave's body as a sort of throwback to more primitive states, such as that of the orang-utan, the 'old man of the forest'.

So much, then, for the fabled symmetry between 'master' and 'slave' in Hegel's *Phenomenology of Spirit*. If we take seriously the reading provided by interpreters from Karl Marx to Kojève, the (false) mutuality of the slave and the master, each needing the other to define his role, is disrupted by Hegel's aesthetic of posture. Indeed, the posture of the slave as antithetical to that of the master seems clear in Hegel's aesthetics. Here Kojève is much closer to Frantz Fanon's reading of the dialectic than to that of the Hegelians: 'I hope I have shown that here the master differs basically from the master described by Hegel. For Hegel there is reciprocity; here the master laughs at the consciousness of the slave. What he wants from the slave is not recognition but work.'[93] In the history of posture, the slave's role is clearly defined and is dependent not on the role assigned but on the very bodies of the slave and the master, on the difference between submissive and dominant posture.

The Enlightenment and its impact, as we can see from Hegel, provide a focus for our modern understanding of posture. While there are constant references to antecedent models of postural meaning, from Greek philosophy to Renaissance art, in the Enlightenment thinkers come to see posture in all arenas of human endeavour. Equally important, they begin to translate theological concepts of human posture into what will become the language of medicine and science. In the nineteenth century, the age of Hegel, this was seen in terms of the warfare between 'theology' and 'science', as in the title of an important book of 1896 by the former American ambassador in Berlin, Andrew Dickson White. If the old saw that science comes to replace theology is only partially true, it is in the vocabulary of posture that we can see this shift most clearly. The ancients are reread and posture is refitted into the needs of modernity. And 'warfare' comes to be not only a metaphor for modernity, but the site where posture becomes most evident in its structural importance.

THREE

Chest Out!
Posture's Military Meanings

T HE ORIGIN OF UPRIGHT posture in the divine is a conceit that centres on the uniqueness of the human being. We reach up towards the gods and seek to become like them, or at least emulate them in our moral and physical constitution. In the Enlightenment people begin both to question such tales of origin and also to recognize how very deeply they are embedded in the modern world. It is striking that posture (always with the hint of imposture clinging to it) comes to be part of a modernity represented by changes in the technology of war, the world of colonial expansion and national reinvention. In this setting, our posture comes to mean how we handle the weapons of war.

The military meaning of posture as 'a particular position of a weapon, or a method of wielding it, in drill or battle', is documented as early as 1611 in William Strachey's *For the Colony of Virginea Britannia: Lawes Diuine, Morall & Martiall*: 'Concerning the training, and cleanly exercising of their Armes, & their postures, the captains shall haue order and directions for the same vnder the Marshals hand.' Very quickly, even the figurative meaning of posture as 'a mental or spiritual attitude or condition' takes on its military implications, as seen in 1642 in the very title of the Puritan divine John Taylor's *An Apology for Private Preaching . . . Whereunto Is Annexed . . . the Spirituall Postures, Alluding to that of Musket and Pike*. Taylor concludes his text with an admonition to engage in 'spirituall warfare' and instructs his congregation: 'in the postures of your Doctrine you will goe neere to suffer, and all the select of us; the first I will instruct you in shall be that alluding to Pike'.

Round heads stand to your Armes.

When Authority is absent, – Disorder your Doctrine.
When present, – Order your Doctrine.
If absent againe, – As you were.
If you conceive you shall have the better on't, Shoulder your
Doctrine and march.
If Authority bee too strong, then (Round-heads) as you were.
If Authority appeare weake. Advance your Doctrine.
If strong, – As you were.
If you get stronger in Faction, – Charge to the you.
But if Authority come in full power, – Faces about.[1]

Indeed, it is striking that thereafter the military meaning colours all future usage. The political meaning of posture as 'a state of being; a condition or situation in relation to circumstances' is also present in English from the seventeenth century, as in a letter from Sir Henry Wotton in 1620: 'We stood thus in a posture of affairs . . . very favourable.' The scientific meaning of posture as it is used in contemporary scientific papers is a twentieth-century use, but there is an obsolete scientific meaning as 'the position of a thing (or person) relative to another; position, situation', documented as early as 1605 in Francis Bacon's *The Two Bookes of Francis Bacon: Of the Proficience and Aduancement of Learning, Diuine and Humane*: 'In describing the fourmes of Vertue and Duty, with their situations and postures, in distributing them into their kinds, parts, Prouinces'.[2] Posture is both the military act and the military mind in terms of how things are positioned antagonistically, having thus had multiple, overarching meanings that exemplify the entangled genealogies inherent in any understanding of the human body.

As complicated as such entangled understandings of posture are, we can see that the idealized upright, static and mechanical posture in the early modern West seems to have originated at least in part in the late sixteenth century with the development and representation of specific forms of military drill formation. It is in Spinoza's Netherlands that this image of posture takes root. He too saw the theological implications of being 'upright', for 'What can give an upright intellect more pleasure in this life than the contemplation of that perfect godhead? For as it is concerned with the most perfect [being] it must also involve in itself the most perfect [thing] that can fall under our finite intellect.'[3] As we have seen in the debates about becoming human in the world of theology and philosophy, the age of Spinoza incorporates the ancient image of warfare as the means of training posture.

Romans and their Military Posture

The idea of physical training was inherent in the notion of shaping the soldier as early as Roman times, but what it entailed and how it was understood were radically different from what early modern warfare imagined. The Roman recruit marched 32 km (20 miles) as part of his training, carrying a heavy pack, as the late fourth-century Roman historian Vegetius (Publius Flavius Vegetius Renatus) notes in *De re militari*:

> The first thing the soldiers are to be taught is the military step, which can only be acquired by constant practice of marching quick and together. Nor is anything of more consequence either on the march or in the line than that they should keep their ranks with the greatest exactness. For troops who march in an irregular and disorderly manner are always in great danger of being defeated. They should march with the common military step twenty miles in five summer-hours, and with the full step, which is quicker, twenty-four miles [38.5 km] in the same number of hours. If they exceed this pace, they no longer march but run, and no certain rate can be assigned.[4]

While there must be order and regularity in the pace of marching, there is no required stance that defines the soldier's marching body as unique. The ideal posture of the soldier while standing was little different from the posture of the Roman citizen at the Forum casting his vote or engaging in *negotium* (business), as contrasted with its opposite, reclining at leisure (*otium*). The habitus of the soldier was standing, but not necessarily standing 'to attention'. This can be seen as ideally present in Roman art, where 'Roman soldiers maintain upright postures and calm expressions, while barbarians most often are prostrate, dead or dying in combat scenes, bound or seated, or cringing or groveling on their knees.'[5] Here again, we must remember

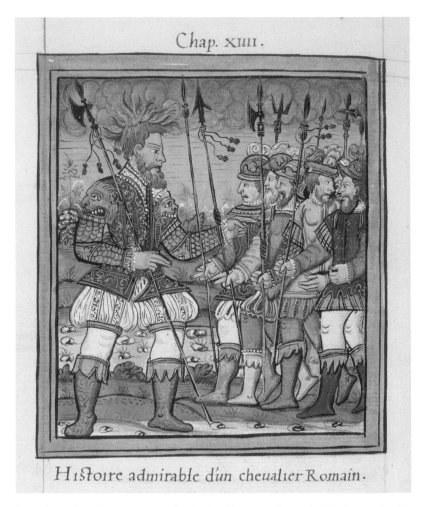

An early modern fantasy representing Lucius Martius, a Roman knight, haranguing his soldiers in order to exhort them to vengeance, from the *Histoires prodigieuses* by Pierre Boaistuau (1560). The image of the soldiers' posture reflects the image of a pre-modern form of slack bodily discipline.

that art presents a model for perfect posture with all its implications, not a reflection of actual practice. What was central was that the image of the Roman soldier's body was different from that of the woman or the defeated barbarian. As Pierre Bourdieu has observed, standing posture itself often signals masculinity, whether that of the soldier or of the citizen, since 'standing was a masculine habitus in the Algerian Kabyle and in modern Western society; a bent posture was appropriate to women.'[6] Masculinity is evoked by such posture, and such male bodies are by their very appearance also brave:

Modern masculinity and modern national consciousness had grown up at the identical time, and while the image of the warrior was needed, the nation itself looked beyond war to an ideal type, a living symbol, that like other national symbols might breathe life into an abstract concept . . . The man who was said to fulfill this role, with some national variations, approximated the masculine stereotype.[7]

Its roots, however, are seen to lie in the ancient world, admittedly a Rome invented in the Enlightenment as the place to locate the antecedents of the understanding of posture.

Yet there is a sense that these soldiers' bodies are different from those of the businessman or the citizen at the Forum: 'The Roman soldiers also became weapons but neither their physical nor their social bodies were enclosed in this rigid total armor. Instead their bodies were *tensed*, as muscles are tensed, the strings of bows drawn taut, and catapult cables wound up for release.'[8] They are neither 'armoured' in the medieval sense nor rigid in the sense of the modern soldier at attention, but they are soldierly in their 'tensed' bodies. This distinction is a historical one, but it is also in line with Bourdieu's view that posture has both a moral and a psychological meaning entangled in it, 'a sense of the equivalences between physical space and social space'.[9] This was little different in ancient Rome.[10] And it is more or less true today, but with very different presentations and manifestations of posture.

The Modern Military Posture Evolves

The break at the early Enlightenment in the meaning of drilling soldiers seems obvious to military historians.[11] The argument is that by the sixteenth century medieval armour, so compromised by the longbow, had been more or less abandoned. The rigidity of armour came to be replaced by other means of standing with a tenser, more 'unnatural' posture, the posture that we associate with a rigid plumb line running from the crown of the head through the body to the feet. The soldier's body had become a 'stereometric figure', as the Nobel Prize-winning thinker Elias Canetti observed, for 'a soldier is like a prisoner who has adapted himself to the walls enclosing him and fights against his confinement so little that the prison walls actually affect his shape.'[12] In Canetti's view of the soldier's body, this internalized rigidity is simply a definition of the soldier, a given rigidity of the body, beyond history, indebted to the rules and orders that shout 'stand up straight!' This is the case with other forms of this argument, such as the image of the soldier's 'muscle physis' as described by Klaus Theweleit concerning the fascist body. For him, it is the internalization of a sense of rigid order, 'wholeness', of the new 'man of steel, to pursue, to dam in and to subdue any force that threatens to transform him back into the horribly disorganized jumble of flesh, hair, skin, bones, intestines, and feelings that calls itself human.'[13] Such global statements are certainly indicative of the bodies of Nazi soldiers, to which both Canetti and Theweleit refer, yet they are the culmination of a process, not inherent in its original form.

Michel Foucault contrasts the pre-modern soldier with that of the modern age. In *Discipline and Punish*, he characterizes the former as 'someone who could be recognized from afar; he bore certain signs: the natural signs of his strength and his courage, the marks, too, of his pride; his body was the blazon of his strength and valour.' Such a soldier has a body that reflects the untaught and natural (according to Foucault's view): 'an erect head, a taut stomach, broad shoulders, long arms, strong fingers, a small belly, thick thighs, slender legs and dry feet'. The modern soldier, who is trained and shaped by the military manual, is quite different: 'By the late eighteenth century, the soldier has become something that can be made; out of a formless clay, an inapt body, the machine required can be constructed; posture is gradually corrected; a calculated constraint runs slowly through each part of the body, mastering it, making it pliable.' The soldier whose body is defined by his posture is one who 'may be subjected, used, transformed and improved.'[14] This transformation is, as we have seen, a product of the institutionalization of body image within the military, but it does not remain there.

We should note that Tobin Siebers, writing from the point of view of contemporary Disability Studies, criticized Foucault's concept of the docile soldier as conceived in the eighteenth century. Foucault distinguished between the pre-modern soldier, seen as healthy and erect, and the docile soldier, a body reshaped by the demands of the modern nation-state. According to Siebers, while Foucault was trying to demonstrate how the state gradually transformed the human body into a machine, he betrayed his own 'purer and fitter conceptions of

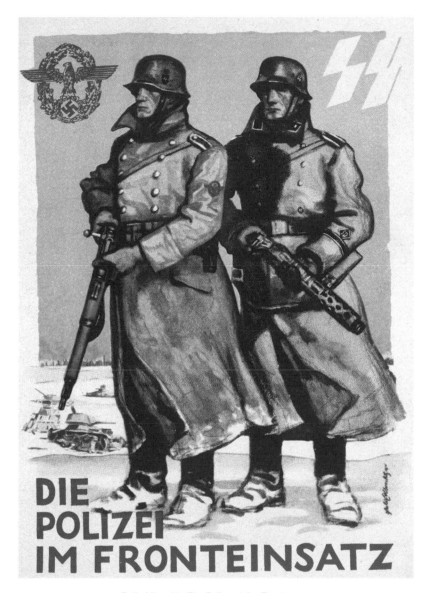

Felix Albrecht, *The Police at the Front*, 1942.

body and mind' in preferring what Foucault defined as the healthy, pre-modern soldier's body; for Foucault, docility begins to resemble disability, and the docile body is a faulty invention of modernity, just like the disabled body.[15]

Yet such a rigid body was established slowly over time, and the rigid, masculine habitus that Canetti describes is the result of the imposition of a greater and greater limitation on the postural presence of the soldier. The soldier's body is shaped by discipline, but it is a quality not simply of the form of discipline but of its very expectation. Standing up straight comes to mean different things over time.[16]

The reason for the final abandonment of armour was the introduction of something new on to the battlefield: gunpowder and early guns. While armour continued to be worn for show and for its ornamental value, as in the famed 'triumphal procession' of the Holy Roman Emperor Maximilian I in 1459, with its highly ornamented

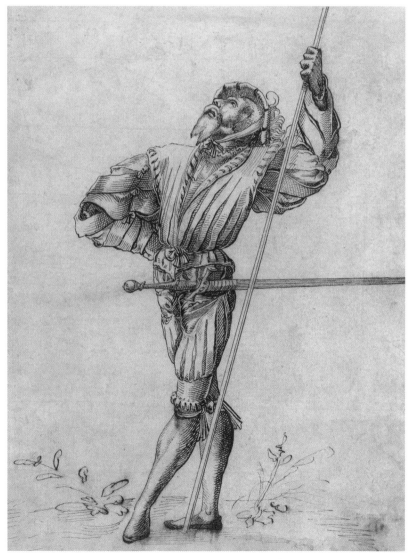

Standing Landsknecht, c. 1520–30, pen and black ink.

armour, it had been replaced on the battlefield by drilled soldiers moving in a more systematic manner in order to maximize the use of new weaponry, and the adaptation of older weapons to these new circumstances. The deportment and posture of the single soldier, however, was nowhere near the later idealized posture imagined in close drill. Indeed, there remained a notion of the individual in the melee, even in the image of the *Landsknecht*, the mercenary foot soldiers actually hired to fight the battles. Maximilian I, in spite of his glorification of horses and armour (or perhaps because of it), formed the first of these mercenary armies in 1487. First trained in hand-to-hand combat, following the model of the Swiss irregulars, these soldiers slowly adapted to the new weaponry of the age of gunpowder, opening them to ever-increasing regimentation and more highly organized military posture. What had been seen as the 'melee' of battle, even with its armoured knights, bowmen and soldiers, gave way to an ordered and structured sense of warfare. Its impact was immediately felt in the soldier's posture.

It is in a single text produced at a single moment that we can see the development of our modern sense of the military body. Jacob de Gheyn's 117 illustrations for *Wapenhandelinghe Van Roers, Mvsquetten, Ende Spiessen* (1607; translated as *The Exercise of Armes*) present images of close-order drill. They visually documented the training methods of Maurice of Nassau, developed with his two cousins, the brothers John II of Nassau and William Louis of Nassau, showing the optimum positions for carrying and shooting or using weapons, in particular the older pike and the very new ambuscade, the forerunner of all our hand-carried guns. The manual broke down the 'loading, shouldering, and firing of the newly developed musket into forty-two simple steps giving matching simplified verbal commands. [The men also] developed the "volley" technique of fire after carefully studying the ancient Roman military methods.'[17] We must note here that the reconstruction of the meanings associated with creating such an archaeology of the warrior's body means that the 'Romans' were clearly understood from the perspective of the sixteenth century. The new weaponry, as well as the different meanings that have been ascribed to Roman imperial history, alters the meanings associated with the upright body. For sixteenth-century Holland, it created an innovation: as each rank fired, a new rank took its place while the first rank reloaded – a laborious process.[18]

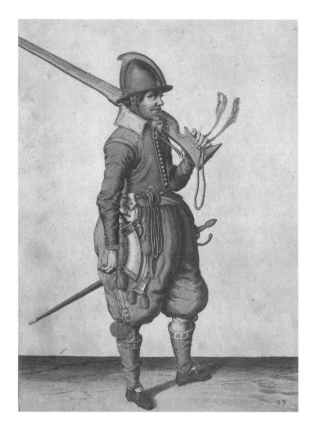

First position for
the soldier with
a caliver. From
*Wapenhandelinghe
Van Roers,
Mvsqvetten, Ende
Spiessen* (The Hague,
1607).

But it is the visual image of the handbook that is central to an understanding of the development of military posture. Most other handbooks of military exercise of the day show

> the regularity imposed upon a mass of individual soldiers . . .
> underscored by the diagrams that illustrate infantry forma-
> tions: grids composed of repeated letters of the alphabet, in
> which the rows of identical symbols correspond to the theo-
> retically homogeneous members of the army. The abstraction
> of the weak, imperfect flesh of the soldier's body into the black-
> and-white regularity of a piece of movable type expresses the
> desire for the homogenization of the potentially disruptive
> combatant into a collective military machine.[19]

This was typical of manuals such as that of Freiherr Johann Friedrich von Flemming, published in 1726, which contains diagrams and lists of simple orders.[20] By then the image of how one held oneself was no longer

First position for the pike man. From *Wapenhandelinghe Van Roers, Mvsqvetten, Ende Spiessen* (The Hague, 1607).

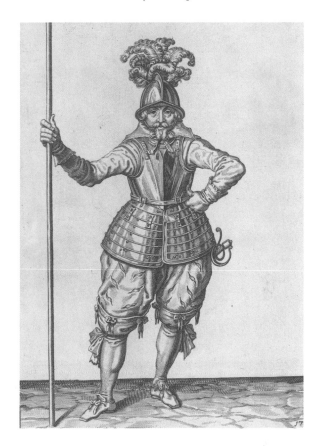

needed. Indeed, even the pike men, so central to the Dutch manual, vanished with the introduction of the bayonet in about 1700. Here we have individual soldiers, not the ordinary soldier in any case, but the extraordinary one, well-dressed, well-armed and obviously well-trained. Indeed, the pike men wear the uniform of Wilhelm's own guard.

The resting position or 'attention' forms the basis of the 'ideal' posture. This is what comes to be 'standing at attention', with a more or less rigid spine, tucked-in chin and feet positioned under the head, which is back but not yet aligned rigidly with the rest of the body. A 'plumb line' running from the top of the head to the feet is present, at least in rudimentary form. All the other positions illustrated by de Gheyn are functional – they instruct the reader or viewer on how to hold the musket (or pike) in a series of positions that enable units of soldiers to volley-fire or charge.[21] Two plates, one of the pike man and one of the soldier with a caliver (a smaller form of the ambuscade), show the initial stage, the soldier at rest.

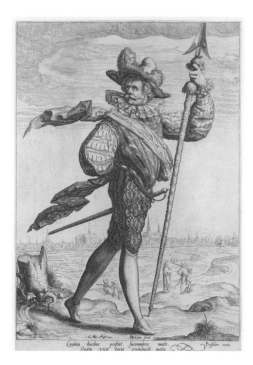

Jacob de Gheyn,
Lieutenant with a Pike,
1589, engraving.

The additional 31 plates for the pike man and 41 for the musketeer present the stages by which the weapons would be used. It is these first plates that are of interest to us, for here we have the military bearing of the soldier at 'rest'. He is not at all rigid in the sense of Canetti's 'stereometric figure', but rather attentively present and aware. Indeed, by showing one foot forwards, it is almost as if de Gheyn is indicating a movement in anticipation, a movement gesturing towards the *contrapposto* (think Michelangelo's *David*, resting on one foot, his body twisted as if he is beginning to move). In one of the later versions of the plates depicting the pike man in movement,

> de Gheyn's soldier has both feet flat on the ground. His air of relaxed stasis is achieved through the visual compression of the body, in opposition to the flamboyant rotation of the lieutenant's body in space. The legs are separated slightly, but the turn of the front foot toward the picture plane denies forward progress.[22]

Examination of the first plate shows us how the body's movement in space is understood: not as a rush forwards, but as an almost contemplative movement towards a specific goal. If the 'passive' plates, which precede the initiation of the action, show the body at rest, at ease, although at attention, the vocabulary of action in this series of images is extensive, including – and this is important – a figure of the musketeer lifting his musket that seems to be taken not from any military parallel but from the world of dance.[23]

The Nassau drill manual was intended to show how to load, shoot and reload in unison or to attack with the pike as a group, and therefore each movement had to be precise and was frozen in time in de Gheyn's illustrations.[24] It was quite different from all the various handbooks on drills, but also very different from the fencing manuals that preceded it, since it encompassed not only the individual fighter but the extension of that individual body into a collective.[25] Thus the most popular fencing guide of the eighteenth century, Domenico Angelo's *The School of Fencing* (1763), stresses only individual posture, not fighters in formation.

The body of the soldier mirrors the rigidity of the weapon, but also shows the action of the use of the weapon. Indeed, the very term for such drill books as that illustrated by de Gheyn is 'posture book'. In

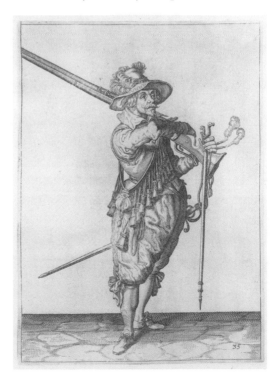

Caliver at rest. From *Wapenhandelinghe Van Roers, Mvsqvetten, Ende Spiessen* (The Hague, 1607).

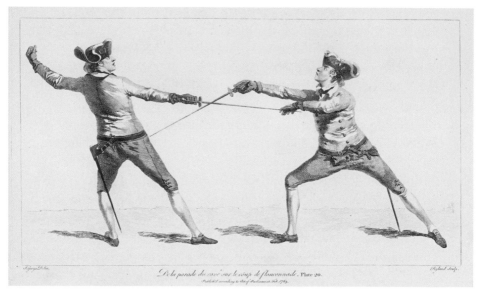

De la parade du cavé sur le coup de flanconnade. Plate 20.
Published according to the Act of Parliament Oct. 1763.

The movement of the cavé, bending one's sword-arm elbow, when a flannconnade, an attack in which the attacker first binds the opponent's blade then glides along the bound blade to deliver a hit to one of the lowlines, is attempted. From the English adaptation of Dominico Angelo's work. This is from the second edition, printed for S. Hooper, *The School of Fencing, with a General Explanation of the Principal Attitudes and Positions Peculiar to the Art* (London, 1765), with a dual-language text in French and English and 47 engraved plates by Ruyland and Hall after J. Gruyn. It was first published in French in 1763, and its influence was not confined to England: Diderot incorporated the plates into his *Encyclopédie* under the heading 'Escrime'.

1631 Ben Jonson, in his drama *The Divell Is an Asse*, has the confidence man, Meercraft, give ironic advice to his co-conspirator, Guilthead the goldsmith, the father of Plutarchus, a young man destined by his parent to a tame life in the country. Meercraft urges Guilthead to buy his son a captain's rank and let him explore the world, rather than merely buying him a 'posture book' and letting him play with mock soldiers in the sporting ground at Finsbury, in east London, in order to seduce his mistress:

> And by the vertue' of those, draw downe a wife
> There from a windo', worth ten thousand pound!
> Get him the posture booke, and's leaden men,
> To set vpon a table, 'gainst his Mistresse
> Chance to come by, that hee may draw her in,
> And shew her *Finsbury* battells.[26]

Jonson's mockery contrasts real soldiers with those who merely drill 'by the book'.

The military view of posture as those drill positions is early present in English. In *The Souldiers Accidence; or, an Introduction into Military Discipline* (1625), Gervase Markham writes of 'the three Postures or words of Command, which are vsed for the Musquet in the face of the enemie . . . 1. Make readie. 2. Present. 3. Giue fire.'[27] By 1691 such use of the term 'posture' comes to be commonplace: 'He learned . . . how to handle the pike and musquet, and all postures belonging to them.'[28] Posture is clearly defined; posture is visually represented; posture is manly, erect and upright, but not rigid. Shakespeare recognizes this when he has Cassius, approached by Brutus to overthrow Caesar, observe:

> Antony,
> The posture of your blows are yet unknown;
> But for your words, they rob the Hybla bees,
> And leave them honeyless. (v.1.33)

Sweet words, he notes, do not presage what is described as a 'particular position of a weapon in drill or warfare'.[29] Posture implies a military position, even when understood as metaphor.

Military Rigidity

During the next century the rest position itself was so altered that by the eighteenth century it is more rigidly 'aligned', with the feet together rather than apart and the spine rigidly erect.[30] By the Enlightenment Denis Diderot and Jean d'Alembert had illustrated this as a given in the first of the military drill plates in their universal encyclopaedia of 1762.[31] Their plates represent the movement of the military focused on the individual soldier, and only the last few exemplify a mass movement of units. The plumb line itself evolved over time, becoming more and more rigid. The plates by the Swiss engraver Christian von Mechel in 1799, in his translation of a French handbook from 1791 of drill positions for the infantry, even included a plumb line in their representation of the correct rest posture. In the note to the first plate, Mechel stresses that the feet must be at an angle at rest (figures 1 and 2), since this distributes the weight of the entire body so that 'the perpendicular line

(C, D) is divided exactly in half.' In motion (figures 3 and 4), 'the perpendicular line (C, D) runs through the head, [and] the torso, when marching, is brought forward.'[32] Note, however, that this image aligns the upper body with the tip of the musket, causing the upper torso to be forward of the pelvis. The more traditional plumb line runs, as we have noted, in an alignment through the ear, shoulder, pelvis and ankle. Here the soldier literally becomes an extension of his weapon, a tension that comes to haunt military images of posture.

This was clearly never a 'natural' position; it was learned, rehearsed and habituated until all soldiers at attention appeared uniform and moved in an identical manner. The position came to define the military body and, through the meanings attached to it, the normal, healthy individual. This has become normalized in military training to the present day. It also always represented not only the soldier's body, but the soldier's psyche – his code as a member of a unit, not as an individual. As the British corporal in the Royal Marines shouts at his raw recruits in Carney Lake's novel *Reflected Glory* (1990),

> You neglected your body. That's why you joined. 'Cos you wanna be strong. And fit. And use the *gift*. That God *gave* you. Your body. And your brain. Mens sana. In corpore sano. You know what that means? A healthy mind. Is in a healthy body . . . You! STANNUP STREAIGHT! YOU DISGUSTIN' CREATURE . . . That's what I mean. Posture! Stand up streaight. The natural way. CHEST OUT. GUT IN . . . You'll learn to take charge of your body.[33]

Carney's introduction to life in the Commandos starts with an admonition about correct military posture, the 'natural' plumb line. It will define his mental state as a commando, as a cog in this new machine.

Other, older qualities continued to play a role in imagining the soldier's body. Indeed, it was clear that the static size of soldiers in the early modern period was as important as their deportment. Vegetius noted:

> we find the ancients very fond of procuring the tallest men they could for the service, since the standard for the cavalry of the wings and for the infantry of the first legionary cohorts was fixed at six feet [1.8 m], or at least five feet ten inches.

These requirements might easily be kept up in those times when such numbers followed the profession of arms and before it was the fashion for the flower of Roman youth to devote themselves to the civil offices of state.[34]

In 1675 Frederick Wilhelm I of Prussia (1688–1740) created an elite unit known as the Potsdamer Riesengarde (Giant Guard of Potsdam), in which all the soldiers were at least 6 Prussian feet tall (6 ft 2 in./1.9 m). He was quickly copied in other imperial capitals, such as St Petersburg. But, while size did not always matter, posture did. That his son Frederick II ('the Great'), king of Prussia from 1740 to 1786, is credited by historians with the development of what we recognize today as the formal and rigid posture associated with close-order drill is a later part of the tale of military posture.[35] This development holds pride of place in Diderot and d'Alembert's *Encyclopédie méthodique*, where they carefully trace the visual history of close-order drill from the Romans

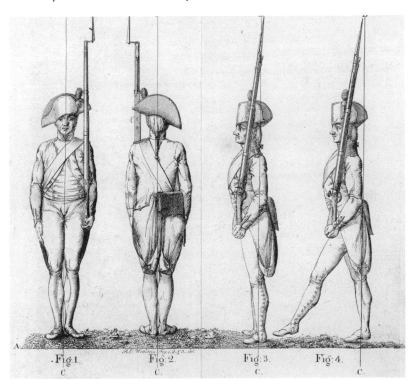

Christian von Mechel, *Soldaten- und Plotons-Schule für die Infanterie, aus dem französischen Reglement vom 1. August 1791*, übersetzt. *Herausgegeben mit 13 meist neu gezeichneten Kupfer-Tafeln* (Basle, 1799).

to the Enlightenment. But posture in this Enlightenment sense also means the development of the sense of the good citizen in the service of the absolutist state. Posture comes to define the new soldier's body as it moves in space.

By the time of Frederick the Great, drill had become formalized and highly structured as a means of training the soldier's body. In the Prussian king's lieutenant-general Friedrich Christoph von Saldern's *Tactical Principles and Instruction for Military Evolutions from the Hand of a Famous General* (1784), not only is the step of the soldier regulated but, reflecting the renewed importance of Roman drill in Prussia, so is his posture in rank. Indeed, posture comes even before the fabled gait of the Prussian soldier, with semi-locked knee and toe-forward precision. Saldern begins his account by noting that 'a body upright and well formed, sets off every man and particularly the soldier, who being under arms, must keep himself upright without stiffness. A forced position becomes painful and fatiguing, but a natural one is easy to every body.'[36] Indeed, such training to stand (before you walk) always begins with the soldier's resting posture:

> The first thing a recruit is to learn, is a good position; that is to say, to keep his body very upright, his head inclined to the right, his eyes turned a very little towards the flank man; by this means his soldiers will be so placed, that one will not be more to the front than the other, which is the main point, and cannot be too carefully observed. He must bring his breast forward, his arms must hang close to his side without stiffness, so that his elbows may come back, and that the seam of his sleeves may be seen, that is to say, to keep his arms so as to touch his thigh with the flat of his hand. His toes must be turned outwards, but not too much.[37]

There is a note here that defines the mechanical and highly symmetrical notion of how ideal posture should be accomplished: '[the] angle is about 60 degrees, consequently the cord AC from one point of the foot to the other, will be nearly equal to the length of the foot AB or BC because ACB is an equilateral triangle.'[38] The body is reduced to anatomical geometry.

These mechanical rules, the so-called Saldern-tactics, were used very successfully to train the Prussian troops. The French, having been defeated by Frederick in the Seven Years War using exactly those tactics, introduced the so-called mixed order of battle, more flexible and less confined, following the new rules espoused by the relatively conservative Colonel Turpin de Crissé in *The Art of War* (1754). While he advocated for traditional forms of battle, including the siege, he also stressed that such approaches must be flexible and respond to the needs of the moment.[39] Flexibility of mass movement and the parallel flexibility of training enabled the Napoleonic forces to overcome the more static and rigid Prussians at the Battle of Jena in 1806.[40]

The British, too, adopted these more rigid ideas of the soldier's posture, and they formed the basis of the British 'Dundas' drill book, *Principles of Military Movements*, written by the future commander-in-chief of the British Army, Sir David Dundas (nicknamed 'Old Pivot') in 1788, mimicking the Saldern-tactics of the Prussian army.[41] The soldier must stand with heels

> nearly close, the toes a little turned out – The arms hang near the body, but not stiff – the flat of the hand touches the thigh – The elbows and shoulders are kept back, and the belly is drawn in, which occasions the breast to be advanced, and the body to be upright, but rather inclining forward – the head should be erect, and not turned (or the least possible) to right or left, as the shoulders would certainly accompany it.[42]

These Prussian tactics led to the ignominious defeat at New Orleans in late 1814, when 11,000 'redcoats' were simply slaughtered by 5,000 American troops and irregulars with almost ten times the losses on the British side.

Both gait and posture are defined by Dundas. The stiffened leg of the rigid but mobile body of the soldier moves with braced knee and rigid pelvis at a more leisurely pace than that of the 'normal' citizen, mimicking what the Germans imagined as the gait of the Roman senators, as opposed to the more laid-back Austrians, who saw themselves as Greeks.[43] That this pseudo-Roman manner of presentation became the norm illustrates how entangled notions of citizenship and nation become with ideas of posture.

Military posture marks the gentleman even out of uniform: James Fenimore Cooper introduces us to Harvey Birch, the protagonist in his novel of the American Revolution, *The Spy* (1821), by contrasting

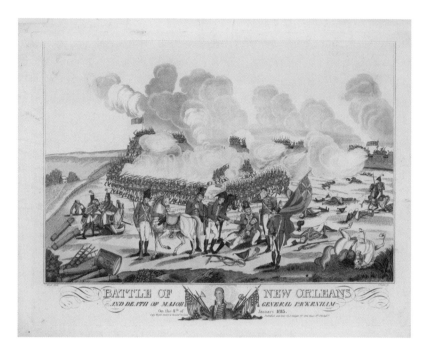

William Edward West, *Battle of New Orleans and Death of Major General Packenham: On the 8th of January 1815*, 1817, aquatint, etching and line engraving. The Battle of New Orleans is seen from the British perspective, as British forces advance on the earthworks or barricades from which the American forces, under the command of Andrew Jackson, repel the attack. The image includes a remarque printed at bottom centre that shows a head-and-shoulders portrait of Andrew Jackson, facing slightly left, with American flags and various weapons.

his disguise as a peddler with the hidden nature of his calling, revealed by his military posture:

> The passage of a stranger, with an appearance of somewhat doubtful character, and mounted on an animal, which, although unfurnished with any of the ordinary trappings of war, partook largely of the bold and upright carriage that distinguished his rider, gave rise to many surmises among the gazing inmates of the different habitations; and, in some instances, where conscience was more than ordinarily awake, to no little alarm.[44]

Victorian literature saw the soldier's body even when it was dressed as a civilian's. Emily Brontë has Nelly Dean recognize the adult Heathcliff, who may well have also fought in the American Revolution, as 'his upright carriage suggested the idea of his having been in the army'.[45]

Sherlock Holmes could immediately recognize Watson as a former officer who had served in Afghanistan by his posture in *A Study in Scarlet* (1887). Watson is puzzled by this revelation at their first meeting, and Holmes later explained that he had 'the air of a military man'.[46] Holmes's competitors knew this trick well. In the 1880s Captain Finden, the protagonist of one of Thomas Wilkinson Speight's 'sensational' murder mysteries, 'had the upright, assured carriage and chivalrous bearing of a born soldier, so that, even when in mufti no trained eye could take him for other than what he was'.[47] In 1912 the Anglican canon Victor L. Whitechurch, a contemporary and competitor of Conan Doyle, had 'A stiffly-upright, military-looking man, with the ends of his fair moustache strongly waxed, dressed in a frock coat suit, walk down the platform'.[48] But Watson's limp and Heathcliff's rigidity reveal little of their real character. The postural body can mask true character, for the expert whose eye can see the military body even in civilian dress cannot extrapolate the former soldier's character from his stance. Heathcliff is thus truly on a different moral plane from Watson in spite of their carriage.

The Mechanics of Movement and Military Posture

Once the military body comes to shape the cultural fantasy of the spine as naturally rigid and as defining load-bearing, the trajectory is clear. By the late eighteenth century, in a gradual but inexorable manner, the military body becomes stiffer and more rigid.[49] The science of the time comes to react to such images by trying more and more to abandon the anatomists' notion of a static body and to see that body's posture in motion.

The brothers Wilhelm Weber, a professor of mechanics, and Eduard Weber, an anatomist, both academics and interested in human gait from rather different perspectives, published their *Mechanics of the Human Walking Apparatus* in 1836.[50] The third brother, who contributed to the greater project, was Ernst Heinrich Weber, an anatomist and physiologist, who in 1827 published a description of stance and the spine that examined how the spine maintained upright balance. Not only using the dissection of corpses but measuring the actual movements of living human beings, he observed the enormous flexibility of the spine as it was constantly able to correct and adjust because of the tractable discs between the vertebrae.[51] In their work on locomotion in the 1830s, the brothers then challenged the claims of efficacy in the existing military rules for upright Prussian posture. Indeed, as at least one historian of drill has observed, the eighteenth-century Prussian 'goose step', so strongly associated with Saldern, was an 'unauthorized aberration on the part of some Prussian drillmasters'.[52] It was a variation of the original sense of military gait, which was slow and regular rather than precise and exaggerated. But it seemed a natural extension of the rigid posture of the soldier. The Webers stressed that the 'body's natural forward motion is lawful, efficient, and self-regulating'. Interested in natural gait as a process, as well as fixed stance, the Webers present scientific materials to stress 'efficient and comfortable posture'.[53]

In linking two aspects of military movement – the soldier at rest (the fixed stance of the soldier) and the moving soldier in the field as a skirmisher – the Webers modified the older, more rigid understanding of posture by stressing it as flexible and mobile. The fixed movement of Saldern-tactics, both in terms of gait and of stance, gave way to a notion of fluidity in both. But they also understood the power of habituation in the training of human posture: 'Thus the inhabitants of the Alps climb their mountains with forward bent bodies and, unlike ourselves, are not exhausted, since we have convinced ourselves that upright posture [*aufrechte Haltung*] is a jewel.'[54] They answered the notion of the 'natural human plumb line' by observing the central problem that the anatomists had had: they were dealing with corpses laid out on a table, and, as they noted, 'it is difficult to understand after death the position that the living body is able to take.'[55] What convinced the Webers of the possibility of a more efficient, more natural posture was the angle of the pelvis. If the military (and the post-mortem) pelvis is rigid and inflexibly straight, as some anatomists claimed, then the 'natural' pelvis of the Alpine mountain climbers, just at the beginning of the explosion of mountain climbing as a sport, proved them wrong. But it was the scientific work of Franz Carl Naegele in 1825 that provided the actual empirical data for the Webers. Naegele was interested not in the *male* body but in posture in pregnant (and uncorseted) women, and he noted that women incline themselves forwards to varying degrees when walking.[56] The woman's body comes to be the litmus test for natural gait and stance. He found that in walking the pelvis is angled at 21 degrees from the vertical; it is not plumb.

Prussian politics follow the Prussian body in complex ways. Once the idea of physical rigidity comes to be questioned, the very notion

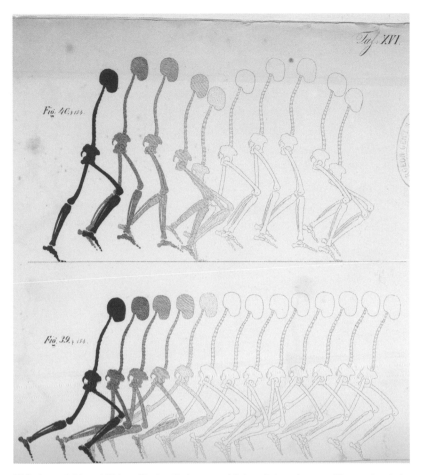

Wilhelm and Eduard Weber, *Mechanik der menschlichen Gehwerkzeuge: Eine anatomisch–physiologische Untersuchung* (Göttingen, 1836).

of rigidity in tactics and in politics follows. The Prussian general Carl Philipp von Clausewitz, in what came to be the major answer to Prussian eighteenth-century notions of both war and the state, employed this as a metaphor in his classic *On War* (published posthumously, in 1832):

Afterwards tactics attempted to give to the mechanism of its joints the character of a general disposition, built upon the peculiar properties of the instrument, which character leads indeed to the battlefield, but instead of leading to the free activity of mind, leads to an Army made like an automaton by its rigid formations and orders of battle, which, movable only by the word of command, is intended to unwind its activities like a piece of clockwork.[57]

Not the body as clockwork but the body as a flexible and responsive identity is his core metaphor for the new army. It is here that Jean-Jacques Rousseau's natural body, augmented by the ideas of the Webers, begins to shift the image of the soldier away from that of Saldern. Yet the reality was that although von Clausewitz recognized the need for both a flexible idea of war and a more flexible body for the soldier, the authoritarian tradition of Prussia carried itself into the late nineteenth century. It was present well into the world of a new state, Wilhelm I's Germany, a state that came about because of the success of the Prussian

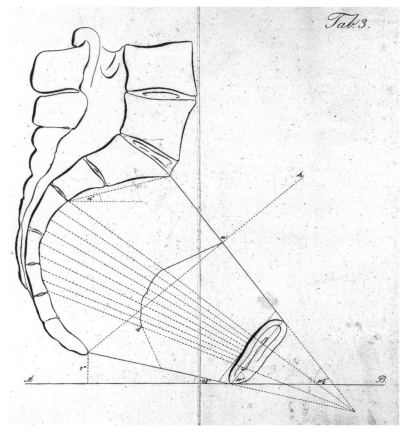

Franz Carl Naegele, *Das weibliche Becken: Betrachtet in Beziehung auf seine Stellung und die Richtung seiner Höhle: Nebst Beyträgen zur Geschichte der Lehre von den Beckenaxen* (The Obliquely Contracted Pelvis: Containing Also an Appendix of the Most Important Defects of the Female Pelvis; Karlsruhe, 1825).

army with older notions of both the function of war and the flexibility of the body. In defeating France in 1871, Wilhelm answered the defeats inflicted on the Prussians by Napoleon. Yet it was not the Prussian soldiery alone that conquered France, but the extraordinary range of modern technology, from the railway to artillery, that extended the meaning of this body. It is no wonder that the unification of the new German state was announced at Versailles, after conquering Paris. By the next decade a novel science of the military body was being laid in the new Germany by disciples of the Webers.[58]

By 1889 the Leipzig anatomist Christian Wilhelm Braune and his student Otto Fischer dropped the plumb line along the now marginal rigid posture of 'standing at attention', further incorporating the study of military posture into the medical literature on kinesiology, a term coined in the early 1890s.[59] (Braune's interest was also personal: he was Ernst Heinrich Weber's son-in-law.) They had begun a decade earlier by examining and anatomizing cadavers to determine their centre of gravity. Accepting and extending much of the Webers' work on natural posture, they retained the plumb line as their base for natural posture. Using chronophotography (sequential, rapid images to record motion), they had photographed the soldiers of the Eighth Royal Regiment Prinz Johann Georg in order to document human motion.[60] The use of photographic evidence for gait was an important feature of the physiological school, and laid the groundwork for the extensive study by Nathan Zuntz and Wilhelm Schumberg, *Studien zu einer Physiologie des Marsches* (Studies of the Physiology of Marching; 1901), which examined all aspects of military drill from clothing to nutrition, but especially the 'pathology of the march' and the complex illnesses resulting from the postures of drill.[61] The 'normal' military body came to be defined by its ability to march without fatigue. Thus their interests lay in those deviations from normal posture that marked the boundary of fatigue. This normal body came to be connected to the plumb line and the appropriate posture of the soldier under every possible physical situation while marching. Braune and Fischer's groundbreaking statistical measurements of body posture remain the basis for all contemporary discussions of the 'straight line inside the body' within the various sciences of posture, from orthopaedics to military medicine.[62]

Rooted in Braune's complex analysis of the centre of gravity in human anatomy, the study of posture is an attempt to translate such knowledge into a mechanical profile of what the upright body can be made

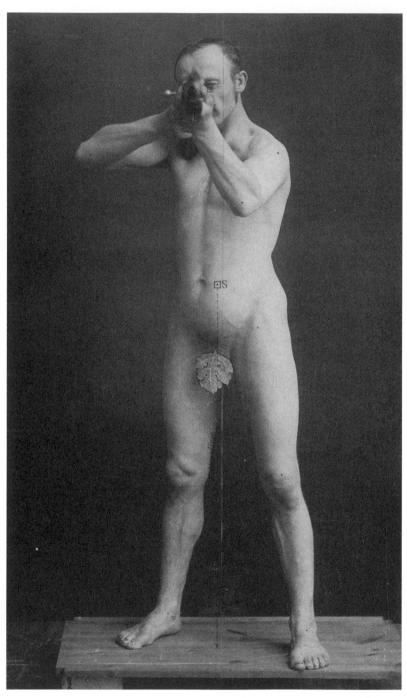

'Firing Stance without Backpack'. From Christian Wilhelm Braune and Otto Fischer, *Über den Schwerpunkt des menschlichen Körpers mit Rücksicht auf die Ausrüstung des deutschen Infanteristen* (Leipzig, 1889).

to do in optimum circumstances, and to define those circumstances. Braune and Fischer understood notions of flexibility and strength with regard to their studies of how soldiers could best move with heavy equipment. Yet the 'Prussian' image of the erect body trumped their own science. They quite easily use the concept of the plumb line, employing an actual plumb bob as a means of imagining the forces moving through the body. For them, the body is always dynamic but must be understood as having a maximum productive stance for specific undertakings.[63] The science of posture results from this moment in military medicine. 'Stand up straight' may not have arisen first in the military (parents might well have that priority), but its first codified and visual documentation is in this world, and the military origin of upright posture informs later discussions of posture as a quality not of men but of human beings.

Seeing Military Posture

In the work of Braune and Fischer, the photograph was more than mere ornament; it served as scientific validation of their theories. Speculation on the objective nature of the scientific photograph was the focus of photography from its origin in the 1840s, with interest in microphotography and medical physiognomy. This realist fallacy was simply part of the scientific discourse of the day. Oliver Wendell Holmes, Sr, wrote in 1859 that

> the Daguerreotype has . . . fixed the most fleeting of our illusions, that which the apostle and the philosopher and the poet have alike used as the type of instability and unreality. The photograph has completed the triumph, by making a sheet of paper reflect images like a mirror and hold them as a picture.[64]

What is seen is true.

The interest in empirical evidence for the nature of correct and corrected gait and posture reached its high point in the 1870s. Seeing the difference was at the core of Eadweard J. Muybridge's huge project in the 1880s documenting virtually every form of locomotion. Having begun in 1871 by freezing the galloping horse of his sponsor Leland Stanford, showing for the first time that horses could indeed trot with all four feet off the ground, Muybridge extended his interest to all forms of 'animal locomotion', including that of the human. He attempted empirically to clarify these questions by using sequential photography to document human gait across class, race and disability in his photographic project on human and animal locomotion conducted between 1883 and 1886 at the University of Pennsylvania. His focus remained on movement in time. Posture came to be defined as the most efficient way that any given body moved over time. His study of 'pathological' as well as 'normal' bodies in motion thus stressed the ability rather than the disability of the subjects. As the essayist Joseph Grigely notes,

> Have you ever seen Eadweard Muybridge's nineteenth-century photographs of humans and animals in motion? If you look closely at the serial photographs of people walking, particularly those of disabled people, you might notice among all of them that the idea of 'walking' is a generalization for human locomotion – of moving one's body from point A to point B using nothing more than one's own physiological reality. Whether the person is a young child or a young man, a woman with multiple cerebro-spinal sclerosis or a young boy with double amputation of the thighs, there is no way to define normalcy except through the abstract idea of locomotion.[65]

Indeed, that is also true of the postures that accompany locomotion in Muybridge's images, especially that of the final plate (562) of his series depicting human locomotion, that of 'lateral curvature of the spine; walking'.

What was vital was that Muybridge, in creating his images with multiple cameras, showed how posture and gait changed from individual to individual, from the young to the old, from the heavy to the thin. The image itself provided a litmus test for the idea of a universal posture that had infinite variations. Among the wide reach of images that Muybridge captured were ten of individuals and couples dancing (plates 187–97), as well as eight of various forms of military drill from "'fix" and "unfix" bayonets' (351) and "'shoulder", "order" and "carry arms"' (352) to 'on guard, walking and turning around' (355); as well as 'lying prone and firing' (357); 'lying on back and firing' (358); and 'charging bayonet' (359).[66] This places Muybridge in the trajectory of the scientists dealing with the military body. His focus is the limitations that the conventions of military posture impose on the movement of the soldier.

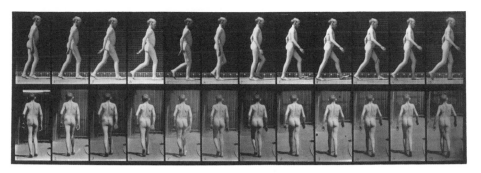

Eadweard J. Muybridge, *Lateral Curvature of the Spine; Walking*, 1887, collotype print. From Eadweard Muybridge, *Animal Locomotion* (Philadelphia, 1887).

Seeing such images today, especially those of the pathological cases probably provided to Muybridge by the Philadelphia physician Francis X. Dercum, may cause us, as it did Sarah Gordon, to comment that 'they also captured viewer's attention in more voyeuristic ways' – often because these figures were captured nude or partially clothed.[67] But this is also the case for the military photographs. Yet such a sense of the realism of the image was counter to its contemporary effect in representing the postural body as an aesthetic object. Contemporary artists took up (and rejected) Muybridge's work. They were convinced that the accuracy of his images vitiated the complexity of posture in the frozen form. Auguste Rodin noted: 'It is the artist who tells the truth and photography that lies. For in reality, time does not stand still. And if the artist succeeds in producing the impression of a gesture that is executed in several instants, his work is certainly much less conventional than the scientific image where time is abruptly suspended.'[68] The Classicist painter and sculptor Jean-Louis-Ernest Meissonier, who met Muybridge in Paris in 1881, argued that 'for the artist, there exists only one category of movements, those which the eye can grasp.'[69] As with virtually all discussions of the differences between aesthetic and scientific representations of posture (and there are substantial overlaps, as this study has shown), the idea of an abstract art seeing the body is more highly valued than 'mere' scientific accuracy. The art critic Georges Guéroult noted in 1882 that Muybridge's images were 'not only ungraceful, but false and impossible in appearance', for 'ideals of posture and grace as embodied in painting and sculpture were simply undone by the encyclopedic motion studies.'[70] They seemed to be better science than art, and therefore violated the conventions of posture, much indeed as classical sculpture had done – but their fault was accuracy.

While indebted to the French chronophotographer Étienne-Jules Marey, Muybridge's work provided the first empirical evidence of human movement in space and time and set claims for all subsequent use of images to document posture and gait. Yet it was Marey's photographic work, using multiple exposures, reducing the movement of soldiers to a graph, that would inspire the first scientific study of human gait in Braune and Fischer's detailed atlas of military posture of 1889. Marey's work provided an abstraction of posture and gait, reducing it to pure evidence, almost without human presence. This was certainly not inherently new, given how the Webers, using drawings, had reduced movement to comparable abstractions. Yet photography, even two generations after its invention, still had the penumbra of the realist fantasy; what you photographed was real in the world. The more innovative the photographic technique, the more such a claim could be substantiated within science. The more it was substantiated within science, which had become the core means of understanding the modern world, the more the arts were forced to wrestle with such

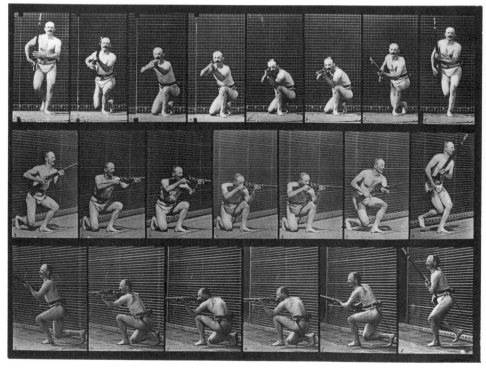

Eadweard J. Muybridge, *Kneeling, Firing, Rising*, 1887, collotype print. From Eadweard Muybridge, *Animal Locomotion* (Philadelphia, PA, 1887).

claims. Scientific epistemology reified the notion of the natural body defined within the rules of military posture.

Think about the quintessential image of the day representing movement in a fragmented time and space, Marcel Duchamp's *Nude Descending a Staircase, No. 2* (1912), which – according to Duchamp – owed its origin to 'chronophotographs of fencers in action and horses galloping (the forerunner of what we today call stroboscopic photography)' that he had seen.[71] Duchamp's Cubism and Muybridge's work gave way to even greater abstraction of movement in the work of painters such as Robert Delaunay and Kazimir Malevich, as well as the Italian Futurists and the English Vorticists, where bodies in motion came more and more over time to resemble Marey's cinematic work. What scientists saw was not the human – that was the purview of artists like Rodin – but the purity of posture and gait in space and time. Such a reduction could have substantial implications for the world of the military, but also began, in the world of modernism, to generate images that were more abstract and therefore truer to the inner image of the human body that those of late nineteenth-century Realism, even a realism as abstracting as that of a Rodin. Given that the Futurist Giacomo Balla used Marey's work as the basis for his own experiments in abstracting the body in movement in 1912, the line between abstraction and science grew blurry. By 1913 Anton Giulio Bragaglia's manifesto on 'Futurist Photodynamism' argued that modern art photography 'constituted a unique and autonomous form of art that must be distinguished from ordinary photography, as well as from Étienne-Jules Marey's chronophotography, which he characterized as providing only static views of external reality'.[72] This is identical to the tension we saw in Rodin's comment.

The idea of upright posture and upright character certainly haunted the new Prussian court, setting the tone for Braune and Fischer's work. Unlike the movement into modernism in the world of late nineteenth-century dance, Prussian postural training demanded rigidity. For rigid posture was a metaphor for adherence to an authoritarian notion of the state for the new Germany. Having abandoned any idea of a constitutional monarchy after the British model well before 1871, the German emperor retained much of the traditional status and power of his former role as the king of Prussia. The plumb line as much as the goose step defined the new state and the new court. The irony is that when Meiji Japan wanted to modernize its army, it turned to Germany after the Franco-Prussian War for its model, with rigid posture and goose-stepping soldiers. Prussia sent General Klemens Wilhelm Jacob Meckel, who introduced German drill and posture during his time in Japan (1885–8). He taught not only tactics but the military's absolute loyalty to the emperor.[73]

Kaiser Wilhelm II, who succeeded both his father and grandfather in 1888, hired the Vienna-based American body culturist Elizabeth Marguerite de Varel Mensendieck (1864–1957), better known as Bess M. Mensendieck, to improve the posture of his courtiers:

> The potbellies of the ladies-in-waiting of the last German imperial court always annoyed Kaiser Wilhelm II. In an effort to appease him, whenever they stood at attention in his presence they folded their hands over their bulging abdomens. This posture made them look like fantastic beer-mugs, a sight which vexed Wilhelm further. Hearing that a sturdy little blonde u.s. esthete named Bess M. Mensendieck taught men & women how to stand and move gracefully, by means of what she called 'functional exercises', he summoned her to do the same for his court. Cried the Kaiser: 'They are the most awkward women in the world. One never sees women at the courts of London, St Petersburg or Rome stand about in the graceless attitudes I see at mine.'[74]

Mensendieck's popular book *Körperkultur des Weibes* (Female Body Culture; 1906) dominated discussions about posture and gymnastics in Germany well into the 1930s, and generated a system of improving movement and posture that still is used.[75] Her books are well-illustrated and provide models of appropriate feminine posture that is efficient and functional, a '"correct" posture of equilibrium'.[76] The sense of correct posture she communicated is one we have seen before:

> When the human animal stands properly erect, an imaginary line should cut the nose, chin, breastbone and crotch. Another imaginary line should drop from the mastoid, in front of the shoulder joint, through the elbow and little finger (palm turned to the rear), side of knee and ankle. This is achieved by standing with feet together, shoulders held back, abdomen tucked in, buttocks clenched.[77]

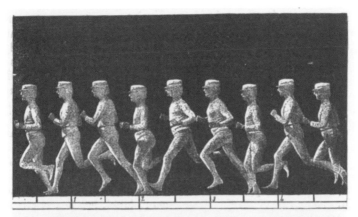

Fig. 3. — Un homme qui court. Reproduction par l'héliogravure d'une photographie instantanée de l'auteur.

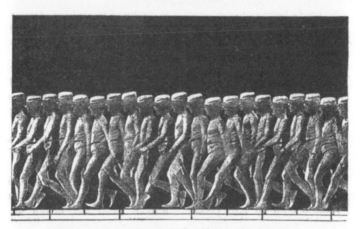

Fig. 4. — Un homme qui marche. Photographie instantanée.

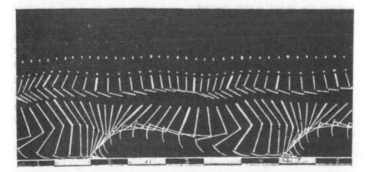

Fig. 5. — Photographie instantanée des bandes de métal brillant appliquées le long de la jambe et du bras d'un coureur.

Étienne-Jules Marey, *Two Images of Running Men Reduced to a Linear Graph of Running Man in Black with White Stripes*, c. 1882. From 'La station physiologique de Paris', *La Nature*, XI/2 (1883).

Goose-stepping, rigid, inefficient soldiers with new weaponry that made them effective on the battlefield were now the models for the posture of the imperial court.[78] Indeed, important political figures such as the Weimar politician and banker Hjalmar Schacht became recognizable by their 'distinctive characteristics – the crew cut, the rigid bearing, the stiffly upright posture'. So much so that one acquaintance of his remarked that he 'managed to look like a compound of a Prussian reserve officer and a budding Prussian judge trying to copy the officer'.[79] But such military postures were inappropriate for middle-class women. Mensendieck's model for training those female bodies rested on the notion that 'simple' people living in non-urban settings had a more natural posture, which she held to be equivalent to the posture of classical Greek sculpture. By examining Greek sculpture (such as the Venus de Milo), she noted, we can see how 'deficient we are in all-round bodily perfection'.[80] But Mensendieck's theory of posture had a clearly eugenic goal. It was concerned with 'building fit mothers for the future civilization, as opposed to the stooping of simian ancestry'.[81] Such postural training would reform the middle-class female body and

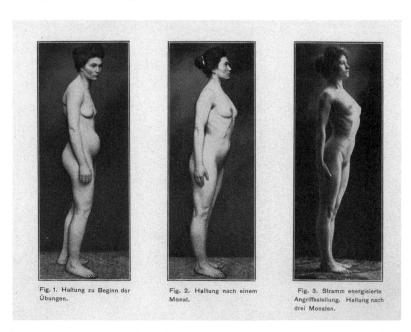

Fig. 1. Haltung zu Beginn der Übungen.

Fig. 2. Haltung nach einem Monat.

Fig. 3. Stramm energisierte Angriffsstellung. Haltung nach drei Monaten.

From a slouching posture at the beginning, to improved posture after one month's training, to the perfect plumb line after three months. From Bess M. Mensendieck, *Körperkultur des Weibes: Praktisch Hygienische und Praktisch Ästhetische Winke* (Munich, 1906).

make it both healthier and more beautiful, and more able to produce healthy boy children for the army and healthy girl children to further the race, as the court itself reflected a more military postural protocol.

This was, however, not merely an aberration of imperial Berlin, where Mensendieck served as a 'scientific adviser' on posture, beauty and health.[82] In mimicry of the Wilhelminian court, the erect body becomes a standard to which a rising middle class (whether in the army or in the drawing room) can aspire, imagining that their bodies are no longer marked as different from those of the elite. Its reform was a type of military retraining of the body for civilian purposes. It made better bodies out of the urban middle class and their slouching postures, since slouching was a sign of innate rebellion against the 'natural'. The 'natural' came to be that which society superimposed on the modern bourgeois body.

FOUR

Medicine as Therapy
for an Unhealthy Posture

P ERFECT BODIES MEANT perfect posture, and that in turn meant perfect moral character. But how do you define, not to mention treat, 'bad' posture? Distinguishing between normal or normative posture and bad or pathological posture is not merely a problem of labelling in medicine. Diagnostic classifications reflect the demands of the physician and the patient for clarification of the definition of illness, as well as the trajectory of any potential therapy. It is clear that if as a patient you do not understand yourself as ill, you will not pursue such clarification. When you do, such classification becomes part of your identity, for better or for worse. Such definitions are reflections of the society in which you function, as well as of your relationship to that society. Thus you can be said to have bad posture only if you internalize the nature of your posture as pathological rather than different. There are many variables that define the healthy and the unhealthy, the acceptable and the unacceptable, the normal and the deformed (all lived and experienced categories). 'Bad' posture remains a good litmus test for examining how these variables interact to define the healthy or normal body.

'Bad' posture has been the subject of Western medicine since the time of the Hippocratic corpus, for posture played a role in diagnostics for the Greeks, as well as in their classification of disease:

> The patient ought to be found by the physician reclining on his right or left side, with his arms, neck and legs slightly bent, and the whole body lying relaxed; for so also recline the majority of men when in health, and the best postures to recline in are

most similar to those of men in health. But to lie on the back, with the arms and the legs stretched out, is less good. And if the patient should actually bend forward, and sink foot-wards away from the bed, the posture should arouse more fear than the last.[1]

Treatment should be given with posture well in mind, because it is one of the basic variables that the physician can control. But diagnosis is more than that, as Carolyn Smith-Morris, in her introduction to *Diagnostic Controversy*, writes: 'Diagnosis is among the first responses to suffering, the one that initiates and organizes all others'; she acknowledges its paradoxes, noting: 'Diagnosis is a necessary and speculative tool for the identification of and response to suffering in any healing system. But it is also an expression and a vehicle of bio-medico-capitalist power.'[2] Even for the Greeks, diagnosis meant being able to predict and measure the difference between successful treatment and the potential for a fatal failure.

Hippocratic texts first described the 'posture syndromes' in the treatise *On Joints*, in which diseases of the spine are classified into visible subcategories of impairment, whether caused by infectious processes (such as tuberculosis), traumatic injury or physical anomalies present at birth.[3] The division of malformations of the spine into pathological postures such as the kyphotic (exaggeration of the thoracic curve) and lordotic (exaggeration of the lumbar curve), the flat back and swayback posture, as well as scoliosis (today defined as lateral shift and rotation of the spinal vertebrae with pathological curvatures of the spine), have their roots in ancient medicine.

Let us focus on one of these Hippocratic diagnostic categories, scoliosis, which has a longer history as part of our understanding of posture. It is important that in the Hippocratic works the term 'scoliosis' was applied to almost every kind of spinal curvature, including those spinal variations resulting from injuries of the vertebrae with or without dislocation of the vertebral bodies. He divides the curvatures of the spine into the swelling or posterior projection, the anterior projection and the lateral curvature. Hippocrates mentions two possible causes of the disease: infection and postural habits; 'all such affections, or most of them, are due to gatherings on the inner side of the spine, while in some cases the positions the patients are accustomed to take in bed are accessory to the malady.'[4] The Roman physician Galen later

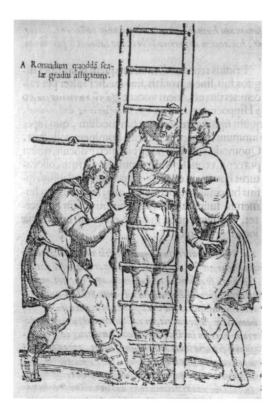

A Rotundum quoddá fca-
lae gradui alligatum.

The Hippocratic mechanism for correcting spinal disorders in order to return the patient to better posture, in an image by Vidus Vidius. Reproduced from Galen, *Opera ex nona Juntarum* (Venice, 1625).

limits scoliosis to a specific malformation of the lateral curvature of the spine.[5] Like Hippocrates, he claimed that such deformities could be caused by the presence of tubercular nodes in the lung, by a spinal injury caused by a fall or other trauma, or as a result of ageing and fatigue of the spine. The mechanism of the deformity, according to Galen, is the formation of tubercular nodes next to the vertebrae as well as intervertebral ligament shrinkage and pulling of the vertebrae towards the nodes. All distort the spine into the curve indicative of scoliosis.

Here, however, we should remind ourselves that the Greeks understood posture as the defining character of mankind in all stages of life. Scoliosis was a medical category of postural anomaly, and as such was also inhabited by a range of cultural meanings. Poor posture, while not barring one from activities, such as serving in the army, did reflect one's character. Homer's scapegoat soldier Thersites, who confronted Agamemnon over the preparations for the Trojan War and was soundly beaten by Odysseus for his trouble (*Iliad* 2.216–19), was 'bandy-legged, lame, and humpbacked'.[6] Plato in *The Republic* has him reborn as an ape, and Shakespeare in *Troilus and Cressida* (1602) does not treat the 'deformed and scurrilous Grecian' (as he is described in the *dramatis personæ*) much better. Postural anomalies marked one as not only visible but vulnerable.

Sophocles, to no one's surprise, makes the riddle posed to Oedipus in his *Oedipus Rex* by the monstrous Sphinx at Thebes precisely a problem of human posture. What, the Sphinx asks, goes on all fours in the morning, on two feet in the afternoon, and on three at night? Answer incorrectly and you die. Oedipus, according to Sophocles' version, drawing on Hesiod, answers correctly that it is mankind that crawls as an infant, walks upright (facing the gods) as an adult and limps with his walking stick at the end of life. (Sophocles only gestures at the riddle and its answer, since his audience knew it all too well to have it spelled out for them. Images of Oedipus and the Sphinx were a commonplace on antique vases such as the Attic red-figured *lekythos* in the manner of the Meidias Painter in the British Museum.) Solving the riddle and destroying the Sphinx enables Oedipus – whose name means 'swollen-footed', because his feet were pierced when he was exposed to die as an infant – to thwart the prophecy that he would murder his father and assume the throne, to continue limping on his fateful journey. Indeed, having already unwittingly killed his father, he then continues into Thebes to marry his mother. Posture and gait haunt the tale and point to limping Oedipus as 'above and also below human beings, a hero more powerful than man, the equal of the gods, and at the same time the brutish beast spurned and relegated to the wild solitude of the mountains'.[7] This inevitable pursuit of fate reveals Oedipus to be morally tainted, to be one of those lame of spirit in soul as well as in body, as recent commentators on *The Republic* have observed concerning Plato's views on postural disability:

those lame in spirit were opposed to those who were agile, quick, steady, on their two legs, *bebaioi*, and those who went straight, *euthus, orthos*. Plato makes a distinction between wellborn souls, made for philosophy, and souls that are 'deformed and lame.' In so doing, he assimilates, as if it were self-evident, intellectual lameness and bastardy of soul, for the *cholos* [lame, defective] is a *nothos*, a bastard, not a *gnesios* [geniune, lawfully begotten] of direct and legitimate descent like the son 'who resembles the father' who has engendered him in a regular

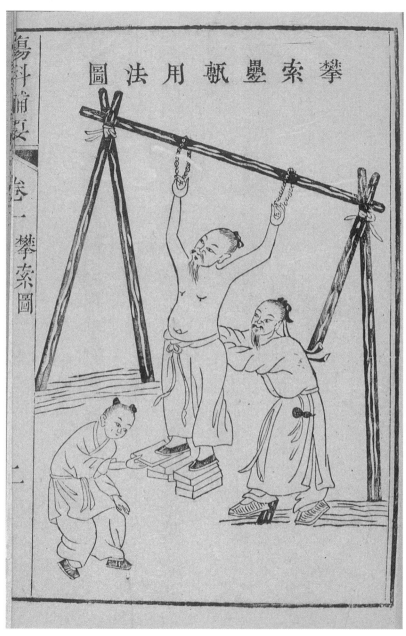

The Hippocratic ladder comes to be adapted as Graeco-Roman medicine enters East Asia via the Silk Road. Woodcut from *Shangke buyao* (Supplement to Traumatology) by Qian Xiuchang, published in 1818. *Pansuo diezhuan* ('holding a rope and standing on a stack of bricks') is an orthopaedic technique in which the patient stands on the bricks, grasping a rope in each hand. The practitioner holds and supports the affected part, while assistants remove one brick from the stack under each foot. It is considered to soothe *qi* and disperse stagnations, raise up prolapsed vertebrae and correct curvature of the spine.

fashion, without deviation or deformity since he is born in a direct, unhalting line.[8]

Scoliosis in Greek medicine is thus framed by the complex meanings associated with posture, represented by the course of human ageing and the curse of lameness. René Girard evokes the 'physical infirmity that the multitude regards as uncanny, such as Oedipus's lameness', as a sign of the social and moral scapegoat.[9] The moral overlay was clear to Sophocles' viewers, and it served to accentuate the double meaning of the corruption of body and spirit associated with postural infirmities. Harold Bloom notes this in rereading Oedipus' answer to the riddle as a foretelling of the protagonist's own life course: 'Oedipus the infant on all fours cruelly wounded so he could not escape; Oedipus the mature man standing tall, two-legged, ruler of Thebes; and Oedipus, the lame and blinded man, wandering into exile relying on a cane.'[10]

Authorities adopted Galen's limited term (with its disguised moral message) in the nineteenth century, as, for example, the surgeon Maximilian Joseph von Chelius (1794–1876). It is only at this moment that Percivall Pott (1714–1788) described spinal tuberculosis in his work *Remarks on the Kind of Palsy of the Lower Limbs which is Frequently Found to Accompany a Curvature of Spine*. Tubercular spondylitis is now known as 'Pott's disease' and is seen as very different in its causation as well as meaning from scoliosis and other such deformities of posture. Before Pott, the various aetiologies of spinal deformity were often confused.

The Hippocratic texts seem mechanically to describe curve progression during the formation of the spine throughout human growth. Hippocrates identified the cause as chronic poor posture, and classical medicine proposed the first recorded treatment, which included an extension apparatus to cause axial distraction, separating the joint surfaces without rupturing their binding ligaments and without displacement. Yet, throughout, the taint of a misspent youth, of Oedipus, remains in the background.

The devices used by Hippocrates for the treatment of spinal deformities were the Hippocratic ladder, the Hippocratic board and the Hippocratic bench. Images are provided by Apollonius of Kitium (first century BC), who commented on the techniques presented by Hippocrates in *On Articulations*. The Greeks understood that bad posture could be cured by introducing technology, and thus the human being returned to their ideal physical and moral state. Such a view of the treatment of postural abnormalities (however defined) became the norm, even in traditional Chinese medicine.[11] For the East, as we shall see, would come to give moral qualities to posture in ways analogous to the West.

The Anatomists' Postural Disciplines

While classical medicine was concerned with the pathology of posture, it was also equally obsessed with the mapping of the body. The commonplace that anatomical instruction came more and more to be the reading of the classical anatomical texts, ignoring the actual body, was for the most part true. The wide dissemination and transmission of these anatomical texts through Arabic and Hebrew translations and adaptations also meant that other anatomical traditions became part of the medieval understanding of the body's posture. By the sixteenth century human dissection, although prohibited, was a regular feature of the artist's if not the anatomist's experience. It was after Sixtus IV's bull in 1482, which clarified the Church's somewhat more benign attitude towards dissection – at least of executed criminals – that artists such as Leonardo and Michelangelo were able to be present at dissections in the monastic hospitals of Florence. The human body came to be explored, but the presuppositions about how that body was supposed to appear and to function changed more slowly than did the ability to measure classical accounts of the anatomist, such as Galen, against observation.

The view of the plumb line as defining normal posture was reinforced by some of the anatomists mapping the body following the atlas by the first modern anatomist, Andreas Vesalius, *De humani corporis fabrica libri septem* (1543). Many of the classic anatomies of the seventeenth century represent the erect and upright body. Thus we can find in Govert Bidloo's *Anatomia hvmani corporis* (1685), with its images of dissected cadavers as well as of the living body in motion by Gerard de Lairesse, greater insight into how upright posture was seen by the anatomists of the age.

The popularity of Bidloo's work can be noted by the fact that William Cowper plagiarized it for his *Anatomy of the Humane Bodies* (1698), which gave no credit to either Bidloo or de Lairesse. The erect body's posture reflects post-Vesalian notions of what the spine should

Gerard de Lairesse, from Govert Bidloo, *Anatomia hvmani corporis* (Amsterdam, 1685).

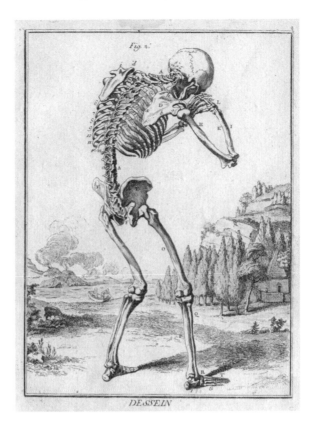

be. Vesalius' sense of the spine was one that reflected his own anatomical fantasy of the body, stressing its architectural solidity rather
than its malleability and the absence of any rigidity through the very
positions that he has his skeleton take. He sees 'a vertebra in the midst
of the back, stable and supported on both ends just as we see builders
place one stone between two others in vaulted and arched buildings,
which is supported on each side though it supports no stone itself,
while all the others support one stone and are received and supported
by another'. He acknowledges the triple curvature of the human spine
without noting that it had been well-known long before Galen.[12] He
illustrated the spine slightly rotated (a practice he often employed in
other illustrations), thereby minimizing the cervical and lumbar
curvatures.

Here Vesalius and his immediate successors break clearly with
the book learning of Galen and the ancients as taught in the medical
schools of his day. Galen had compared the spine to a vault in *On the
Use of the Parts*, and had explained that, 'in order that the whole

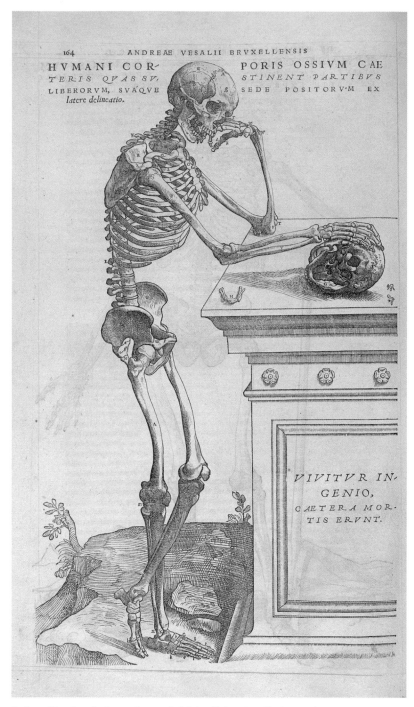

Andreas Vesalius, *De humani corporis fabrica libri septem* (Basle, 1543).

Claudius (Pseudo) Galen, 'Muscles Man', showing the muscles and spine without the triple curvature of the spine, back view, on an anatomical diagram from the mid-15th century.

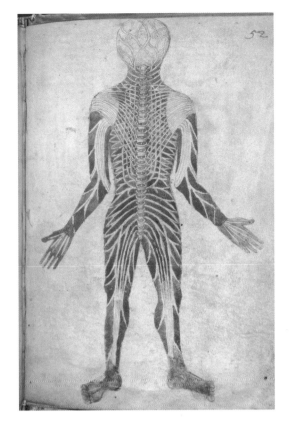

spine might bend uniformly it was of course necessary for the middle vertebra to remain in place while all the others withdrew gradually from one another and from it, the upper ones retiring upward and the lower ones down.'[13] Galen had based his description on his own dissection, not of a human body but of the Barbary apes, which, because they do not hold an erect posture, have only a single curvature in their spine.[14]

By the mid-eighteenth century the military body had begun to shape the anatomist's understanding of posture. In 1747 Bernard Siegfried Albinus's *Tabulae sceleti et musculorum corporis humani*, with illustrations by Jan Wandelaar, presented a 'natural' form of the body, where erect posture is represented by the evocation of the military plumb line.[15] The pelvis is fixed and the body is as perpendicular as possible. The Leyden anatomist was presenting his concept of a 'Homo perfectus', the ideal body of the ideal man. His desire was to show perfect human skeletons without blemish and without pathology. The skeleton itself had to be perfect, and 'he chose a skeleton that showed all signs of strength and agility, one that was elegant but at the same time not too delicate, that showed neither juvenile nor feminine roundness and slenderness nor uncouth roughness and clumsiness; in short, one whose parts were all beautiful and pleasing to the eye. It was a "naturae exemplum ex natura optima".[16] But that was not sufficient, for Albinus and Wandelaar's images should also 'convey an expression of beauty true to life and a vitality based on grace, strength and harmony. Therefore, a lean man of equal height was placed beside the skeleton as a living model while Wandelaar was drawing it. The man had to take the same posture as the skeleton, as a further help towards orientation for Wandelaar.'[17]

Now if indeed Albinus undertook such a procedure to correct the skeleton with the actual form of the living human being, he falls into what one can call the Vesalian paradox, an error of perception attributed to Vesalius.[18] Why, historians of anatomy have asked, did not Vesalius, whose groundbreaking anatomy relied on examining the corpses of hanged criminals rather than repeating the errors in the textbooks of the ancients, see the Fallopian tubes? The answer is clear. While he believed himself to be seeing into the body in an unmediated fashion, the fact is that he too saw human reproduction through the eyes of Graeco-Roman medicine, of Galen and his academic predecessors. Ancient anatomy demanded symmetry between male and female anatomy when it came to reproduction. Vesalius' flawed understanding of male anatomy, taken from Galen, was simply projected on to the anatomy of female reproduction. A generation later Gabriele Fallopius saw them because he had a different model for reproduction in mind. Likewise, Albinus' rigid skeleton was the ideal – military plumb line incarnate. Lying on the table or suspended for examination, the pelvis falls into a line from the ear to the ankle. Thus Albinus was much closer to Aristotle's understanding of anatomy than to that of Vesalius (or indeed of Fallopius). The images are not of potential bodies with their slightly asymmetrical posture, but of ideal bodies:

> For him, this meant ideal beauty, strength and health. If the symmetry was disturbed, such an imbalance reflected disease because the symmetry in all parts of the body determined their proper functioning. Consequently, Albinus eliminated all structures, which disturbed the symmetrical balance. Crests and grooves of the bones, holes for nerves and blood

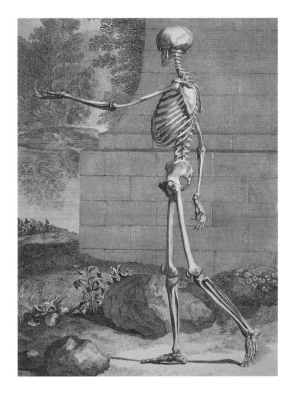

Jan Wandelaar, articulated full skeleton, side view, 1747. From Bernard Siegfried Albinus, *Tabulae sceleti et musculorum corporis humani* (Leiden, 1747).

vessels were systematically obliterated or relocated if they did not fit symmetry and the corresponding notion of beauty and balance. In line with this, he also strove for a congruence between left and right, asking Wandelaar to draw only one half of a bone and copy the other half after folding the paper. By this procedure, Albinus paradoxically eliminated vital structures for the sake of symmetry – in his view a symbol of vitality – and sacrificed the vitality of form to the wholly dominating consistency of the pencil strokes.[19]

Albinus's spine is the body in its imagined symmetrical military posture. Human beings could indeed become habituated to such postures, but it is also clear that Albinus saw this as the natural form of the body at rest.

Posture and the Moral Imperative for an Upright Carriage

The anatomists' reimagining of ideal (read 'normal') posture parallels medical interventions for pathologies (read 'abnormalities') of posture.

Scoliosis is a term that becomes part of the intrinsic vocabulary of abnormal posture in the nineteenth and twentieth centuries.[20] In the West, the anxiety about the medicalization of slouching persisted even after the Hippocratic aetiology of scoliosis in tuberculosis and other infectious diseases had been abandoned or at least mitigated in the early twentieth century. (That this shift was very gradual can be seen in our discussion of Maria Montessori's work later, when we turn to education and posture.) What is striking is the gradual accrual of moral meaning to postural variations defined as diseases. The Greeks seemed to have defined postural variations such as scoliosis as physiological variables with moral overtones. By the early modern period the moral qualities ascribed to such variations, embedded in a Judaeo-Christian reading of postural variation, come to be part of medical theory. The biblical edict banning such people from serving at the Temple because they were 'haram' comes to haunt the practice of medicine.

The disease that now threatened posture was 'idiopathic scoliosis', a spinal irregularity for which the physiological cause was unknown. What had been part of a disease process had gradually become a cultural abstraction. Suddenly an absolute definition of upright posture, which was understood in terms of the plumb line, was used to define the healthy spine and normal posture. All other deviations came to be pathological. By 1905, after Robert Koch's description of the infectious nature of tuberculosis became widely accepted, the Society of Medical Inspectors of the New York Health Department instituted a system of physical examinations of posture that specifically targeted physical disabilities rather than contagious disease. In 1925 a physician at Columbia University estimated that more than 20 per cent (four million children) had orthopaedic deformities.[21] Public schools physically examined their pupils once at the beginning of the school year and then again at the close, to judge the improvement in the children's posture. The newest technology was employed to define deviations from the norm, as well as to treat them. X-rays, developed by Wilhelm Roentgen in the 1890s, were widely accepted by the beginning of the century as scientific proof of the status of the body.

The Harvard orthopaedist Joel E. Goldthwait used X-rays to show how a slouching posture cramped the lungs, pinched off circulation and caused the vital organs of the abdomen and chest to descend. Poor posture wrought havoc on the physiological functioning of the body, he concluded, thus weakening an individual's ability to fight off infectious and chronic disease: 'irrespective of the type, the postures, which are assumed as the body is used determine very largely whether the individual is to be well or ill. The most perfect, anatomically, may have the poorest health, while the most imperfect, anatomically, may have good health.'[22] In his Shattuck Lecture of 1915 before the Massachusetts Medical Society, he had presented images of what he labelled 'the normal human type' standing at plumb-line attention. He provides a taxonomy of the various classifications of poor posture, in which variations from the norm are catalogued as anything from 'congenital visceroptotic' to 'macrocelous' to 'narrow-backed.'[23] But he sees all these as redeemable through early education, since 'this is the great opportunity and responsibility for the educator.'[24]

Medicine could be accused of merely perpetuating the ability of those with poor posture to reproduce: 'the splendid work of our profession along preventative medical lines was a curse to the race by preserving the lives of the slender or delicate physical type, which Nature, in keeping with the law of the survival of the fittest, would have thrown off.' But if postural education by teacher and physician 'recognizes these facts and applies the natural principles for the proper development of these individuals, the result must be inevitable – a stronger and finer race'. For what postural education does is 'gradually [to] remove the weaker elements, which if perpetuated would surely lower the vitality of the race as a whole'. Goldthwait argues strongly *against* mere natural selection, stressing positive eugenics as man's ability to shape the posture of the race, and thus its future: 'In the moral choice man is given great responsibility and the physical responsibility is none the less great, unless the human family is to be governed by the same law of survival of the fittest and natural selection which has governed the development of the lower forms of life.'[25] Posture defines human potential in the age of eugenics as a means to shape the body into those forms best suited to modern life.

The ancients had seen tuberculosis as a cause of scoliosis, while the moderns saw postural insufficiency as the underlying cause of infectious diseases such as tuberculosis. Thus Irving Fisher, professor of political economy at Yale, and Eugene Lyman Fisk of the Life Extension Institute wrote in their best-selling study of posture and its discontents,

One of the simplest and most effective methods of avoiding self-poisoning is by maintaining an erect posture. In an erect posture the abdominal muscles tend to remain taut and to afford proper support or pressure to the abdomen, including the great splanchnic circulation of large blood-vessels. In an habitual slouching posture, the blood of the abdomen tends to stagnate in the liver and the splanchnic circulation, causing a feeling of despondency and mental confusion, headache, coldness of the hands and feet, and chronic fatigue or neurasthenia, and often constipation. A slouching attitude is often the result of disease or lack of vitality; but it is also a cause.[26]

Fisher attributed his own tuberculosis to his 'consumptive stoop'.[27] This was a commonplace of the debate about the cause of tuberculosis throughout the nineteenth century. The idea that a too narrow chest, a stooped posture or a weak body predisposed one to or indeed even caused tuberculosis continued well after Koch's discovery of the tuberculosis bacillus in 1882.

In addition, the eugenic argument almost always evoked race. Even though the common belief was that Jews had a higher resistance to tuberculosis than other groups, by the early twentieth century and in light of the Jewish mass immigration to the United States, Fisher and Fisk were also arguing for clear racial distinctions in terms of what are healthy and normative bodies:

> The robust Indian and the Negro, whose races, until the last generation or two, roamed in the open, fell easy prey to tuberculosis as soon as they adopted the white man's houses and clothes. The Anglo-Saxons who have withstood the influence of indoor living for several generations have, probably by the survival of the fittest, become a little better able to endure it, while the Jews, a race which has lived indoors longer than any other existing race, are now, probably by the same law of survival, the least liable to tuberculosis, except when exposed to especially unfavorable conditions of life.[28]

Race is evoked over and over again, even in texts where it is not present overtly, to reflect on the normal and healthy 'American' (or 'German' or 'English') body, as opposed to the weak and corrupt posture of those seen as inherently different. The new immigrants to New York City, the now reservation-bound Native Americans, the former slaves in the age of Jim Crow all suffer from illnesses marked on their bodies by their posture. The only question that remained was: could such bad posture be redeemed by intervention, or were such bodies inherently corrupt?

As with the Hippocratic interventions, technology came into play to correct scoliosis as a marker for such postural deficiencies. The Milwaukee brace and other versions of the full upper-body brace echoed the Hippocratic interventions. But also unlike them, given the broadened definition of scoliosis, was the demand that schoolchildren be regularly screened and treated. As with so many questions after the First World War, the claim that at least 10 per cent of American draftees had postural deformities made such intervention a means of securing healthy citizen soldiers.[29] The obsession with the perfect spine and perfect posture continued in the United States at least until the end of the twentieth century. Elsewhere in the world, scoliosis as the disease entity that links posture, medicine and education has waned, and the radical interventions recommended for treatment have given way to a more nuanced understanding of the limits of 'normal' posture.

Rickets and the Bad Posture of the Poor

Scoliosis is clearly a disease entity that begins with ideas of alterations of posture owing to various forms of bodily 'corruption', from tuber-culosis to fractures to the effects of poor posture. The medical cate-gories of healthy versus ill posture may well have had their roots in the medical understanding of correcting 'poor' posture in cases clearly defined as pathological posture, such as the posture that results from vitamin-deficiency diseases such as rickets (which is caused by a lack of vitamin D). But, as with scoliosis, such views come to reflect on the character as well as the body of those with poor posture. Beginning with the first modern treatise on rickets, Daniel Whistler's *Disputatio medica inaugurales de morbo puerili Anglorum quem patrio idiômate indiginae vocant the rickets: quam Deo suppetias ferente* (Inaugural Medical Disputation on the Disease of English Children which is Popularly Termed the Rickets; 1684), there has been a focus on the posture of the sufferer. As early as Ambrose Pare, military surgeon and medical innovator of the sixteenth century, braces – in his case made

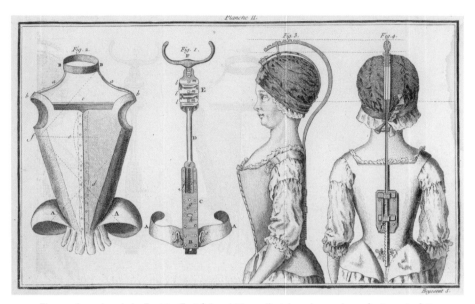

Thomas Levacher de La Feutrie, *Traité du rakitis, ou l'art de redresser les enfants contrefaits* (Treatise on Richitis; or, the Means of Correcting Disabled Children; Paris, 1772). The Greek word 'rachitis' (ῥαχίτης) meaning 'of the spine' was adapted in the 17th century as the scientific term for rickets not only because it was a homophone but because of the association of spinal diseases with poor posture.

out of metal – were used to correct the poor posture associated with rickets. In his *Traité du rakitis, ou l'art de redresser les enfants contrefaits* (1772), Thomas Levacher de La Feutrie provides both exercises and implements to correct such pathology.[30] He suggested a restraining bed echoing the Hippocratic tradition, but without traction, as well as an innovative 'Minerva' corset to correct the scoliosis associated with rickets. The corset, especially with the introduction of the 'patented improvements' of spring steel stays in the early eighteenth century, came to be a primary form of medical intervention for reshaping postural deficiencies.[31] As early as 1734, London makers of corsets, generically called 'truss makers', such as James Lane in Fleet Street, were advertising 'steel stays . . . to prevent Children being crooked' or to *correct* any problem that might have already arisen 'from any Cause Whatsover.'[32]

The general sense is that rickets (called 'the English malady') presents a manifest misshaping of the limbs in knock knees or bowed legs and in the earliest stages a so-called tailor-like posture, which is seen to mirror the position a tailor takes in sewing. In some cases, kyphosis

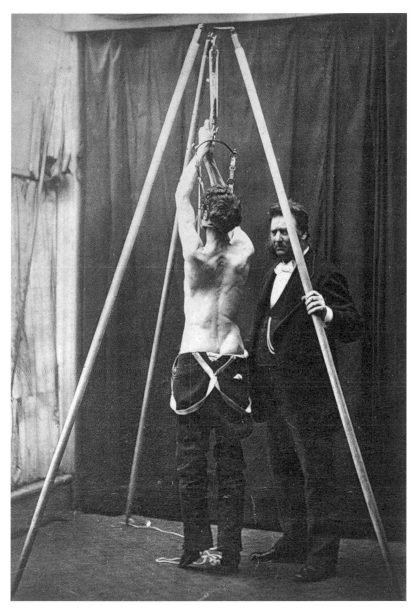

Lewis A. Sayre, *Spinal Disease and Spinal Curvature: Their Treatment by Suspension and the Use of the Plaster of Paris Bandage* (London, 1877).

(hunchback) is also present. The very image of the child with rickets now having its body reformed, straightened and corrected comes to define mechanical interventions in orthopaedics, a medical discipline that uses instruments regularly to correct the body's malformation and ideally allow it to stand up straight.

By the modern period, rickets was 'considered by many to be a most prolific cause of scoliosis'.[33] Bad posture in this sense is disability, and correction is demanded to return the disabled body to the plumb line. In doing so the claim is that the disabled body is made productive and returned to a meaningful role in a capitalist society in the form of an erect body.

By the end of the nineteenth century such horrors of posture came to have social significance as 'the twisted legs of malnourished working-class children signalled the ravages of rickets' and were the subject of social commentary. This narrative is part of the muckraking accounts of the cities at the beginning of the twentieth century, when 'the thousands of rickety infants to be seen in all our large cities and towns, the anaemic, languid-looking children one sees everywhere in working-class districts, and the striking contrast presented by the appearance of the children of the well-to-do bear eloquent witness to the widespread prevalence of underfeeding'.[34] Yet physicians of the time, even those recognizing that 'bad food and, what is probably of much more importance, want of sunshine' are causal in developing rickets, claim that these 'operate with greater force on children who have

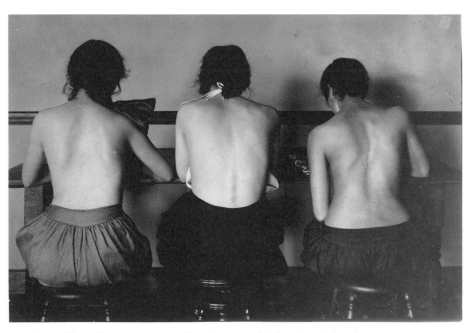

Lewis Hines, 'Incorrect sitting position for postural deformity and dorsal curvature cases. Scoliosis. Stooping, lopsided or humped over position. Work in this position is harmful. Need for advice of examining physician' (Boston, 1917).

inherited from either parent a constitution unduly prone to be affected by their influence'.[35] Neither poor hygiene nor nutrition trumps poor inheritance, leading to entire families of children with severe symptoms, including 'the rickety chest, the pot belly, and in addition, a marked dorso-lumbar kyphosis'. We see your moral failings on the bodies of your child, the physician notes, and the suicide of the father of the five affected children seems further proof.

Posture defines class and demands reform. At the same moment the psychoanalyst Alfred Adler noted that the 'inferiority complex' may be the result of early childhood inhibitions in movement:

> When a child takes an unusually long time to learn to walk, but can walk normally once he has learned, it does not mean that the child must develop an inferiority complex for the rest of his life . . . There are many children who at one time had rickets and who, though cured, still bear the marks of the disease; crooked legs, clumsiness, lung catarrh, a certain malformation of the head (caput quadratum), curved spine, enlarged ankles, feeble joints, bad posture, etc.[36]

The child's situation, he continues, 'is an unhappy one'. Adler's notion of the inferiority complex was rooted in his early work on 'organ inferiority', which reflects his concern with bodily compensation for weaker organs or limbs. It was rooted, too, in his own experience as a child with rickets and his lower-middle-class Jewish upbringing on the fringes of Vienna.

Posture and psyche are equally shaped by the experience of disease, and psychoanalysis recognized this in cases of rickets. In the 1950s the émigré psychoanalyst William Niederland notes that

> When the illness persists beyond the first year, thoracic changes as well as marked cranial deformity are frequently found, the head being enlarged out of proportion to the rest of the body. The English word 'rickety', which originally meant affected with rickets, clearly denotes the state of severe musculoskeletal weakness and general helplessness produced by the disease. There can be little doubt that at the time the child learned to stand or walk – though nothing definite about this period became known during the treatment – the interference with

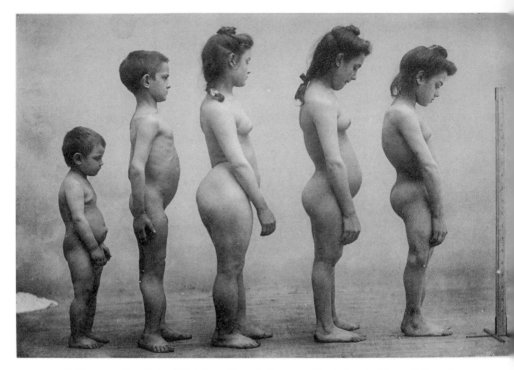

A. Zimmern, 'Familial rachitis'. From *Nouvelle iconographie de la salpetriere; clinique des maladies du systeme nerveux* (Paris, 1901).

both the development and function of normal skeletal and muscular activities must have been considerable. It seriously disturbed the integration and development of the body ego.[37]

Posture deformed deforms the psyche. The therapy needed is psychotherapy, in addition to physical therapy. It is therefore not at all surprising to find images of children with rickets in the most prestigious journal presenting the iconography of the psychiatrically ill and neurologically disabled at the turn of the twentieth century.

The physician and psychologist William James was convinced of this as he noted that erect posture keeps up the sprits and tends to banish fear, despondency and depressing thoughts. He was convinced that posture influenced the emotions:

if we wish to conquer undesirable emotional tendencies in ourselves, we must assiduously, and in the first instance cold-bloodedly, go through the *outward movements* of those contrary dispositions which we prefer to cultivate . . . Smooth the brow, brighten the eye, contract the dorsal rather than the ventral aspect of the frame, and speak in a major key, pass the genial compliment, and your heart must be frigid indeed if it does not gradually thaw![38]

Both twentieth-century claims evolved at the close of the nineteenth century.

The Moral Machines of Posture

By the end of the nineteenth century there was an entire medical sub-speciality that defined the healthy body and treated the ill body based on notions of acceptable posture (think of this as a plumb line from alternative therapies such as Swedish gymnastics to German medical *Krankengymnastik* to modern gym culture, in addition to medical specialities such as orthopaedics). The only question was the format: would it be rigidly performed activities or more 'natural' approaches to bodily movement that could reform poor posture? Or indeed, did it demand orthopaedic intervention, with braces and halters and machines of all types to stress and stretch the body? But older therapies are also evoked. When Karl Friedrich Koch opened his institute for gymnastics in Berlin in 1828, gymnastics was dependent on medicine or, more precisely, dietetics, as Heikki Lempa notes. In order to correct medical dependency Koch suggested that they 'reinstitute the art of dancing' to improve the bad posture of the 170 students trained in gymnastics.[39]

The range of representations is almost always one that generates an image of the ideal posture, then moves to pathological postures and finally to the military posture as an exaggeration of the ideal norm. Diagrams of the time show the position of head (skull), neck (cervical vertebrae), thoracic and lumbar vertebrae, pelvis, leg (femur, tibia, fibula) and foot. Those are the anatomical features that define natural versus pathological posture, just as the bright line defines the pre-human and the human in terms of their upright posture.

Yet, as we have seen, bad posture is not only a sign of physical pathology but of moral degeneration. The form of the external body reflects character as well as psyche. By the time of Daniel Gottlob Moritz Schreber's *Die ärztliche Zimmergymnastik* (Medical Indoor Gymnastics; 1855), the line between physical state and moral position had become completely blurred (if it was ever clear). For Schreber, a strong spine, 'the central force in maintaining the body', prevents a range of illnesses from hypochondria to hysteria.[40] Schreber, who was an orthopaedist in the tradition of the French school of the late eighteenth century, advocated both his 'systematic remedial exercises' and countryside exercise for urban youth to overcome the problem of physical and moral degeneration. But he was also committed to an allopathic medical model for the treatment of what he defined as pathologies. From 1844 onwards he directed an orthopaedic and physiological clinic in Leipzig, where a wide range of interventions were undertaken.

Schreber was a firm believer in medical gymnastics, but his allegiance to the power of restraints and corseting was unquestioned. Corseting comes to have a double significance, both in the history of orthopaedics and in the competing history of fashion. In both it reflected on the meanings read into the character by the form of the body, although in widely different contexts.

Schreber begins his *Medical Home Gymnastics* with a paean to *mens sana in corpore sano*, a healthy mind in a healthy body, the phrase from Juvenal's *Satires* that became the motto of the *Turnverein*. These political as well as gymnastic organizations were developed by the advocates of a new nationalistic gymnastics as the proper place for a 'new German' body for a yet non-existent pan-German state. Indeed, in 1845 Schreber was one of three physicians to found the Leipzig *Turnvereine*, which was supposed to provide a space for political and moral development through gymnastics.[41] In his *Medical Home Gymnastics*, he maintained that 'man is, so to speak, a double being, consisting of a wonderful, intimate union of mental with a bodily nature. He is destined to activity in both ways – to the full use of his mental and bodily powers: his whole being is so arranged. The sluggish of mind or idle of body long in vain for the full enjoyment of mental or bodily pleasures.'[42] For Schreber, body and character are firmly bound up in his goal of creating a new 'healthy people'.

During the mid-nineteenth century the term *Volksgesundheit* (people's health) was coined to reflect the inherent relationship between body and spirit. But how does one achieve both a healthy mind and a healthy body? There was of course the military training of the body, but in the age of industrialization machines that could cripple the body were also turned into devices for its reform. In Germany, the very late appearance of the Industrial Revolution demanded that popular culture see the machine as an intervention to correct bad posture. In what comes to be his most detailed account of how the machine can alter posture, in his handbook on bodily reform, *Die schädlichen Körperhaltung und Gewohnheiten der Kinder: Nebst Angabe der Mittel dagegen* (Poor Posture and Habits of Children: With the Means to Change Them; 1853), Schreber documents how implements and corsets can alter children's bodies to prepare them to become healthy citizens.[43] (He went on to write other handbooks on childhood bodily reform.[44]) In it he advocates exercises and postural training but also the use of mechanical devices, crafted by Johannes Reichel, the local mechanic in Leipzig, from whom you could buy a '*Geradehalter*' (a steel upright brace with either a mobile [11] or fixed [12] steel crossbar that could also be fixed to a table surface) and the necessary leather bands for only '4 Thaler and 5 New Groschen'.[45] The optimum age for such devices would be between eight and sixteen years.

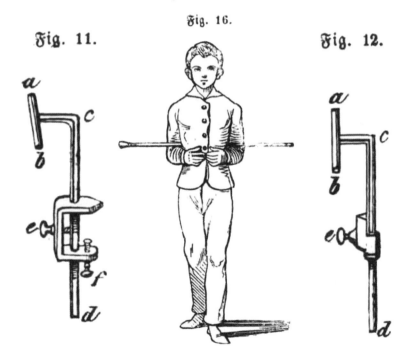

Schreber's two types of steel brace, and his means of training good posture in a form well-known from the 18th century. From Daniel Gottlob Moritz Schreber, *Die schädlichen Körperhaltung und Gewohnheiten der Kinder: Nebst Angabe der Mittel dagegen* (Leipzig, 1853).

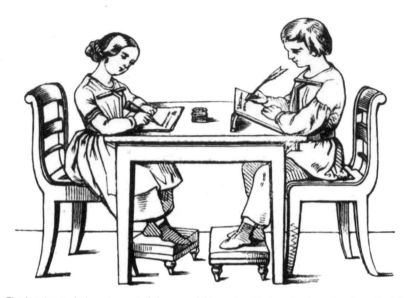

The bracing technique to control the way children sit while learning to write. From Daniel Gottlob Moritz Schreber, *Die schädlichen Körperhaltung und Gewohnheiten der Kinder: Nebst Angabe der Mittel dagegen* (Leipzig, 1853).

Such restraints were used, as we can see here, to correct posture while the child was sitting and learning to write, but also while they were sleeping, moving or simply standing. This movement away from the more traditional posture boards and gymnastic training to restraints and even braces is part of the general merger of various forms of bodily reform. It is bodily reform as much now a part of education and medicine as nationalism and popular culture. The slippage in Schreber's world is evident, but it is not unusual in the history of posture. Thus it is not only exercise and training that correct bad posture and bad minds in all these realms, but machines.

Schreber's braces, corsets and machines become important for a further reason that haunts our present sense of the relationship between posture and the psyche. In 1910 Carl Gustav Jung, the Swiss psychiatrist, suggested to his then friend and colleague Sigmund Freud that a self-published account of a case of paranoia might provide some insight into the state of the severely disturbed human psyche. Through this, Daniel Paul Schreber's *Memoirs of My Nervous Illness* (1903) became 'undoubtedly the best-known example of schizophrenia – and one in which the diverse bodily symptoms . . . are exhibited', according to Thomas Szasz.[46] It remains one of the standard texts by the mentally ill that shape our understanding of severe mental illness. (Schreber, who was Daniel Gottlob Moritz Schreber's son, was diagnosed as having dementia praecox; Freud labels it dementia paranoids, one of the diagnoses that morphed into schizophrenia at the time.) Freud's monograph on him, published in 1911 and based solely on his reading of Schreber's account of his first two attacks of mental illness, came to hold a central place in the medical and popular literature on mental illness. Schreber, formerly a judge, wrote his account to prove that he was competent to be released from the Leipzig asylum, since 'insane people' were not believed to be able to undertake such a task.

As the critical literature on Freud and Schreber has made substantially clear, especially since the work of Morton Schatzman in 1974, central to Schreber's paranoid fantasies were his father (who reappears in a number of guises, from God to the asylum director) and his father's multiple forms of restraint.[47] Schreber's comments on how his 'physical posture' was of significance in the world he inhabited, as well as his observations on the posture of others in his mental universe, allowed his father's preoccupation with postural control to bubble up into the text.[48] In a later addition to the text he adds that he is now 'completely bent and can hardly walk upright'.[49] Schreber senior's implements for the correction of the spine of his patients reappear in his son's narrative as the 'compression of the chest miracle', which 'consisted in the whole chest wall being compressed, so that the state of oppression caused by the lack of breath was transmitted to my whole body'.[50] Freud had immediately connected Schreber's illness with the medical role that the father had played in the son's frightening fantasies, as he wrote to Jung in 1910: 'Don't forget that Schreber's father was – a doctor. As such, he performed miracles, he miracled. In other words, the delightful characterization of God – that he knows how to deal only with corpses and has no idea of living people – and the absurd miracles that are performed on him are a bitter satire on his father's medical art.'[51] The 'miracles' to which Freud referred, employing Schreber's term, were the bodily transformations that Schreber felt he was forced to undergo. In Schreber's account we have a sense of how extremely powerful the very notion of postural reform could be within the complex map of the relationship between the body and the status of the psyche.

The 'people's health' became a focus not only of allopathic medicine (and its patients in and out of the asylum) but, as we have seen with Schreber *père*, of the popular fascination with bodily reform. Everything

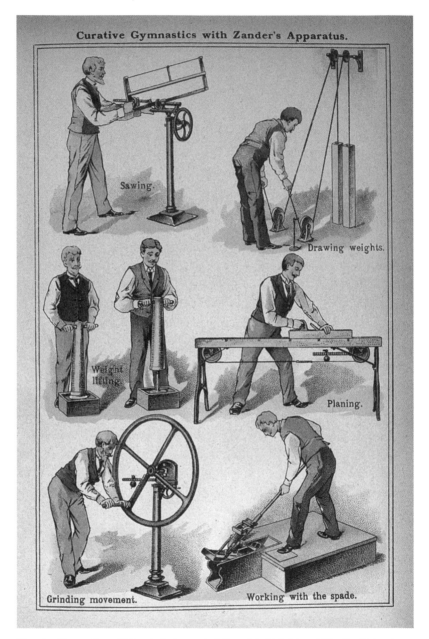

'Curative Gymnastics with Zander's Apparatus'. From Friedrich Eduard Bilz, *The Natural Method of Healing: A New and Complete Guide to Health* (Leipzig and New York, 1898).

from Indian clubs to complex forms of exercise machinery were developed to aid in the social movement to reform the body in order to make better citizens and neighbours. By 1917 more than two million copies of *Das neue Naturheilverfahren* (The Natural Method of Healing; 1888), written by the German exponent of self-cure Friedrich Eduard Bilz, were sold to middle-class readers in Germany who were convinced that they had to learn to stand up straight.[52] Bilz was a former weaver who 'advocated a lifestyle of joyous moderation' and was able in 1892 to found a popular sanatorium that treated 1,500 patients in 1900 alone.[53] 'Pathological' or 'poor' posture was now clearly linked not only to machines that corrected posture but to machines that mimicked work. 'Naturopathy' became alternative medicine yet remained concerned with posture both as symptom and as aetiology.

Bilz's popular text advocated for those machines that mimicked factory or farm work. Developed by one of the major innovators in physical therapy, Gustav Zander, they began at the end of the nineteenth century to replace manual manipulation for postural pathology. (Think of these as the forerunners to our contemporary gym equipment that mimics bicycle-riding or stair-climbing.) Zander was so renowned in his day for having developed machines that could use double tension to train the body that he was considered for the Nobel Prize in medicine in 1916.[54] (It was never awarded because of the war.) Zander had been a disciple of Pehr Henrik Ling (1776–1839) (who was followed by his son Hjalmar Ling (1820–1886), continuing his father's tradition). Ling's system also had a therapeutic connection, advocated by alternative and allopathic practitioners and seen as a forerunner of physiotherapy; his 'Swedish gymnastics', however, was a direct answer to Friedrich Ludwig 'Turnvater' Jahn's 'German gymnastics', which shaped nationalistic discourse in nineteenth-century Germany. (Indeed, Ling's influence was so powerful that the German term for his approach, *Krankengymnastik*, was altered to the more international *Physiotherapie* only in 1994.) For Bilz, this was clearly an alternative non-medical therapy for posture problems. Such views became dominant, even permeating the therapeutic regimens in John Harvey Kellogg's sanatorium in Battle Creek, Michigan. Not through the Hippocratic 'ladder' but through good, honest German work could the body be reformed.

What had been alternative medicine, as Kellogg notes, became mainstream during this time: 'The history of medicine shows that it has constantly been enriched by therapeutic contributions from sources outside the recognized medical authorities . . . Physiologic medicine is making marvelous progress in recent years.'[55] 'Good' posture was accomplished by such imitated work; the citizen with good posture was the citizen who could contribute to society by work or war. This became codified within the medical sub-speciality of physical therapy at the close of the nineteenth century, but also remained part of counterculture with the work of a wide range of body therapies, from that of the Australian actor Frederick Matthias Alexander (1869– 1955) to Joseph Pilates, whose system was developed with the dance therapist Rudolf Laban. Postural training was ubiquitous.

Mens sana in corpore sano

The ancient claim – best articulated, as we have noted, by Juvenal – that a healthy mind demands a healthy body has a very specific posture in mind as an indicator of a disturbed psyche. The interrelationship between physical and psychological states is revealed by posture. In the Old Testament book of Daniel (4:33) the Babylonian king Nebuchadnezzar is damned for disobeying God and sinks into madness: 'he was driven from men, and did eat grass as oxen, and his body was wet with the dew of heaven, till his hairs were grown like eagles' feathers, and his nails like birds' claws.' If, according to later interpreters of the book of Genesis, man was created after the animals of the field and made upright to face God, then the image in Daniel is one of regression. This image of a madman driven to abandon upright posture comes to define gait and posture as a quality of sanity.[56] Nebuchadnezzar reverts to the moment before he is upright and becomes a four-legged beast of the field.

In my study of the visualization of mental illness, *Seeing the Insane* (1982), I traced the image of the 'depressed' posture from Albrecht Dürer's engraving *Melencholia I* (1514) through to Vincent Van Gogh's *Sorrow* (1882) and beyond.[57] Such images of the seated depressive, head in hands, elbow on knee, become so embedded in Western culture that public health posters in the 1980s reflecting on the isolation of people with AIDS incorporate them as a visual icon.[58] In the course of the nineteenth century, the cues read into the posture of the mentally ill continue to factor in a broad range of psychiatric diagnoses as well as popular images of deviant or pathological character.

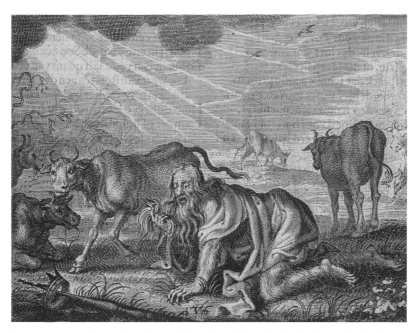

Nebuchadnezzar, Gone Mad, Grovels Like a Beast of the Earth; He Gropes for his Crown,
c. 17th century, Dutch line engraving.

Phrenological handbooks, such as that by a student of the pioneer neuroanatomist Franz Joseph Gall, Johann Spurzheim – the man who coined the term – stressed the reading of the totality of the body, especially such aspects as posture and gait, as the key to character. Spurzheim's stepson the French artist Hippolyte Bruyères provided a wide range of such images in his handbook of 1847.[59]

In *Physiognomy Illustrated* (1887), Joseph Simms sets out a series of gaits and what they indicate about mental states. The 'toddling gait', for example, indicated a helpless, childish man: 'the toes of his shoes are much further out of repair than the heels; . . . there are seldom all the buttons on the garments, and . . . both a glove and an umbrella have just been lost; occasioning the necessity for trying to recollect every place Mr. Toddler has been.'[60] He is contrasted with 'Miss Mary Frisk'. There was also a 'plunging gait' with a very exaggerated up-and-down motion, which Simms linked to alternating states of depression and buoyancy:

The form of those so affected is quite in accordance with the up and down or undulatory appearance of the walk. Alternately you will find them in high spirits, full of hope and jubilant;

again in deep depression, soon to rise into the opposite extreme. Hence the life of the plunger is one of fear and dread, hope and joy. His countenance most truthfully indicates this.[61]

With regard to human 'self-esteem', the leader and spokesman of the British phrenological movement George Combe notes in 1826 that 'when very large, the individual walks generally in an erect posture, and by his reserved and authoritative manner, induces the impression in others, that he considers himself infinitely above his fellow men.'[62] Through the course of the nineteenth century

an emergent technology of surveillance, physiognomy[,] was frequently discussed as a weapon against dissimulation. For

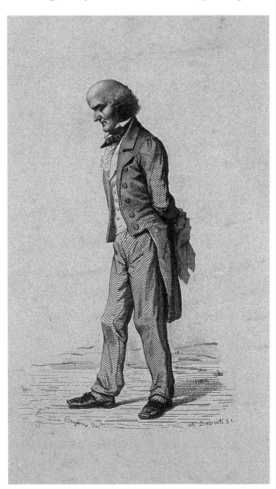

A. Devrits, after H. Bruyères, *Phrénologie, causalité, le penseur profond* (Phrenology, Causality, Deep Thought), 1847, steel engraving. A man with a large, protruding head walks with a heavy gait, illustrating the reflective faculty in phrenology.

those whose economic and social capital were most threatened by dissimulation – particularly the genteel elite – the logic, if not practice, of physiognomic distinction offered a means to establish moral character, embody social origin, and restrain the mobility enabled by the cultural capital of civility alone.

The link between character and postural training was thus a question of preserving (or expanding) elites.[63]

Medical textbooks admonished students of psychiatry to take a comprehensive history that would examine: 'the *conduct, attitude, manner, gait, posture, complexion, expression, gestures,* and *individuality* of the person . . . This observation becomes in time a trained, almost automatic, faculty, so that minute details subconsciously apprehended at the time can be readily recalled.'[64] Human physiognomy when seen in the configuration of the insane shows inadequate posture, as Frederick Peterson – president of the New York State Commission in Lunacy; professor of psychiatry at Columbia University; consulting alienist at Bellevue Hospital; manager of the Craig Colony for Epileptics at Sonyea, New York; and president of the New York Neurological Society – noted: 'Idiots all show deficiency in their general appearance. There is always something ungracious, uncouth, ugly in their figures, faces, attitudes, or movements. Very common among them are misshapen or asymmetrical heads, dwarfishness, lack of proportion of the limbs, stooping and slovenly postures, deformities of the hands or feet, and awkward and wobbling gait.'[65] Posture, he maintained, is an indicator of mental disease.

The standard psychiatry textbooks of the day, such as that by the Munich clinical psychiatrist Emil Kraepelin (1896), also explained unnatural posture as a defining characteristic of mental illness. Kraepelin, a student of the psychologist Wilhelm Wundt, was one of the creators of psychophysical research into posture. He argued, against the views of pure physiologists such as Christian Wilhelm Braune and Otto Fischer, that posture was not merely a question of internal training and the limits of human fatigue, but responded to the external influences, which he labels toxins, that limit physical endurance. Thus even in the best of all possible cases, such as soldiers in training, human posture was dependent on the environment in which the individual functioned. When he looked at pathological cases, yet another level of influence could be seen. For, as a contemporary British psychiatrist

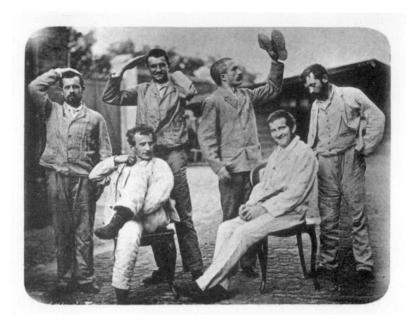

Patients exhibiting catatonic posture. From Emil Kraepelin, *Psychiatrie: Ein Lehrbuch für Studierende und Ärtze*, 5th edn (Leipzig, 1896).

noted, the postures of the mentally ill may be an indication of earlier evolutionary development with 'attitudes of crouching like a beast without moving, standing or sitting in fixed poses which had an insane or delusional significance'.[66] Thus the frozen catatonic posture is unnatural not only because it is frozen and unmoving over time but because the positions themselves are pathological (that is, the patients do not 'stand up straight').

For Kraepelin this symptom, defined as a stereotypic *Haltung* (posture), is also a hallmark of other forms of mental illness, such as dementia praecox, his term for schizophrenia, which can also have a catatonic component: 'The catatonic form of dementia praecox is especially characterized by stuporous states with negativism, hyper-suggestibility, and uniform muscular tension; excited states with stereotypy and impulsiveness; leading in most cases, with or without remissions, to mental deterioration.'[67] With Kraepelin the independent diagnostic category of catatonia is folded into dementia praecox. Posture remains a significant factor in the diagnosis of schizophrenia well into the twenty-first century.

In the 1940s the Dutch phenomenological psychiatrist Henricus Cornelius Rümke created the idea of the so-called praecox feeling.[68]

Experienced mental-health professionals who work with the mentally ill, he argued, are able to sense 'intuitively' those who suffer from schizophrenia. Rümke's belief was that after time the experienced professional simply could see who was schizophrenic. What is actually 'seen' by the medical professional is the subtle shifts in non-verbal communication in certain forms of schizophrenia. The idea that one could see the schizophrenic quickly became associated with a notion of a schizophrenic posture. Researchers argued that there was some type of vestibular involvement that could be used to explain the perceived S-curve of schizophrenic posture. Such schizophrenic postures, along with other physical signs such as a shuffling gait, inflexibility of the neck and shoulders and a resting posture, were explained, much as with Kraepelin, as a regression to primitive labyrinthine reflex, characterized by flexion, internal rotation and adduction.[69] Another explanation of the schizophrenic posture, if indeed there actually is one, credits the impact of visual acuity in schizophrenia, seeing posture as a major component of how schizophrenia presents itself, if only in the most subliminal manner: 'The hypothesis is that the "praecox feeling" might be linked with loss of natural gracefulness of body movements, which is reflected to disintegration of visual information on postural control.'[70] Even if the source of the poor posture is not the loss of acuity in the visual field, the argument is that posture remains a marker for the syndrome. For such 'abnormalities of postural control in schizophrenia are poorly understood . . . abnormalities could lead to subtle clumsiness or lack of plasticity which characterizes a proportion of patients with schizophrenia, including those never medicated.'[71] We should add that with the introduction of psychotropic medication for schizophrenia, such as chlorpromazine in the 1950s, the problem of posture was also related to the development of tardive dyskinesias, the involuntary movements of the tongue, lips, face, trunk and extremities that occur in patients treated with long-term dopaminergic antagonist medications. Even if we recognize the impact of medication on the patient's posture, posture never vanishes completely from discussions of schizophrenia. The most recent systematic account of mental disorders still notes concerning schizophrenia that one hallmark of the syndrome is 'catatonic behavior . . . [with its] marked decrease in reactivity to the environment. This ranges from resistance to instructions (negativism); to maintaining a rigid, inappropriate or bizarre posture; to a complete lack of verbal and motor responses (mutism and stupor).[72] There is no crediting any specific aetiology for catatonic posture.

Rümke's view was that, after having seen enough patients, one becomes subconsciously attuned to this posture. For him, neither the expression of the illness nor its perception was in any way 'hardwired'. It was a purely learned awareness, and it might even be a learned awareness not of a specific pathological presentation of schizophrenia but of the cultural patterns by which those suffering from mental illness can express their symptoms. This quickly becomes an inherent feature of the neurological underpinnings of schizophrenia by the organic psychiatrists who followed in Kraepelin's wake. Posture, so vital for the ancients, seems remarkably central even today.

But what posture comes to mean in medicine had already begun to expand in the 1920s with the shift from dementia praecox, the fatal brain disease as diagnosed by Kraepelin, to schizophrenia, a treatable disorder of the psyche as reimagined by Eugen Bleuler in 1908. Posture comes to be a secondary product of the schizophrenic, as we see in modern studies, rather than a diagnostic criterion of the underlying aetiology of the disease. Indeed, in a lecture to the Vienna Psychoanalytic Society the year before he published *The Artistry of the Mentally Ill* (1922), the Heidelberg psychiatrist Hans Prinzhorn 'pointed to the interrelation of primitive art and that of mentally deranged patients particularly with reference to the hermaphroditic figures, the stiff posture, and the grotesque traits. Some of the pictures would cause one to hesitate in deciding whether they are made by savages or by mental patients.'[73] Rigid posture even permeates the creations of the severely mentally ill.

If we return to these links between neurology and posture in the late nineteenth century, it is clear that one of the dominant theories is that of the origin of hysteria in the 'railway spine'. That people could be horribly maimed in the ubiquitous train accidents of the day was clear; that they could be paralysed without any overt lesion presented a puzzle to physicians and insurance companies alike.[74] In 1864, after a series of catastrophic accidents, the British Parliament made the railway companies financially responsible for the health of their passengers. Two years later the Scottish physician John Eric Erichsen published seven cases of this condition, which he dubbed 'railway spine', an early theorization of what came to be called traumatic neurosis, a term coined by the Berlin neurologist Hermann Oppenheim in 1889. Erichsen defined the origin of these phantom lesions as being the result of 'The shake or jar that is inflicted on the spine when a person jumping from a height of a few feet comes to the ground suddenly and heavily on his heels or in a sitting posture'.[75] That these patients were paralysed was not in question – or was it?

Were these individuals dissimulators, or were they actually damaged? Was the result of such accidents to be associated with bad character, or was it some type of postural defect that predisposed one to paralysis? Here the spine, character and malingering are so intertwined that the seeming ubiquity of 'railway spine' demanded a more compelling answer from neurologists. The answer came to be the idea of a traumatic neurosis caused by experiencing a train accident, as outlined by Herbert Page in his classic work on *Injuries of the Spine and Spinal Cord* (1883) and accepted in toto by the most important neurologist of the day, Jean-Martin Charcot, in his work on the neurosis of fright or shock. 'Railway spine' was thus merely the direct (brain or spinal-cord lesion) or indirect (shock) result of physical trauma. That such lesions could not be found post-mortem – and the neurologists tried – meant only that they were so infinitesimal as to be invisible even under the most powerful of microscopes. Here the confusion between the models of traumatic neurosis evolved by Charcot and the British neurologist John Hughlings Jackson must be stressed. For the 'traumatic' event causes hysteria only in those who are predisposed to being hysteric (Charcot), but the lesion caused by trauma also releases those subterranean aspects of our earlier evolution held in check by the highest order of neurological organization (Hughlings Jackson). Charles Darwin's shadow was always present when posture was evoked. Did invisible lesions or shock make those who became paralysed revert to earlier, pre-bipedal states? But why were not all individuals who were involved in railway crashes paralysed? This question was answered in part by the neurologist Charles-Édouard Brown-Séquard, who had argued as early as 1860 that there were hereditary transmissions of acquired injuries, as in the case of 'animals born of parents having been rendered epileptic by an injury to the spinal cord'.[76] This view of reflex theory quickly became a standard one in the literature on 'railway spine'.[77] One could revert to earlier pathological forms if one was constitutionally weak because of one's degenerate inheritance. Spines were thus a constant focus of the neurologists trying to provide physiological explanations for psychogenic disorders. By the end of the nineteenth century these views about spines, posture and damage came to form the underpinnings of the cultural obsession with hysteria. Who was crazy? And why were they crazy? Both questions came to be linked to the spine and postural damage.

Yet posture as a symptom of mental illness is used in a very different context as evidence of the maltreatment of the mentally ill. Reformers such as the Victorian Quaker Daniel Hack Tuke, whose great-grandfather had become one of the creators of the British reformed asylum in founding the York Retreat in 1796, wrote about the creation of a posture of insanity as a result of the maltreatment of the Victorian insane:

> Lord Ashley quoted a letter from one of the Commissioners, written in Wales, in which it was stated, 'We have met with one case which we think most atrocious. A. B. was sent to the Hereford Asylum from near Brecon on November 28, 1843. She died on January 30th. She was in such a shocking state that the proprietor wished not to admit her; she had been kept chained in the house of a married daughter. From being long chained in a crouching posture, her knees were forced up to her chin, and she sat wholly upon her heels and her hips, and considerable excoriation had taken place where her knees pressed upon her stomach. She could move about, and was generally maniacal. When she died it required very considerable dissection to get her pressed into her coffin! This might be taken as a sample of Welsh lunatics.'[78]

For the Victorians and their Continental cousins, madness entailed a specific deformation of upright posture. How it was read was clearly determined by the ideology that defined the aetiology and potential treatment of the insane. Posture defines bodily as well as psychological health and the normative body and mind implied is a cultural ideal, which, like posture, could be displayed as a form of public education.

Hygiene and the Exhibition of Posture

At the Paris World's Fair in 1867, more than six hundred exhibits were devoted to health and hygiene; in 1882 the German Association for Hygiene held its first World's Fair in Berlin. Posture and the correction of posture were a theme in both. By the time of the International Hygiene Exhibition held in Dresden in 1911, health, gymnastics and sport comprised fully one-fifth of all the exhibits. Also introduced at the exhibition was the means of defining and treating posture through technology: the world's first motorized treadmill for people, developed by the physiologists Nathan Zuntz and Curt Lehmann in Berlin in 1889, first appeared in Dresden in 1911.[79] (They had initially developed it to test the respiration of dogs and horses under stress.) Such devices were introduced, as were other means of measuring effort but also treating pathology. Posture continued to play a prominent role in early twentieth-century health fairs, which became part of popular culture, captured at various events such as the state fairs across America. What had once been agricultural and industrial exhibitions became, in part, public health fairs.

Eugenics came to play an ever-greater role in the understanding of posture. Sir Francis Galton (Charles Darwin's cousin), who coined the term, noted in 1905 that

> eugenics is the science which deals with all influences that improve the inborn qualities of a race; also with those that develop them to the utmost advantage. The improvement of the inborn qualities, or stock, of some one human population will alone be discussed here . . . A considerable list of qualities can easily be compiled that nearly everyone except 'cranks' would take into account when picking out the best specimens of his class. It would include health, energy, ability, manliness, and courteous disposition.[80]

Discussions of race, here meaning 'collectives', are haunted by race in the sense of racial difference. Thus the novelist H. G. Wells responded directly to Galton:

> At the risk of being called a 'crank', I must object that even that considerable list of qualities Dr. Galton tells us that everyone would take into account does not altogether satisfy me. Take health, for example. Are there not types of health? The mating of two quite healthy persons may result in disease. I am told it does so in the case of the interbreeding of healthy white men and healthy black women about the Tanganyka [sic] region;

the half-breed children are ugly, sickly, and rarely live. On the other hand, two not very healthy persons may have mutually corrective qualities, and may beget sound offspring. Then what right have we to assume that energy and ability are simply qualities?[81]

Positive eugenics – sexual selection for advantageous qualities – was a theme in the public sphere, and healthy baby exhibitions competed with presentations of healthy posture at fairs at the most distant points of the compass. By the time of the First World War, in the United States,

'Fitter Families for Future Firesides' contests [that] had their origins in 'better baby' contests [were] held sporadically at state fairs during the 1910s. Whereas these earlier contests empha-sized infant health, the Fitter Families competitions sought to stimulate 'a feeling of family and racial consciousness and responsibility' . . . They probed participants' physical and mental health by measuring posture and strength, peering into eyes, ears, and throats, and taking blood and urine samples.[82]

Postural health was racial health.

Health presentations from the beginning of the century onwards were surrogates for how one could not only improve one's own life but that of the 'race' in all senses of the word. Galton noted late in his life about the Jews: 'It is a praiseworthy feature of the Jewish religion that, as a religion, it enjoins the multiplication of the human species. But it is still more important to determine that the children shall be born from the fit and not the unfit.'[83] Among the unfit were those with poor posture, and these were thought by many, but not Galton, to include the Jews.

At the Minnesota State Fair in 1922 there was an exhibition of posture, with lectures on correct posture:

Not only does correct posture concern physical bearing but affects the circulation, digestion, relieves constipation, but gives the heart and lungs freer action. While people who stand straight, sit up straight, as a rule are better able to resist disease and have better brain and muscles, good red blood freely coursing through the body. The erect position not only affects the eyes and the voice, but gives harmony to all the organs of the body; prevents curvatures of the spine and a lot of other things. Children in school cannot do good work all bent over. Parents, see that your children are erect.[84]

Correct posture is correct health. But the exhibitions also presented the ideal, normative body, in the form of a transparent human whose perfect posture spoke to the ideology of health and hygiene in the 1920s.

Late nineteenth-century fascination with health and posture focused on notions of hygiene. In 1911 the pharmaceutical manufacturer Karl August Lingner, whose mouthwash Odol, introduced in 1892, was the first broadly successful German product for personal hygiene in the age of bacteriology, sponsored the first International Hygiene Exhibition in Dresden as an attempt to further the cause of 'hygiene'. (The American product Listerine, named after Sir Joseph Lister, one of the heroes of this age, was created in 1879 but not sold over the counter until 1914.) The Dresden exhibition presented a wide range of displays, including a statue of the ideal German working man by Kurt Hermann Hosaeus, the creator of the Mozart Monument in Dresden (1906/7). Bare-chested and erect in a dramatic military posture, a sledgehammer over his naked shoulder, the statue represented the postural goal in this age of hygiene.[85] Also central to the exhibition were anatomical images that made the workings of the body transparent: 'The adult human body was, in its entirety and in parts, shown in the natural state, in the form of models, paintings, drawings, all displayed in the most artistic form by artists of the first order, the high walls and high windows admitting a flood of light and rendering inspection thorough and easy.'[86] Seeing the human body in its perfection was an educational objective. These images provided an idealized model for all observers to strive to attain. By 1912 such an ideology had morphed into the German Hygiene Museum in Dresden, which covered all forms of hygiene, from public health to eugenics.

The exhibition of 1911 was a worldwide success, and in 1924 the health exhibition to end all health exhibitions was held in Dresden, called 'Gesolei' (*Gesundheitspflege, Soziale Fürsorge, und Leibesübungen*; Health Care, Social Care and Exercise). It covered in detail the care of health and bodily fitness through positive eugenics. Central to it was

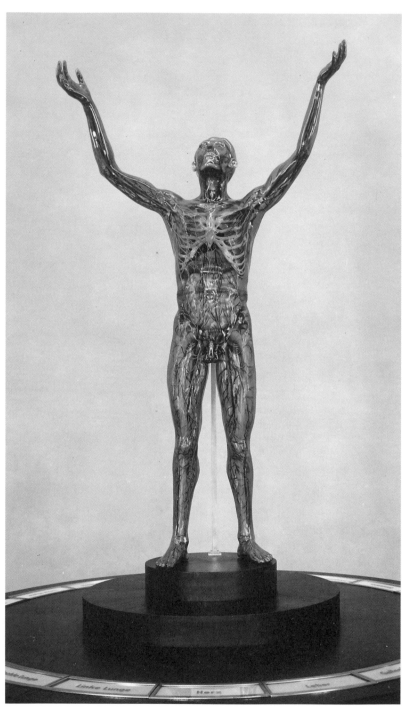

The 'Transparent Man' in 1930 with arms erect, facing the divine and being the ideal body of the German world of hygiene.

Franz Tschackert's amazing 'Transparent Man', which had been first displayed in 1911 and later in Düsseldorf in 1921, as the catalogue explained:

> As the Transparent Man first came to be 're-awakened' in 1921, it could not be denied that age had already taken its toll and that he could no longer escape critical contemporary review. Since that time, however, he has benefited from continuous recovery, rejuvenation, and growth, and in this process he has evolved in the fashion of a truly well adapted organism. The enthusiasm of the inspired exhibition-concept creator has indeed linked the medium intimately to the message, the exhibition of the model of man, to man. Our new and most recent jewel in the crown *is* the 'Transparent Man'.[87]

He was modern in every way, including in terms of his upright posture: not the worker with his sledgehammer confronting the toils of daily life, but the worshipping figure of upright man. For this 'Transparent Man', who eventually stood in the very centre of the Hall of Man (opened in May 1930) at the Hygiene Museum in Dresden, stood upright and looked towards the heavens.

A recent historian of science commented on the figure:

> The symbolism of the model was expressed by its position within the inner sanctum of the museum, by its bearing, and finally by the material itself. Bruno Gebhard, who had been scientific collaborator in the setting up of the museum, refers to an illustrious prototype of the figure, the Greek statue 'Adoring Youth', that is ascribed to Boedas of Byzantium (*c.* 300 BC) [a student of Lysippus]. In fact, the fine arts of the nineteenth and twentieth centuries have long been influenced by the model of the erect figure with outstretched arms. That prayer stance (erect, arms bent or stretched out, palms open, gaze directed obliquely upward) conveys to the viewer, even to one not versed in the canons of religious gesture, a consciousness of appeal to the superhuman-divine.[88]

While Boedas most probably did not make the model for this figure, it was one of the most important figures in the collection of ancient

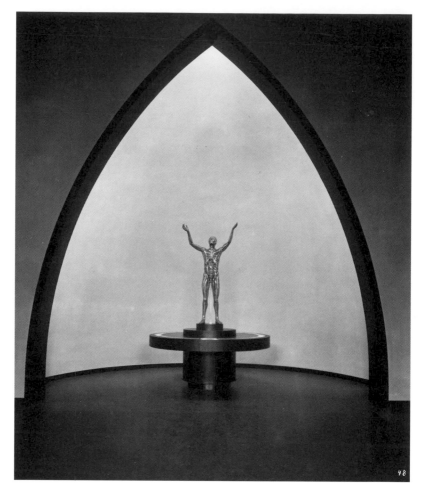

The temple-like setting in which the 'Transparent Man' was housed in 1930.

antiquities at the National Museum in Berlin. Originally sculpted for ritual purposes in Rhodes in about 300 BC, it had been taken to Paris in the seventeenth century. Frederick the Great purchased it from the French in 1747 and had it taken to Sanssouci, his palace in Potsdam, where it stood on a terrace until 1786.[89] All the antiquities in the royal collection were moved to a public space, designed by Karl Friedrich Schinkel, in 1830. In the course of the early twentieth century it was discovered that the uplifted arms did not belong to the original figure, but are instead a skilful restoration done while the statue was in France, probably during the reign of Louis XIV. It was one of the favourite figures in public Berlin museums, including Schinkel's museum, and one of the major features of the new capital of the German Empire, as

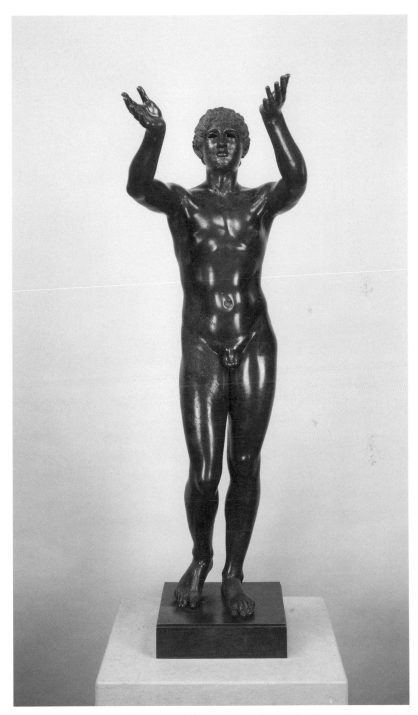

Attributed to the school of Lysippos of Sicyon, *Bronze Statue of a Young Man: So-called Praying Boy*, c. 300 BC.

much because it had been seized from the collection by Napoleon and repatriated to Berlin after his defeat. It served various political purposes in the iconography of upright posture.

One can note here, as mentioned earlier in the discussion of Hegel and classical posture, that such sculptural bodies did not reflect the reality of human posture. Idealized forms of posture had, since Johann Joachim Winckelmann and the Enlightenment, served as models not only for human posture but for the moral and ethical dilemmas confronting the human being. Certainly, G. E. Lessing's reading from 1766 of the tormented bodies in the classical *Laocoön Group*, first excavated in 1506, pointed at the merging of systems of postural representation and moral claims.[90] As early as Darwin, the anatomical absurdities of their physiognomy were made apparent.[91] Statues, we repeat, are not people.

Transmogrified into the 'Transparent Man', the 'praying boy' became a global symbol of the new eugenics and the normative reading of posture as a reflex of race. The 'Transparent Man' made his American debut at the Chicago World's Fair in 1933, the Century of Progress Exposition, and reappeared in the main hall of the American Museum of Health at the New York World's Fair of 1939.[92]

The 'Transparent Man' (and his companion, the 'Transparent Woman') symbolized the ideal of what came to be Nazi racial ideology, much as Hosaeus' figure of the worker in 1911 exemplified the evolving racial ideology of the new German Empire. Paul Schultze-Naumburg, in what was the official aesthetic line about race, commented in 1937 on the meaning of posture and the German body, a product of the mixing of the higher races:

> German civilization has clearly established an internalized standard for the epitome of beauty . . . Upon closer examination of this phenomenon, we find that this standard for the epitome of beauty unmistakably follows the outline of that race that has assumed leadership in all the great epochs of German history. And that is the Nordic race . . . Even in light of the diverse admixture evident in the German *Volk*, it is easy to see that high-level achievements occur primarily when there is sufficient or even a surfeit of Nordic blood present in the population.[93]

Posture is merely one variable, but it must be taken into account in understanding racial hierarchies, as Schultze-Naumburg claims. The 'Transparent Man' came to represent this epitome of the Aryan race. A version was purchased by the Buffalo Museum of Science from the German Hygiene Museum in 1935 (and returned because of its associations with Nazi eugenics in the late 1980s).

We, of course, recognize this as the model of upright posture from the ancient world to the modern. Modern, healthy humans have upright posture not only as a guarantee of health but as the inheritance of the divine inscribed on the modern body, although the divine in the 1930s may no longer signal the myth of Creation in the Garden of Eden. It may instead reflect the racial ideals that inhabited notions of hygiene, and that were present in virtually all the hygiene exhibitions from the very beginning of the century. Such views are certainly tied to fascism in all its forms, but they pre-date these political movements and also clearly outlive them.

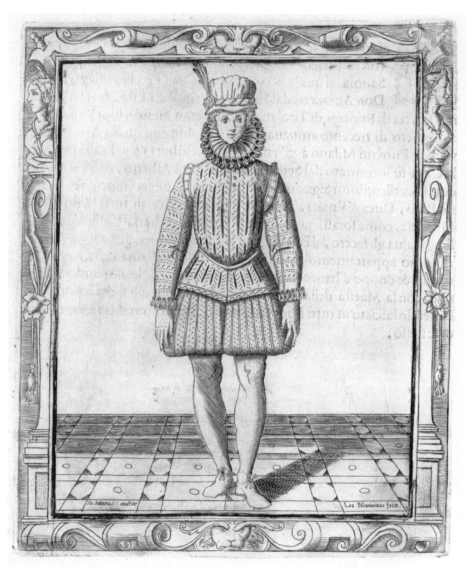

'The first position'. From Cesare Negri, *Nuove inventioni di balli* (Milan, 1604).

FIVE

Dance and the
Social Taming of Posture

I N AN ODD WAY, military posture and the posture of dance are closely linked. The military positions of the courtiers are also those of the dance: clearly 'unnatural' and having a specific function only within the movements required for their specific undertaking. You can't imagine goose-stepping or waltzing down your office corridor except in the most anxiety-provoking nightmare. Yet such postures, in the appropriate setting, become quickly routinized and habituated.

Posture in dance and the military seem to be interrelated not, as the noted historian William H. McNeill claimed, because such organized effort reflects the intuitive imperative of the beating heart translated into movement, but because both define what is acceptable in any given setting through normative positions of functional posture. While McNeill is interested in movement to music and the heart as metronome, his own project has yet another source. He writes of his experience of 'swaggering in conformity with prescribed military postures' and of this leading to a 'strange sense of personal enlargement; a sort of swelling out, becoming bigger than life, thanks to participation in collective ritual'.[1] Drill and drill position have meaning; the military posture comes to define collectivity in very specific ways. The sociologist of manners Norbert Elias evokes dance as exactly such a quandary: for him, social processes are sorts of 'mobile figurations of individuals on the dance floor' as a means of understanding 'states, cities, families, also capitalist, communist and feudal systems, as figurations'.[2] But the rules are taught; they are not only habituated, but become part of the way that such individuals relate to one another. This is not merely metaphor, however, for the dance itself becomes a contested space in modernity in which 'good' and 'bad' bodies are contrasted and rules for human interaction are defined.[3] The norms of military posture are integrated quickly into the very moves of the dance. Thus in 1724 Kellom Tomlinson, in his classic handbook on Baroque dance, notes that certain dance moves are

> much the same as when, in Fencing, we put ourselves in a Posture of Defence; but, this Posture being probably unknown to the Ladies, I shall endeavour to give an Explanation of it . . . The Posture of Defence most usually is to the right Hand, the whole Weight of the Body being on the left Foot, and the right stepped out sideways to the same Side of the Room.[4]

For the men dancing, such a posture is known; it must be elucidated for the ladies if they are to learn the 'Chasee'. Dance and the military are spaces of habituation of the body and the constant redefinition of posture.

Imperial court posture is a military posture, but it is also an answer to one other manifestation of modern life in Germany: modern dance, with its new and radical ideas of posture. The rise of modern dance at the beginning of the twentieth century paralleled the height of gymnastics (both in the German and Scandinavian varieties) as physical therapy and physical improvement. By the end of the nineteenth century even ballet, with all its institutionalization in the courts of Europe and on the theatrical stages of the colonial world, had come to be seen as having a corrective or moral quality.

Foucault's 'docile bodies' are the bodies of the modern state, but they have also long been the bodies of the theatre.[5] Foucault's 'military dream of society' served to regiment national cultures to preclude war, and thus its goal was to train not only the body of the soldier but that of the citizen. Yet it used other institutions – Foucault refers to Jesuit education – as a means of permeating society. (Think of the Jesuits as Ignatius of Loyola's 'warriors of God'.) But it also used the world of the theatre and specifically the world of dance as a means of creating new bodies through the imposition of ideas of regimented posture.[6]

In 1650, at the end of his life, the polymath René Descartes, according to tradition, may well have written a ballet libretto called *La Naissance de la paix* for the Swedish court theatre, in which he called war a 'ballet for the birth of peace'.[7] A recent critic noted:

By likening war to ballet (rather than ballet to war), Descartes reversed the analogies of the sixteenth century. This reversal draws attention to a transformation that occurred between those first *ballets de cour* [court ballets] and the mid-seventeenth century: warfare became more balletic. Any who turned out to watch pitched battles . . . might have observed a new precision in the open field, where foot soldiers could fall into a variety of formations, hold together in battle, and execute complex maneuvers in synch. The discipline observed in ballet was eventually implemented in battle.[8]

This can certainly be seen in Jacob de Gheyn's illustrations for *The Exercise of Armes* reproduced in Chapter Four. But dance itself had a rather national and military turn; 'as the *Ballet des provinces* [where in 1573 sixteen dancers representing the provinces of France performed to a martial tune] suggests, the "military dream" was more easily nurtured in the theatrical hothouse of court spectacle than out in the open field of battle.'[9] Dance is war and war is dance, and the irony of that was not lost on the people of the seventeenth century.

When we look at court dance manuals of the late sixteenth century, at the time of the first drill manuals, we see parallels between both images of posture, specifically to de Gheyn's drill book.[10] We can turn to Cesare Negri's *Le gratie d'amore* (The Graces of Love) of 1602 (re-published in 1604 as *Nuove inventioni di balli*, New Inventions of the Dance) for illustrations of the meaning ascribed to posture in formal dance.[11] Negri's texts are famed today (even though they were less visible in his day) as the first formal presentation of the five basic positions in ballet, which require that the feet be turned out and flat on the ground. But the images also reveal the ideal posture for the dancer. Negri begins, as does de Gheyn, with neutral position, the feet at a 45-degree angle, the back straight and the chin erect. Leo Palavicini's plate illustrating Negri's text shows this clearly (p. 144). Compare de Gheyn's plate of the pike man at rest (p. 73). (The irony is that this posture is close, but not identical, to the sixth position introduced into ballet by Serge Lifar after the Second World War, with parallel feet, as in *pas couru sur les pointes en avant* or *en arrière*.[12])

For Negri, *aiere* (posture) is one of the fundamental qualities of dance. *Aiere* became a technical term for the dance in fifteenth-century Italy. Initially it meant 'an aspect, a presence or appearance of a man or woman', but also the air one breathes.[13] It was the manner by which you 'naturally' appeared, as natural as breathing. But it quickly takes on a specific aspect of the dance itself. According to the famed Italo-Jewish dance master Guglielmo Ebreo da Pesaro (1410–1481), *aiere* was 'an act of airy presence and elevated movement, with one's own person showing with agility a sweet and gentle rising movement in the dance'.[14] It is what makes the dance aesthetically appealing.

By the sixteenth century 'posture' comes to signify the rest position. Dance quickly adapted posture as the final moment: after the five-step pattern taken in six beats, the dance ended with a jump and a 'posture' or resting pose.[15] Negri specifies a great deal about the posture of the dancer for these jumps: 'The arms are lowered moving them a little, since always holding them distended would be an ugly sight, with the hands somewhat closed. The body is carried straight, the head raised, the eyes that watch more often a little lower than high but not fixed in one place.'[16] All these are part of a totality of 'the beautiful actions and gracious movements and beautiful good manners . . . that are requisite as much to men as to the women, in the virtue of dancing'.[17] Beauty is defined clearly by Negri:

> In order to go well above the body with that utmost grace and composure that others can honor means to go well with the body straight and the arms at the sides, moving them a little, and the toes of the feet a little out, so that the legs and the knees remain very straight, and in passing one foot ahead of the other, it has to be a distance of two fingers; observing that according to the part and to the body one must do the step forward at a length of a little more than a palm.[18]

Negri's *aiere*, in fact, *is* the definition of what the beautiful posture in dance must be.

Posture, Contortion and Class

It is important to note that such posture defined the dancer's character as well as the dancer's body. In Baldassare Castiglione's *Book of the Courtier*, reflecting the practices of Urbino in the second decade of the sixteenth century, posture when dancing was a courtier's natural way of moving. It was not a posture adopted only while performing a dance and then cast aside when the performance was over. The rules according to which courtiers were expected to move on the dance floor applied to every other part of their lives: a noble and temperate bearing helped to distinguish them from those who did not belong to the elite.[19]

Central to this notion of dance is the fact that the habituation of the courtly dancers during the dance becomes the definition of the normal posture of the elite: 'Their carriage and demeanor when on the dance floor did not change once they finished dancing: it remained with them, as it was their normal posture.'[20] Posture training became interchangeable with dancing. Indeed, the image of the courtier gives way to that of the bourgeoisie over the course of the Enlightenment, but dance and posture training come to be interchangeable concepts.

Learn to dance and you will quickly become the captive of posture training. By the eighteenth century such beautiful postures were the stuff of parody. In 1760 the artist John Collett provided a look at the power of dance to shape the very idea of the citizen, in two prints.

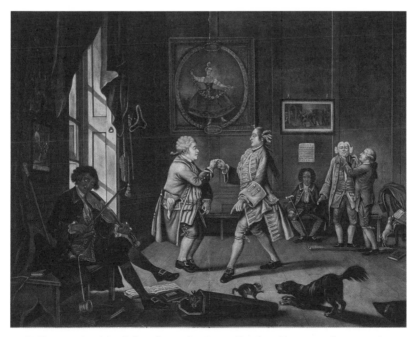

B. Clowes, after John Collett, *Grown Gentlemen Taught to Dance*, c. 1760, mezzotint.

One, *Grown Ladies Taught to Dance*, shows a young dancing master instructing a stiff and ungraceful elderly woman to dance. Two small girls look on, laughing at the woman's clumsy attempts. On the wall is a parody of this scene illustrating a monkey teaching a cat to dance. In his parallel satirical mezzotint, *Grown Gentlemen Taught to Dance*, Collett shows country bumpkins 'taught to dance & qualify'd to appear in the most brilliant assemblies at the easy expence of 1£ 11s 6d'. The music seems to be as tortuous as the dancing, since an ear trumpet rests against the hard-of-hearing musician. A dog is seen reaching up to snatch a paper labelled 'A Treatise on the Antiquity & Dignity of Dancing'. Neither dignity nor grace is to be found here. Not only are these bumpkins being trained to dance but, as we can see from the second figures to the right, they are trained in good posture and thus in good deportment. On a bench in the background, a poor fellow awaits his postural instruction. His feet have been placed in a form to encourage their proper (turned out) position for the minuet. Such postural aids are needed to reform untrained adult bodies.

The key to Collett's irony about masculinity and dance is in the leftmost painting, labelled 'Scalinger performing [the] Pyrrhic dance before the emperor'. When the scholar Julius Caesar Scalinger was twelve years old, in 1496, he became a page at the fabled court of his kinsman Maximilian I, Holy Roman Emperor. The calumny that he had danced in a frenzy before the emperor was one of the attacks on the aged scholar. Everything in the image is a satire, but the reference to the court evokes the military image of the pomp of Maximilian's 'triumphal procession'. Dance defines bodies negatively as well as positively. These are the bodies of almost gentlemen, the nouveau riche, the country squire, the untrained body (untrained in military bearing as well as social grace). It should be noted that more than class plays a role here. Most of the dance masters of the time were French and were represented 'in literature and on the stage . . . [as] ugly, thin-waisted and effeminate . . . [men] who seldom stood straight and never still, [their] form and posture embodying cultural degradation'.[21] As Richard Leppert notes, 'Needless to say this fact forced adult English men and women into permanent subservience to their French instructors, compounding the problem of cultural pollution with that of a perpetual teacher–pupil relationship in which the "natural" social order was reversed'.[22] These are bodies waiting to be formed and thus reformed by those seen as socially marginal – indeed, those who slouched.

The age of Collett was the age of the satiric representation of the military (or at least the militia): 'representation of militiamen became more socially specific, clustering around four main "types": corpulent old gentlemen; foppish young officers; social climbers from the middling sorts; and ragged lower ranks.' Prints such as these 'intended to amuse with social comment rather than to pursue a specific political cause.'[23] Yet note the posture of these dancers: they are clumsy in any and all of their roles. Theirs are untrained bodies. The military drill books of Collett's time 'placed great emphasis upon the contrast of motion and stillness.'[24] The images they contained stressed not only the world of the soldier but, more centrally, the soldier's posture: 'Some manuals . . . were lavishly illustrated with diagrams of weaponry, parade formations, and postures for drill. Similar illustrations were also reproduced on cards, handkerchiefs, and diaries.'[25] The silent contrast to these dancing gentlemen was clear.

Such satires of the rigid dancing body are more than merely commentaries on the foibles of a rising middle class. They also reflect a response to rigid posture that reflected a new aesthetic of flexibility, incorporating the idea of a mobile or natural posture as the definition of a perfect body. Such an aesthetic dialectic became itself, without doubt, a fixed way of seeing acceptable posture. This was encapsulated in William Hogarth's view in his *Analysis of Beauty* (1753): 'There are also strong prejudices in favour of straight lines, as constituting true beauty in the human form, where they never should appear. A middling connoisseur thinks no profile has beauty without a very straight nose, and if the forehead be continued straight with it, he thinks it is still more sublime . . . The common notion that a person should be straight as an arrow, and perfectly erect, is of this kind.'[26] Hogarth continues, reflecting on dance as a defining moment of posture:

> If a dancing-master were to see his scholar in the easy and gracefully turned attitude of the Antinous [the Greek youth, lover of Hadrian, who was made into a demi-god after his death and became the subject of many classical sculptures; see figure 9 on p. 152], he would cry shame on him, and tell him he looked as crooked as a ram's horn, and bid him hold up his head as he himself did.[27]

What is striking is that Hogarth not only famously advocated the serpentine line of beauty (think an 'S') as the basis for a new aesthetics, but demanded that such a rejection of the 'erect' (think an 'I') be an aspect of a new understanding of posture. The eclectic first plate accompanying the volume presents the 'line of beauty' (figure 49) but also, in its central panel, a collection of classical sculptures (*Hercules Farnese, Antinous, Torso del Belvedere, Laocoön, Venus de Medici, Apollo Belvedere*) that define the perfection of the 'S' posture. In contrast, Hogarth places the foppish gentleman of the day with his rigid, upright posture next to the statue of the classically beautiful figure of Antinous, one of the most frequently portrayed figures in Roman sculpture, in a pose emphasizing the line of beauty. While all the numerous sculptures of Antinous 'share distinctive features – a broad, swelling chest, a head of tousled curls, a downcast gaze – that allow them to be instantly recognized', one can add that, for Hogarth, Antinous' posture was his defining quality.[28]

Hogarth continues: 'This tendency to beauty in one, is not owing to any greater degree of exactness in the *proportions* of its parts, but merely to the more *pleasing turns, and intertwistings of the lines*, which compose its external form; for in all the three figures the same

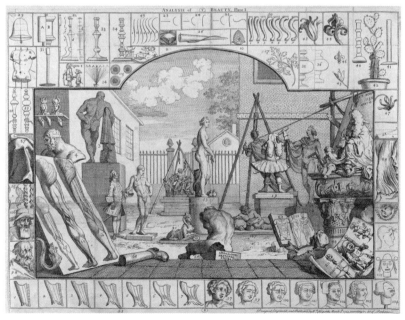

'A Statuary's Yard'. The first plate from William Hogarth, *Analysis of Beauty, Written with the Idea of Fixing the Fluctuating Ideas of Taste* (London, 1753), engraving.

proportions have been observed, and, on that account, they have all an equal claim to beauty.'[29] For symmetry is analogous to disease: 'legs much swoln with disease are as easy to imitate as a post, having lost their *drawing*, as the painters call it; that is, having their serpentine lines all effaced, by the skin's being equally puffed up.' All these are represented in the first plate. And the cure of the oedema of uprightness and straightness is the serpentine line.

Hogarth's rejection of the stiff, upright line is more than an analogy for rigid posture. He continues with a gesture towards the notion of natural posture in the training of children, a theme that would become central to the educational philosophy of the Enlightenment:

> the awe most children are in before strangers, till they come to a certain age, is the cause of their dropping and drawing their chins down into their breasts, and looking under their foreheads . . . it is apt to make them bend too much in the back; when this happens to be the case, they then have recourse to steel-collars, and other iron-machines; all which shacklings are repugnant to nature, and may make the body grow crooked. This daily fatigue both to the children and the parents may be avoided, and an ugly habit prevented, by only (at a proper age) fastening a ribbon to a quantity of platted hair, or to the cap, so as it may be kept fast in its place, and the other end to the back of the coat of such a length as may prevent them drawing their chins into their necks.[30]

Hogarth's rejection of the new innovations in bracing, which arrived in the early eighteenth century with the ability to produce tempered steel, is parallel to the rejection of the shackling of the insane during the Enlightenment and its replacement with the 'English straight-waistcoat.'[31] Yet Hogarth follows this with an acknowledgement that social structures, such as dance, that teach posture (often badly) are not possible during the child's formative years: 'But till children arrive at a reasoning age it will be difficult by any means to teach them more grace than what is natural to every well-made child at liberty.'[32] For Hogarth, the artificiality of such an attempt conflicts with his notion that there are ideals of beauty that the human being can achieve. Thus, at the bottom of his first plate are a series of whalebone corset stays, which can either deform or enhance the (female) body. It is the moderate one, the one in the middle, that provides a 'perfect, precise, serpentine line' in contrast to the 'deviations into stiffness and meanness on one hand, and clumsiness and deformity on the other'.[33] By this moment in the eighteenth century, as Lynne Sorge-English observes, such stays 'have been cut with a sinuous s-curve or "serpentine line" referred to by William Hogarth as "the line of beauty" . . . When the front curved seam of these stays was joined to a straight seam of the side piece, the result was an accentuation of the narrowness of the waist and the fullness of the breasts, thereby recreating in the garment a variation of Hogarth's line of beauty'.[34] This was at the moment when the nascent field of orthopaedics was beginning to advocate for corseting to reform deviant posture. Thus the move to an aesthetics of the serpentine line of beauty is part of a debate about the naturalness of postural traditions in the Enlightenment. But such a move does not remove human intervention (and artifice) from the shaping of the body.

It is striking that the corset, linking fashion and therapy, shatters the very notion of the aesthetic object. Hogarth is quite clear about this. Immanuel Kant in the *Critique of Judgment* (1790) later claims that it is the subjective notion of coherence that creates the aesthetic. But, Hogarth asks, what happens when the beautiful is fragmented, wearing a brace to correct poor posture? Tobin Sieber's thought experiment is apposite: what happens when we suddenly see the broken arms of the Venus de Milo covered in blood?[35] What happens when the aesthetic is suddenly revealed to be flawed to a viewer who defines beauty in terms of their own sense of bodily integrity? Ato Quayson has coined the term 'aesthetic nervousness' for such a moment.[36] Hogarth's world is full of such nervousness.

The Posture Masters

The world of Hogarth and Collett was very much that of the 'posture master'.[37] For the very look of people undertaking such posture discipline lent itself to public mockery. Posture became a shorthand way of speaking about contorting the body. In addition, 'posture masters' appeared daily on the streets and in the theatres of London. Samuel Johnson's dictionary defines him (and they all seem to have been men) as 'one who teaches or practices artificial contortions of the body', citing *The Spectator*.[38] His reference is to an essay by Addison and Steele of 19 February 1712 (no. 305) on the creation in Paris of 'a new Academy for Politicks, of which [Jean-Baptiste Colbert,] the Marquis de Torcy, Minister and Secretary of State, is to be Protector'; to be followed, it was rumoured, by a 'seminary of petticoat politicians' organized by Madame de Maintenon, the second wife of Louis XIV. According to *The Spectator*, Colbert's academy was intended to teach young gentlemen all the arts of governance – that is, how to subvert the state. They are first taught 'in State Legerdemain, as how to take off the Impression of a Seal, to split a Wafer, to open a Letter, to fold it up again, with other the like ingenious Feats of Dexterity and Art'. Then they are 'to be delivered into the Hands of their second Instructor, who is a kind of Posture-Master. This Artist is to teach them how to nod judiciously, to shrug up their Shoulders in a dubious Case, to connive with either Eye, and in a Word, the whole Practice of Political Grimace.' Their tutelage makes them into the perfect French courtier, as least to the satiric eye of *The Spectator*, unlike the British, who are trained in the

> Coffee-houses [that] are, indeed, very good Institutions, but whether or no these our British Schools of Politicks may furnish out as able Envoys and Secretaries as an Academy that is set apart for that Purpose, will deserve our serious Consideration, especially if we remember that our Country is more famous for producing Men of Integrity than Statesmen; and that on the contrary, French Truth and British Policy make a Conspicuous Figure in NOTHING.[39]

On the streets of London the posture master is a bit more pedestrian, which is certainly why the reference in *The Spectator* is so ironic. The vogue for such body training began with the visit to London by Tiberio Fiorillo, a Neapolitan actor known for his interpretation of Scaramouche, at the end of the seventeenth century. The London posture master was both a contortionist, someone who could twist their body into extraordinary forms, and someone who was self-conscious about their movements. He is advertised in various guises on the boards of London's theatres, such as at the Yeates's Medley in *The Beggars' Wedding* in August 1729.[40]

Among the various sights on the streets of seventeenth-century London was the home-grown posture-maker Joseph Clark. He was

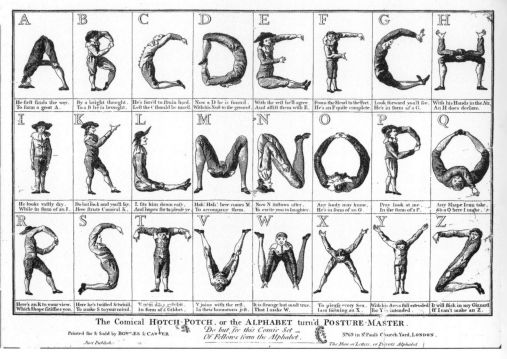

The Comical Hotch-potch, or The Alphabet Turn'd Posture-master (London, 1800).

one of those depicted as early as 1688 in *The Cryes of the City of London Drawne after the Life*. Clark's contorted body became a staple of the long-running 'street scenes of London', images that were reproduced well into the nineteenth century. Yet it is also clear that he was not merely a contortionist but one who lived from his simulacrum of bad posture. His posture was commented on in a report to the Royal Society in 1753, which mentioned his ability to

> appear in all the Deformities that can be imagin'd, as Hunch Back'd, Pot Belly'd, Sharp Breasted; he disjointed his Arms, Shoulders, Legs and Thighs, that he well appear'd as great an Object of Pity as any; and he has often imposed on the same Company, where he has been just before, to give him Money as a Cripple; he looking so much unlike himself, that they could not know him.[41]

He had trained himself as a child to dislocate his limbs. In a later account it was observed that, 'though well-made, and rather gross than

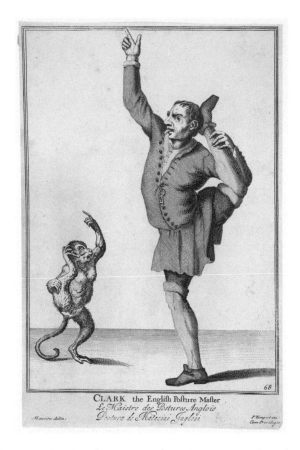

Marcellus Lauroon,
*Clark, the English
Posture Master*, c. 1688.
From *The Cryes of the
City of London Drawne
after the Life*, edn
unknown (first published
c. 1688).

CLARK the Englifh Pofture Mafter
Le Maietre des Posture Anglois

thin, he exhibited, in a most natural manner, almost every species of deformity and dislocation . . . He dislocated the vertebrae of his back, and other parts of the body, in such a manner that Molins, the famous surgeon, before whom he appeared as a patient, was shocked at the sight, and would not even attempt his cure.'[42] Not disabled, quite able indeed to have 'normal' posture, his image becomes that of the comic posture-shifter.

How Clark came to be seen can be judged by the fact that a monkey mimics his positions. In an eighteenth-century novel recounting the education of another animal, a cat, the posture masters teach such mimicry. The cat 'was next tried in the begging attitude, but in this too he excelled all the quadrupeds that ever came within the jurisdiction of this German posture master, so that in his second lesson, he surprised his master as agreeable as before, and actually followed a piece of meat, which was conducted before him, by way of precedent, more erect than many of his bipedal fellow-creatures.'[43] The posture-maker remains within British society at least until Sir Walter Scott's novel *Kenilworth* (1821), 'where a gentleman may break his neck if he does not walk as upright as a posture-master on the tight-rope'.[44] Artificial and highly shaped bodies are no longer limited to the dance floor, but are found now on the streets as well as in better society, if only as the object of amusement.

The Posture Girls

It should be noted here that the parallel to the 'posture masters' in the popular culture of the eighteenth century were the 'posture girls', such as 'Posture Nan', mentioned in the pornographic text *The Royal Rake, or the Adventures of Prince York* (1762).[45] 'Posture girls' such as the generic Nan exposed their callipygous charms for the titillation of London's gentlemen.[46] As David Stevenson explains, 'In the late seventeenth and early eighteenth century "posture girls" were popular there, hired to adopt ingenious poses and display their genitals.'[47] They appeared on stage but also in brothels and private parties, exposing themselves in various postures[48] – using 'Peer-Glasses for the Women to see how they can shew more Postures, when naked, than were ever seen acted by lewd Women at the Celebrated Bawdy-Houses', to quote a source from 1722.[49] These were pornographic precursors of the *poses plastiques* ('flexible poses'), virtually nude *tableaux vivants*, the sort of living pictures so beloved as bourgeois entertainment in the nineteenth century. In *The History of the Human Heart, or, The Adventures of a Young Gentleman* of 1749,

> their Ceremony [was described] which these Wantons went through. They each filled a Glass of Wine, and laying themselves in an extended Posture place their Glasses on the Mount of *Venus*, as every Man in Company drinking off the Bumper, as it stood on that tempting Protuberance, while the Wenches were not wanting in their lascivious Motions, to heighten the Diversion. Then they went thro' the several Postures and Tricks made use of to raise debilitated Lust, when cloyed with natural Enjoyment.[50]

Acrobatic posture tricks indeed, although quite different from those of their male counterparts.

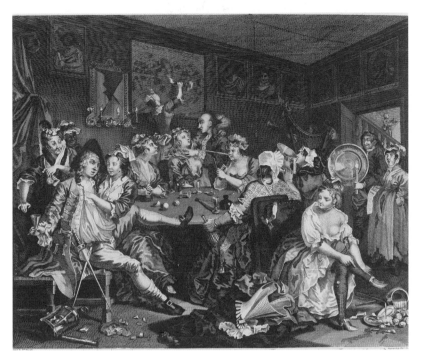

T. Cook, after William Hogarth, *A Rake's Progress* [1735], 1796, engraving.

'Arentine' the 'posture-woman' ('*Posituren-Macherin*') appears in the third plate of Hogarth's *A Rake's Progress* (1734) showing her charms to Tom Rakewell, at least according to the philosopher Georg Christoph Lichtenberg, who undertook a long and detailed series of interpretations of Hogarth's plates beginning in 1784 and concluding only in 1799.[51] The third plate is set at the Rose Tavern, a notorious brothel in Covent Garden. On the walls of the chamber are a variety of pictures. They are inscribed 'Polly Peacham', 'Capn Mackheath' from John Gay's *Beggars' Opera*, 'Tiberius Caesar', 'The Famous Seven Wonders of the World', 'Caesar Augustus', 'Julius Caesar', 'Sarah Malcolm' (the notorious British murderer also portrayed by Hogarth) and 'Nero'. One of the whores kisses the portrait of Dr Henry Sacheverell, the ultra-conservative Anglican theologian. Arentine (whose name echoes that of the notorious sixteenth-century inventor of modern literary pornography, Pietro Aretino) sits front right, very much parallel to Tom Rakewell's dissolute figure on the left. Her corset lies on the floor next to her, and she is rolling down her stockings, preparing to perform her posture act. A porter is bringing a tray upon which the disrobing woman will soon perform the naked contortions for which she is famous, feats that supposedly involved unmentionable deployments of the candle that he also bears.

From the 1770s onwards Lichtenberg was a regular visitor to London, where he was elected a member of the Royal Society. He may well have experienced such shows in his pursuit of somewhat higher culture: he was an admirer of the theatre of the day and especially of David Garrick. Lichtenberg mentions the great plate on which Arentine performed. At the end of her routine, he observed, she was semi-clad in the costume of a chicken (Plato's human?) with a fork stuck in her breast, a living meal, waiting to be consumed by the onlookers. (Remember Thomas Middleton's suggestive bon mot in his *The Old Law, or A New Way to Please You* of 1656, 'though a piece of old beef will serve to breakfast, yet a man would be glad of a chicken to supper.'[52]) About what happens then, Lichtenberg is silent. He found such a postural display revolting, comparing Arentine's viewers to the vermin of the metropolis willing to pay any price for such experiences. That is, of course, why Hogarth included her in *A Rake's Progress* – to chart Rakewell's decline towards his state in the final plate, where he is an inmate at Bedlam, the madhouse.[53] Yet the 'posture girls' were found in the most distant reaches, in towns such as Anstruther in Fife, Scotland, the sort of place from where Rakewell could have originated, as well as in Hogarth's corrupt London, where he was led to perdition. Moral lessons, as both Hogarth and Lichtenberg teach us, are never far from ideas concerning posture and sexuality.

Posture and the Morality of Dance

The tension between training in good posture and the frivolous or even dangerous nature of dance had already been reflected in Puritan America. The Boston preacher Increase Mather saw dance instruction, by a 'Grave Person', as a means 'to learn a due Poyse and Composure of the Body'. A generation later, in 1700, his son Cotton Mather 'implied [in his preaching] that lessons in posture and carriage, from a dance master, had become customary'.[54] Yet both are clearly opposed to social dancing and see it as an evil. In the much more social Southern colonies, such as Virginia, dancing came to define society as much as the Church did in Puritan Massachusetts. 'Virginians are of genuine blood – they will dance or die!' notes Philip Vickers Fithian, a New Jersey visitor to Virginia, in his diary on 25 August 1774.[55] The previous year, on 17 December, Fithian had noted that his lack of training in such social conventions meant that he was truly a Northern barbarian: 'I was strongly solicited by the young Gentlemen to go in and dance. I declined it, however, and went to my Room not without Wishes that it had been a part of my Education to learn what I think is an innocent and an ornamental, and most certainly, in this province is a necessary qualification for a person to appear even decent in Company!'[56] Dance or you are not fit company for gentlemen (or ladies)! Social posture and dance posture are one and the same thing.

In England John Locke, certainly *not* a Puritan in his orientation, in his *Thoughts Concerning Education* (1693) had recommended dance training by a fit dancing master. He believes that children should be taught dance as soon as possible, and although dance 'consists only in outward gracefulness of Motion, yet, I know not how, it gives children manly Thoughts, and Carriage more than anything'.[57] 'But you must be sure to have a good Master,' he continues, 'that knows, and can teach, what is graceful and becoming, and what gives a Freedom and Easiness to all the Motions of the Body. One that teaches not this, is worse than none at all: Natural Unfashionableness being much better than apish affected Postures; and I think it much more passable.'[58] Natural posture as opposed to unnatural and affected posture is the key.

Central to Locke's thought is his reworking of Juvenal's claim in the *Satires* that one must have a healthy mind in a healthy body (*mens sana in corpore sano*). Indeed, this is the opening line of his essay: 'A Sound Mind in a sound Body, is a short, but full Description of a Happy State in this World.'[59] Such a mind is reduced to mere imitation in understanding the proper posture of the body for keeping 'the Body in Strength and Vigor so that it may be able to obey and execute the Orders of the Mind'.[60] Indeed, 'some Exercise of the Body, which un-bends the Thought, and confirms the Health and Strength', is necessary for mental health.[61] As we shall see, the claims about 'natural' posture are central to ideas of posture in education. Here Locke links education and dance, since for him dance is a form of education, for good or for ill, of the body. But education is not limited to students. Ministers, too, should mind their posture. If posture could be trained to reveal as well as conceal, ministers were perhaps most at risk of unequivocally exposing their true intentions through their posture.

By the late sixteenth century and well into the seventeenth, dancers as performers for the world of the elite, the corps de ballet, come to

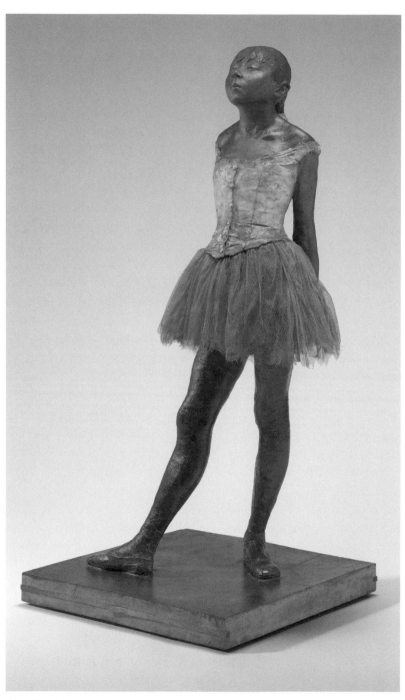

Edgar Degas, *Little Dancer Aged Fourteen*, 1878–81, pigmented beeswax, clay, metal armature, rope, paintbrushes, human hair, silk and linen ribbon, cotton faille bodice, cotton and silk tutu, linen slippers, on wooden base.

mimic the postures of the courtiers but now reflect the aesthetics of a new form, rather than the character of the court. Posture remains a means of control, but the moral character shifts radically. By the nineteenth century the posture of the ballet dancer, as captured, for example, in many works by Edgar Degas, defines quite the opposite of the moral claims of the early modern period.

In a review in 1886, Joris-Karl Huysmans, the novelist of decadence, noted in a volume entitled *Certains* (Certain People) that 'Monsieur Degas . . . in his admirable dance pictures had depicted the moral decay of the venal female rendered stupid by mechanical gambols and monotonous jumps . . . In addition to the note of scorn and loathing one should notice the unforgettable veracity of the figures, captured with an ample, biting draftsmanship, with a lucid and controlled passion, with an icy feverishness.'[62] For Huysmans there is no aesthetic of dance in the ballet, only the spectre of 'moral decay'. How this comes to be written on the dancers' bodies in Degas' work is perhaps best seen in this sculpture of an 'opera rat', a member of the corps de ballet, specifically Marie van Goethem, who had celebrated her fourteenth birthday in June 1879. When exhibited at the Impressionist exhibition in Paris in 1881, it was greeted with horror. The critic Elie de Mont was disgusted by its crudeness: 'I don't ask that art should always be elegant, but I don't believe that its role is to champion the cause of ugliness.' He compared her to a 'monkey, an Aztec'. The diminutive figure, the only sculpture Degas exhibited publicly, was described variously as 'repulsive', 'vicious' and 'a threat to society'.[63] She is assumed to be corrupt, or at least corruptible; indeed her physiognomy, redolent of caricatures of working-class girls of the day, pointed to that.[64] Paul Mantz reviewed the piece, noting:

> The piece is finished and let us acknowledge right away that the result is nearly terrifying . . . The unhappy child is standing, wearing a cheap gauze dress, a blue ribbon at the waist, her feet in supple shoes, which make the first exercises of elementary choreography easier. She is working. Back arched and already a little tired, she stretches her arms around her. Formidable because she is thoughtless, with bestial effrontery she moves her face forward, or rather her little muzzle – and this word is completely correct because this poor little girl is the beginning of a rat . . . Degas is no doubt a moralist; he perhaps knows things

about the dancers of the future that we do not. He gathered from the espaliers of the theatre a precociously depraved flower, and he shows her to us withered before her time.

The viewers were overwhelmed, he continued: 'The bourgeois admitted to contemplate this wax creature remain stupefied for a moment and one hears fathers cry: "God forbid my daughter should become a dancer."[65] Yet we must stress her extraordinarily upright posture, her head held high, as she stands in the fourth position. She is not at all (yet) a sign of 'moral decay', but possesses in her stance a self-awareness that contrasts with the extraordinary number of Degas' images of 'moral decay', as Huysmans observed. These mixed signals of morality at the edge of collapse, such as in William Holman Hunt's *The Awakening Conscience* of 1853, are present in her upright posture. In Hunt's painting, the young woman, in the process of being seduced, leaps upright from the lap of her seducer, signalling her awareness of the danger of moral decay. The posture of the young dancer here is too ambiguous for its audience. Degas's response to the reception of this most ambiguous of figures was never to show her again during his lifetime.

Good posture was encouraged by social dancing, even those dances that at any given moment were considered radical and new. The formal waltz, introduced in the mid-eighteenth century, was first seen to be a radical break with traditional formal dancing, in that the male held his partner around the waist. In her novel *Die Geschichte des Fräuleins von Sternheim* (1771), Sophie von La Roche observed that 'when he put his arm around her, pressed her to his breast, cavorted with her in the shameless, indecent whirling-dance of the Germans and engaged in a familiarity that broke all the bounds of good breeding – then my silent misery turned into burning rage.'[66] By the late eighteenth century the waltz was the rage of upper-class Vienna, and was spreading through the continent.

One learned to waltz, as with other 'ballroom' dances, as a form of socialization in Elias's sense.[67] It was posture training. But it was also therapy. By the end of the nineteenth century, according to a noted historian of the cinema, 'occasional mentions were also made of ballet training becoming more common as a way for city girls and young women to learn how to be graceful or to correct "poor posture, knock-knees and flat feet".'[68] Dance is moral therapy for the working class, raising them to the posture of the modern bourgeoisie.

Modern Dance and the Therapy of Posture

The trajectory (and impetus) of modern dance in its wider implications as body culture (*Körperkultur*) comes to include both the aesthetic and the therapeutic. If there is a clear collateral relationship between dance and the soldier's body, then the overlap between modern dance and therapeutics is a reflex of the late nineteenth century. This is the age that read poor posture, indeed hunched posture, as a sign of a weak will: 'Almost without exception', writes an author in the body reform magazine *Die Schönheit* in 1907, 'one can make the observation that people who are unable to maintain an upright posture . . . are also underdeveloped mentally: they speak slowly and have trouble thinking.'[69] How does one restore both the healthy mind and the healthy body? Movements such as Rudolf Steiner's (1861–1925) eurhythmy, a system of postural training that clearly incorporated both dance and therapy into his system of medical anthroposophy, attempted to address this question. In France the singing teacher François Delsarte (1811–1871) had already developed a form of body training for actors that stressed a system of gestures and postures. These were for him 'natural' gestures and postures that were reflections of the emotions of the actor or singer.

Actors added to this mix of postural reform as a way of dealing with modernity. Certainly the best known at the time was the Australian actor Frederick Matthias Alexander (1869–1955), who developed a theory of posture in the 1890s out of his own struggle with breath control as an actor; it came to have worldwide circulation and impact. His first published work, *Man's Supreme Inheritance* (1910), stressed the correct alignment of head, neck and back. The cry 'long spine' resonated from Alexander studios across the world, correcting breath and body. Alexander notes in the introduction to his complete edition of 1918 (which included two further texts) that his method of postural therapy successfully treated 'the failure of many kinds of treatment, of rest cures, relaxation cures, hypnotism, faith cures, physical culture, and the ordinary medical prescriptions.'[70] Yet, as with virtually all such postural interventions of the time, it is not merely physical therapy. John Dewey, the education theorist, notes in his introduction to the edition of 1918 that 'this whole book is concerned with education . . . He [Alexander] is aware of the perversions and distortions that spring from that unnatural suppression of childhood which too frequently passes for school training.[71] Thus Alexander's system stands against the postural rigidity of the school, but, as Alexander also notes, it is a therapeutic intervention against the plumb-line thinking of the military. Every year 'hundreds of soldiers have to leave the British army' because of the 'strains and rigidities' of the drill sergeant. 'These same soldiers will start on a long route march with chest "well set" and stiff. The strain of marching inevitably brings them later into an easier slouching position, which makes continuance possible and at its worst is not so positively harmful as is the tension of the other posture.'[72] The result of this is exhaustion and depletion, he continues, and school and army are institutions that corrupt posture through their stress on rigidity and discipline:

> For ten years past I have drawn the attention of medical men to . . . the evils wrought by the physical training and the 'stand-at-attention' attitude in vogue in the army, and also to the harmful effects of the drill in our schools, where the unfortunate children are made to assume a posture which is exactly that of the soldier, whose striking characteristic is the undue and harmful hollow in the lumbar spine and the numerous defects that are inseparable from this unnatural posture.[73]

As deleterious as the military and the schools is the teacher of dance, Alexander observes, and postural training in dance contributes to the corruption, not the therapy, of the body. Becoming 'drunk with music', children burst into the lascivious dances of the day, helping only to deform and corrupt their posture: 'it was very obvious to me that all these little dancers were more or less imperfectly co-ordinated; that the idea projected from the ideomotor centre constantly missed its proper direction.' The result was

> that subconscious efforts were being made that caused little necks to take up the work that should have been done by little backs; that the larynx was being harmfully depressed in the efforts to breathe adequately . . . ; and that the young and still pliable spines were being gradually curved backwards and the stature shortened when the very opposite condition was essential even to a satisfying aesthetic result.

What is worse, this improper mode of dance was actually encouraged by their instructors:

> And when we realise that the teachers who witness these lessons are entirely ignorant of the ideal physical conditions that are proper to children, and so are woefully unaware of the dangerous defects that are being initiated by these efforts to dance, we must admit that, as practised, this particular form of free expression is being encouraged at a cost that far outweighs any imagined advantage.[74]

Bad dance instruction leads to poor posture; postural reform leads to healthier and more stable lives. Only through the self-awareness of Alexander's method of postural therapy can such a violation of both body and spirit be overcome.

Indeed, the crossover between posture training and dance is marked. Kaiser Wilhelm ii's 'posture master' Bess Mensendieck is credited by a leading historian of physical culture as a 'harmonic gymnastics advocate' who helped to integrate 'strands of American Delsartism' into German modern expressionist dance.[75] One should add here that the system developed by Delsarte in the mid-nineteenth century and systematized only by Genevieve Stebbins in her *Delsarte System of Expression* (1885) was a means of connecting emotion with gesture for actors and singers. Only at the very end of the century, through its import into the United States, did it become a form of therapeutic gymnastics. Having said that, it is clear that the widest range of modern dancers, such as Isadora Duncan and Ruth St Denis, as well as body therapists such as Rudolf Laban, saw themselves as continuing Delsarte's project.[76]

Mensendieck had studied Delsarte practices with Stebbins, a student of Delsarte, and went on to teach dance at the New School for Social Research in New York in 1930s.[77] (She was a contemporary there of the dance teacher Gertrude Lederer, the widow of the founder of the 'University in Exile', whose image of Ursula Falke is to be seen below.[78]) When Delsartism was introduced into America in the 1920s, it was also a means of 'improving one's health and posture, and add[ing] to one's natural grace.'[79] As we have seen, Mensendieck's approach was remedial in training the body, but at the same time it was always therapeutic.

Modern dance was therapy, but therapy as much for disorders of society as of the body. Modern dancers of the 1920s and 1930s, such as Marguerite Agniel, stressed the notion that dance was indeed therapy for both functional and psychological conditions.[80] A noted historian of the period has observed that, for the dancers of the day, the 'significance of body symmetry and movement stemmed from eugenic anxiety about regressive primate tendencies'.[81] Indeed, dance 'claimed to correct spinal deficiencies and reproductive problems, preparing women's bodies for childbearing'.[82] It came to be seen as a eugenic reform of society through the body, not purely as medical therapy for the body and the psyche (although that, too, through anthroposophic medicine, also made claims on the more limited and defined realm of therapeutics). Here it impinged on other late nineteenth-century forms of alternative postural therapy, from chiropractic therapy (developed by D. D. Palmer in 1895) to osteopathic medicine (developed by Andrew Taylor Still in the 1890s) to forms such as the Alexander Technique developed in the 1890s. All focused on some type of postural therapy to cure the body, the psyche and society, and modern dance came to function within this matrix of postural therapy.

Remember the outrage at the waltz in the late eighteenth century. By the early twentieth century the waltz is the epitome of grace and elegant posture. In the 1920s 'the elegant, erect posture of previous couple dances gave way to the slouched, hunched-over gait of a lumbering animal, and the smooth circular motions of the waltz gave way to the jerky movements of ragtime trotting'.[83] As with the antithesis between the posture of the soldier and that of the guerrilla, the answer to the perceived rigid posture of both ballet and ballroom dancing at the close of the nineteenth century comes to be modern dance and ragtime.

The posture of late nineteenth- and early twentieth-century 'modern' dance, perhaps exemplified by Loïe Fuller (1862–1928) and Isadora Duncan (1877–1927), is 'defined by a dancer's sense of center, gravity, and ground. Pulling the body into spiral positions around a central axis, using the contraction and release as the guiding impulse'.[84] Duncan 'saw no beauty in conventional postures and over-developed muscles'.[85] Drawing on positions in classical Greek sculpture and painting, Duncan and her disciples – including Mensendieck – understood 'that the body can express mental processes by means of posture and movement'.[86] As the American dancer Martha Graham later writes:

'there is only one law of posture I have been able to discover – the perpendicular line connecting heaven and earth.'[87] More than just a gesture at the transcendental, which seems to be built into modern dance as an answer to the rigidity and immorality associated with other older forms of dance at the time, it gestures at a sense of the body as not only infinitely flexible but therapeutic.[88] Not only modern dance at the time but modern art, at least the Surrealists, such as Salvador Dalí and Georges Bataille, shifted the manner of representing human posture. In his 'Manifesto of Futurist Dance' (1917), F. T. Marinetti states that it will be 'anti-harmonic, ill-mannered, anti-gracious, asymmetrical, synthetic, dynamic, free-wordist.'[89] In turn, the Surrealist mechanism of dance rotated the axis that was 'proper' to man – 'his verticality, a station that defines him by separating his upright posture from that of the beasts – onto the opposing, horizontal axis.'[90] Through such alterations new senses of bodily posture are awakened in the dancer as well as in the viewer.[91]

One of the most fascinating figures in northern Germany to combine dance and the therapeutic during the *fin de siècle* was Ursula Falke (1896–1981), who worked with some of the most influential figures in European modern dance, including Laban, Mary Wigman and Kurt Jooss.[92] The daughters of the renowned German impressionist writer Gustav Falke, who lived and wrote in Hamburg, she and her sister Gertrud Falke (1891–1984; later Gertrud Falke-Heller) were part of the north German cultural elite at the turn of the century. But it was also an elite compelled into the world of bodily reform and therapy by the notion of physical and psychological transformation. It was the world of the Danish bodybuilder Jens Peter Müller (1866–1939), whose approach dominated north German *Körperkultur*. He abjured the use of apparatuses such as Indian clubs and spring dumbbells for special sandals to improve posture and handbooks on sexual hygiene. The new 'laws of hygienic aesthetics', as Michael Cowan notes, became the goal of a 'body culture that sought to put the science of orthopedics to work in the systematic education of the populace in the public performance of beauty.'[93] And this was just as true in modern dance. The culture of the time believed that bodily transformation was not only possible but necessary if one were to become a modern man or woman.

Between 1916 and 1918 Ursula and Gertrud formed the famed dance duo known as the Falke Sisters.[94] The two women had been trained as members of the Austrian music educator Émile Jaques-Dalcroze's first professional class at his experimental institute at Hellerau in 1910.[95] It was with the Dalcroze method that dance and gymnastics merged to structure the early developments of pioneers of modern dance, including the innovations of Wigman.[96] Central to Dalcroze's method, which he developed while teaching at the conservatoire in Geneva, was the expression of abstract musical concepts through body movements. He wrote: 'Bodies trained in the refined realization of rhythmic sensations must learn to assimilate thought and absorb music.'[97] His goal was to teach the musicians' bodies actually to move in real time and space, stressing pitch, rhythm and dynamics. What he quickly realized was that the last two defined motion in time and space in analogy to dance (and military drill). He called this blend 'eurhythmics'.

Dance was not only the natural expression of music in time and space, according to Dalcroze, but was also quickly seen to be simultaneously therapy – psychotherapy as well as therapy of the body – by his collaborators, including the Freudian neurologist and child psychologist Édouard Claparède in 1906.[98] It was thus an alliance of psychoanalytic psychotherapy and eurhythmics as an offshoot of gymnastics that claimed to create 'a healthy mind in a healthy body', since it dealt with both the psychic component of physical symptoms and the integration of bodily awareness into the psyche.

The Marxist philosopher Ernst Bloch, writing in American exile in the 1930s, reflected on these

> new schools of dance developing from Dalcroze, [that] attempted to demonstrate a more beautiful image in the flesh; whereby they certainly began the building from a high roof, and consequently had to be extremely 'ideological' . . . It [Dalcroze's method] looked at the beautiful animals with their superbly fit stride well-suspended within them. It was intent on breaking down from top to bottom the purposely concealed or frozen posture, which the master-servant relationship brought with it. The limbs were encouraged, in courses which no longer wished to have anything in common with the learning of manners.[99]

It is striking that Bloch sees the intent of modern dance as a blow against the subservience built into formal dance as a postural discipline. He defines this, as we have seen in our discussion of the philosophy

The sisters Falke performing in the 1920s. From the first systematic attempt to document German modern dance in photographs, Hans Brandenburg, *Der moderne Tanz* (Munich, 1921).

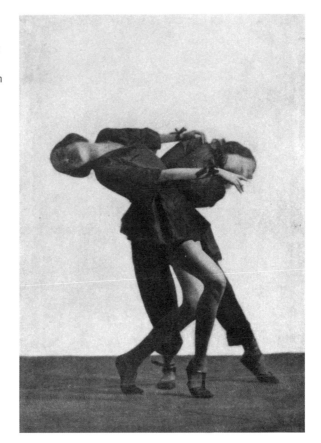

of posture, as a means of overcoming Hegel's master-slave dialectic. For Bloch, the social project of modern dance masked the gradual collapse of modern, capitalist society as it attempted to reform posture beyond the constraints of societal convention. In that way it was at least better than such dance crazes as the 'coarser, nastier, stupid' postures of American jitterbug, 'an imbecility gone wild', which seemed only to be a radical break with the past.[100] Modern dance may desire to be truly utopian in its desire to free the body from postural constraints, but it is in the long run condemned to fail, or so Bloch argued (as did, also in American exile in 1941, Theodor Adorno).[101]

Certainly in Germany and beyond the development of a bodily hygiene also had a clearly political agenda – not just on the right but on the left. Movements of the 1890s such as the *Jugendbewegung* (Youth Movement), with its emphasis on physical activity, music and movement, and sexual enlightenment, were political as well as aesthetic in their intent. That movement seems in retrospect avant-garde, but, like many of its most important figures such as Hans Blüher (1888–1955), it was rooted in a nationalist ideology stemming from the worship of nature in German Romanticism and which provided an underpinning for Nazi views of 'Blood and Soil' (*Blut und Boden*). In the 1910s Blüher – who had once been an advocate of Freud – was a strong supporter of the German youth movement the *Wandervogel*, stressing all its homo-erotic overtones. Returning to nature, camping by an open fire and strumming their guitars, they advocated a new, anti-bourgeois freedom for bourgeois youth. By the 1920s Blüher had broken with psychoanalysis over Freud's Jewishness, which he saw as contaminating the very soul of a 'German' movement. Blüher stressed the superficiality of the Jew's Westernization. For him, the Jews remained 'Orientals', no matter how they seem to have physically transformed; he maintained that they regress to what they have always been once they are removed from Western society. Blüher's text evokes in a powerful manner the idea of a Jewish racial type: 'The Jews are the only people who practise mimicry. Mimicry of the blood, of the name, and of the body.'[102] Here Blüher simply picks up the rhetoric of such 'scientific' thinkers of the time as Werner Sombart, who argued in *The Jews and Modern Capitalism* (1911) that the Jewish body and its posture is inherently immutable, an argument that we shall later see contested through Zionist advocates of Jewish physical reform. Such racial views permeated popular as well as scientific culture across the globe in this age of obsession with posture. All return to an explicit contrast between healthy German posture and the degenerate posture of the Jew.

The rise of contemporary youth movements and radical innovation in all the arts was seen as an attempt to overcome the decadence of the late nineteenth century bourgeoisie, of the world of ballet. In 1920, in a monograph on Expressionism (the newest of the arts), Ernst von Sydow observed that such innovation had powerful psychological as well as postural goals: 'as soon as we speak of decadent people, we have a clear complex of depressive feelings . . . The decadent person can have so many good and pleasant experiences in life that a healthy person would never cease to rejoice – still the wrinkles of worry visible on his forehead will not smooth out; his posture will not become upright.'[103] The source of such degeneracy was left open; was it merely corrosive bourgeois culture or something even more malevolent? The new arts could reform the decadent soul and body of the healthy German or indeed, if race was not a determinant, those of the healthy

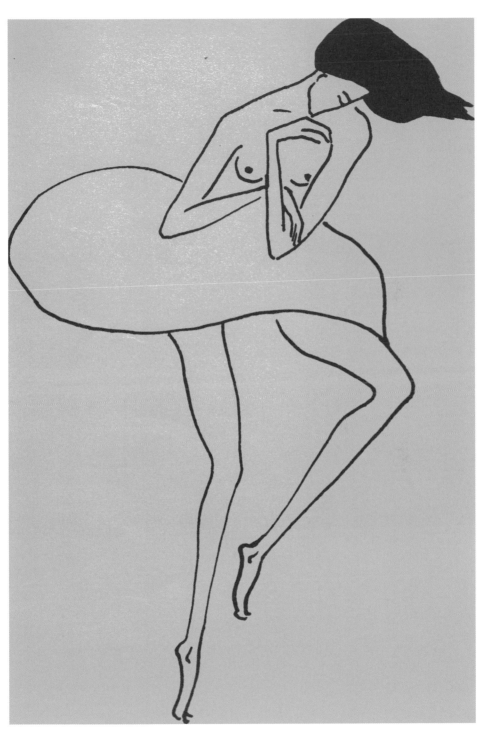

Gertrude Lederer, *Ursula Falke*, c. 1925, pen and ink drawing.

cosmopolitan. The future implications of such views could not be foreseen, but one must note that Ursula Falke, who married the anti-Nazi *Jugendstil* artist Richard Luksch in 1924, was able to remain in greater Germany during the Third Reich, while her Jewish friend Gertrude Lederer was forced to flee to New York in 1938.[104]

Dalcroze's followers studied the relation of movement exercises to musical rhythm in the form of what he called 'Rhythmic Gymnastik'. Such therapies could reform the body as well as the soul. Following their work with Jaques-Dalcroze, the Falke sisters opened the first modern dance studio in Germany. Held in the fabled artists' centre the Curio-House in Hamburg (the site of war crimes trials of ss officers after the Second World War) and having as many as 150 students, it quickly became an important base for experimental dance during the period before the war.[105]

In the summer of 1914 the sisters went to study with Laban in Monte Verità, Ascona. Monte Verità, founded in 1900, had become a gathering place for 'disaffected . . . *Bildungsbürgertum* (educated bourgeoisie)' to escape the pressures of metropolitan existence. It was based on the principle of living life 'close to nature'. It was the home of avant-garde body culture, including vegetarianism, communal living and 'free love'. It was a middle-class variant of the *Wandervogel*, the movement advocated by Blüher. Sexual hygiene was part of physical improve-ment.[106] In its scope, if not its membership, it was allied with the various movements of the turn of the century (from Marxism to Zionism to proto-Fascism) that believed strongly in physical as well as ideological transformation. The sisters also found further contact there with Wigman, whom many credit with making modern dance culturally accessible in Germany, and whom they had met earlier at Hellerau.[107] The three women even worked together in 1920, on a dance piece that unfortunately was never performed; they also taught together for a time, the Falkes giving joint improvisation classes and Wigman teaching technique.[108] The Wigman technique developed out of this collaboration. Performances of the Falke sisters have been described as evoking a clearly aesthetic quality ascribed to the gymnas-tics of the day. According to Kurt Peters, what they lacked in 'uninhibited vitality' (a feature looked for in gymnastic competition) they compen-sated for in an 'understated style' that was 'unforgettable'.[109] The action photographs of their dances from the 1910s and 1920s reveal this in detail.[110] Indeed Hans Brandenburg, who had introduced them to

Laban, featured many photographs of them in his influential study of modern dance.[111] The drawing above is from this early period and reflects the visual merger between dance and gymnastic movement. A contemporary critic described their performance *Versunkene Kathedral* (1918), where Ursula was dressed in silky black trousers and moved as the shadow of Gertrud in a short dress with legs exposed, as 'languid arabesques and eerie mirror movements [constructed] out of the delicate intertwining of their bodies'.[112] The sisters 'cultivated an attitude toward the body unprecedented in its modernity, intensity, and complexity'.[113] Although Ursula incorporated elaborate costumes into her dance in the 1920s, following the Bauhaus model, as in her *Der Prinz* (1925), here it is the physical position that is determinate.

Bodily movement was a key to cultural and social transformation. Rejecting ballet meant rejecting the plot lines with their often fairy-tale quality, as well as the Romantic music that accompanied them. (Think Tchaikovsky's *Nutcracker Suite* of 1892 with Marius Petipa's choreography.) Instead, themes of Greek tragedy accompanied by atonal music, or, indeed, the abandonment of music completely, come to define modern dance at the *fin de siècle*. The extensive number of photographs of her dancing illustrate this notion of fluidity and bodily control in Ursula Falke's early dances. Yet within this developing tradition the rejection of rigidity and artifice meant imagining a reformed bodily posture.

Modern dance uses anti-rigid posture as its key. If the artifice and corruption of the ballet, its loss of aesthetic and moral sense, are key to an understanding of what had happened to formal rules of posture by the end of the nineteenth century, the rise of modern dance redefined the notion of bodily flexibility and the rejection of rigidity. Modern dance is thus not only a form of posture reform but one of postural therapy. It is of little surprise that it not only becomes self-evident in the world of Steiner and his eurhythmy but permeates the very notion of modern posture. We are how we move, whether in the world of William Hogarth or the movement studios of the Falke sisters.

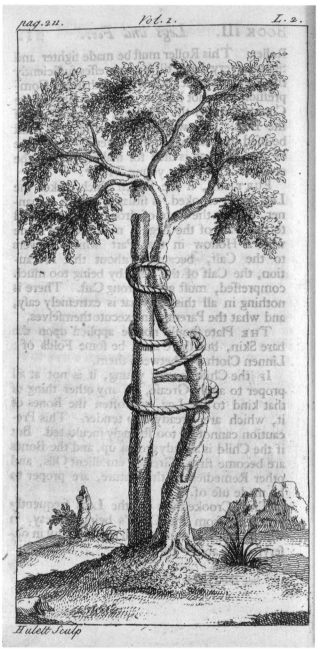

James Hulett, 'Crooked Trunk of Tree Being Straightened by Tying it to a Pole with Rope'. From Nicolas Andry de Bois-Regard, *Orthopedia or the Art of Correcting and Preventing Deformities in Children* (London, 1743).

SIX

Education Shapes a Healthy and Beautiful Posture

I F DISEASE RESHAPES the normal body and destroys healthy posture, then the underlying assumption is that normal posture is 'natural'. This is the argument underlying the relationship between medicine in all its sub-specialities and correct posture. But the very ideas of 'normal' and 'healthy' are themselves always convoluted and often contradictory. From the Enlightenment onwards (one might actually argue from the ancient Greeks, since Enlightenment thinkers placed themselves in a genealogy that they traced back to the ancients), the idea that the civilizing process destroys natural posture is present. In 1741 the aged former dean of the faculty of medicine at Paris, Nicolas Andry de Bois-Regard, then 82, published his *L'Orthopédie, ou l'art de prévenir et de corriger dans les enfants les difformités du corps*, arguing that most of man's ills were caused by the poor posture he developed in childhood. Andry also suggests instruments for treatment, such as a gradual straightening of a malformed tibia: 'you must put a large Compress under the Bandege, on that Part of the Leg. In a word, the same Method must be used in this case, for recovering the Shape of the Leg, as is used for making streight the crooked Trunk of a young Tree.'[1]

Andry believed in the inherent symmetry of the body. When a person had a short torso, he believed, such a body would be compensated with long legs: 'even in Deformity, Nature has observed such an exact Symmetry. Hence we may learn, that we ought not to regard those Deformities of the Body which are seemingly so, as real ones, because that frequently what we look upon as a Deformity, is in truth a Perfection.'[2] While remedying nature meant upsetting the body's 'exact symmetry', he also recognized the need to alter what he and his profession saw as radically pathological postures in the child. In the eighteenth century, especially for medical specialists such as Andry, the manipulation of the body could have a double function: to correct or to enhance, thus entering into a debate that had haunted aesthetic surgery from the seventeenth century onwards. For the orthopaedist, the use of methods of enhancement in medicine that seemed too similar to those in civil society, such as the corset, was anathema. However, the new, modern technology of spring steel, which was introduced in the eighteenth century and slowly replaced whalebone in corsets, came to be seen as an innovation that would more scientifically reform the body.

Andry was an advocate of 'natural' whalebone stays to correct what he (and the new field of orthopaedics) began to call pathologies of posture, including 'crooked-back'.[3] Such new technology set the medical corset, correcting postural deficiencies, on a different moral plane from fashion. The struggle against reshaping the body for fashion's sake is the centrepiece of Jean-Jacques Rousseau's theory of education. Rousseau, along with a great number of Enlightenment physicians and commentators, also condemned corseting for fashion's sake, a condemnation that became an intrinsic part of medical practice during the nineteenth century as corseting for orthopaedic purposes became common.[4] The more the orthopaedists (and many other medical specialists) used corsets and restraints, the less likely they were to see as acceptable such restraints used for the purposes of reshaping the body for 'mere' fashion. This mirrored the struggle in the eighteenth century between the emerging (male) field of gynaecology and the demonized world of the (female) midwife.

Andry's image has a long reach in our imagining posture. In *Discipline and Punish*, Michel Foucault, where he discusses the body of the soldier, uses an uncaptioned version of Andry's bound tree as an icon of disciplinary power. As one critic notes, 'The image raises questions of agency, since it is unclear who exactly bound the tree . . . the image therefore accorded with Foucault's understanding that the operation of these principles was invisible and pervasive.'[5] That they may have been, but the image of the bound tree in the garden was both pervasive and very visible in various attempts to advocate for or against postural reform.

While the bound tree in the garden is an ancient trope, its Enlightenment form is slightly different. In Eucharius Rodion's mid-sixteenth-century book on childbearing, it is used to advocate for swaddling in terms of shaping the body of the not yet self-conscious child: 'A young tree, if it is kept straight and bent, keeps the shape as it grows. The same happens with children, who, if they are well and properly bound in their little bands and swaddling clothes, will grow up with straight body and limbs.'[6] By the Enlightenment it comes to be associated with formal education. Thus the actual precursor of Immanuel Kant's image of the human being as 'crooked wood' comes not solely out of philosophy but out of orthopaedics. The remedy for postural ailments such as rickets is medical intervention. Humans may be 'crooked' (a term that carries heavy moral as well as postural implications), but they can be corrected.

Train and shape or reform the child's body and you will have a healthy, upright man. But is medicine, with its corsets and braces, the best way? Or should we think about the body as 'crooked wood', needing, as Kant proposed, reshaping through other social institutions, such as education? The notion that education was a pathway to postural reform and that such reforms were also a means for moral and rational development has ancient precursors.

To educate for good posture was already perceived in the classical world as vital, since the Greeks and the Romans esteemed correct posture. Cicero in his late, anecdotal *De officiis* (On Duties) stressed decorum and social behaviour, including learning the posture appropriate to the *genus vitae* – the style of life – as necessary for the educated citizen. His text is a mainstay of medieval theories of postural education (St Augustine read and admired it). It reappears as well in early modern notions of education and the role that posture plays in it (to Erasmus and beyond). Yet Cicero's notion of the centrality of posture is different from those of both his Greek forerunners (such as Plato, whom he cites) and his later Christian interpreters. For it is shaped not by any direct obeisance to the gods, but rather by an acknowledgement of the importance of posture, of uprightness, of man as *erectio* (uplifted), in contrast to the base sensuality of the beast.[7] This is the core of the human that is needed in training the citizen. Cicero notes, following Plato, according to one recent commentator, that it is 'upright posture which distinguishes human beings from beasts and gives access to higher realms'.[8] Yet he does not actually evoke the gods to explain the difference between man and beast. His concern is the shaping of the citizen of the Roman Empire, not elucidating how the human arose.

In the Renaissance the basic qualities of the human are transformed into specific qualities of the citizen. Erasmus, who notoriously still echoed Plato's notion of the human as featherless and upright (but certainly not a chicken), picks up on this thread in his amazingly popular *De civilitate morum puerilium* (On Good Manners for Boys; 1530). (At least twelve editions appeared in the year of its publication.) In this handbook aimed at young readers, Erasmus offers an entire chapter on the technical aspects of posture with a clearly moral twist: 'Letting the neck droop forward and hunching one's shoulders betokens laziness, while tossing the head back from the body is a sign of haughtiness. It should be held gently erect, and the neck should incline neither to the left or to the right (for that is the gesture of mimes) unless conversation or some such thing requires it.' The 'mime' is of course what by the seventeenth century comes to be called the 'posture master'. Erasmus continues paraphrasing the classics, including Cicero's *De officiis*, that such postural training is part of a pattern of formal education: 'If neglected in boyhood, bodily habits of this sort become ingrained and deform the natural posture of the body.' Note that the acquired hunchback, not the spinal disability discussed in the introduction, is a moral failing, but the notion that all failures of posture are signs of a secular immorality haunt these images. At this point in Erasmus's argument this view is supported by the classic metaphor for secular education, that of the tree in the garden of education: 'Young bodies resemble young shoots, which come to maturity and acquire the fixed characteristics of whatever you determine for them with a pole or trellis.' Fashion is no excuse, for 'what accords with nature and reason is a ready guide to decency; the taste of fools is not.'[9] The secular body is trained by human education, but is not to be deformed for fleeting fashion.

In the *Dialectic of the Enlightenment* (1944), Max Horkheimer and Theodor Adorno note that there was a shift from the Greeks (and by implication the Romans):

> With the complete transition of power to the bourgeois form mediated by trade and communications, and still more with the rise of industry, a formal change occurred. Instead of to the sword, humanity enslaved itself to the gigantic apparatus, which to be sure, ultimately forges the sword. The rational purpose of enhancing the male body thereby disappeared; the

Romantic attempts to achieve a renascence of the body in the nineteenth and twentieth century merely idealizes something dead and mutilated.[10]

While there were transformations of meaning and posture, these shifts were never without their own substance or their own pitfalls. Certainly such shifts often evoked the past as models, especially the classical past, but they had their own lives and their own echoes.

Postural Education and its Path

The rediscovery in the Renaissance of posture as an intrinsic quality of the educated and chivalrous human rests on the rereading of such classical writers as Cicero. No greater exponent of posture can be found in the Renaissance than Baldassare Castiglione, whose *Book of the Courtier* (1528) centres on posture as a key element in the correct education of the courtier. In his reading of the reception of this book, Peter Burke stresses that central to the education of the courtier is modesty: this includes his behaviour, appearance, gestures and posture (*lo stare*), which constituted education into grace (*grazia*), the idea with which Castiglione has been identified across the centuries.[11]

For Castiglione, posture defines both the positive and the negative aspect of character. In its positive forms, it links the military and dance:

> here is a man who handles weapons . . . if he nimbly and without thinking puts himself in an attitude of readiness, with such ease that his body and all his members seem to fall into that posture naturally and quite without effort, – although he do no more, he will prove himself to everyone to be perfect in that exercise. Likewise in dancing, a single step, a single movement of the person that is graceful and not forced, soon shows the knowledge of the dancer.[12]

The negative is the absence of masculinity, the posture of the effeminate male:

> I would have our Courtier's aspect; not so soft and effeminate as is sought by many, who not only curl their hair and pluck their brows, but gloss their faces with all those arts employed

by the most wanton and unchaste women in the world; and in their walk, posture and every act, they seem so limp and languid that their limbs are like to fall apart ... they should be treated not as good women but as public harlots, and driven not merely from the courts of great lords but from the society of honest men.[13]

Posture thus defines masculine grace as opposed to feminized affect.

What frames such conceits is the anxiety associated with false displays of posture. Gardens, at least as a metaphor, play a role in training the young courtier in such dangers. He is admonished that life is but a remembered garden where

in old age the sweet flowers of contentment fall from our hearts, like leaves from a tree in autumn ... of bygone pleasures naught is left but a lingering memory and the image of that precious time of tender youth, in which (when it is with us) sky and earth and all things seem to us ever making merry and laughing before our eyes, and the sweet springtide of happiness seems to blossom in our thought, as in a delightful and lovely garden.[14]

Gardens, too, are private spaces and thus not to be sullied with public acts that reflect on the display of one's posture. Castiglione tells the tale of 'a young cardinal we have in Rome [who] does better than that; for out of pride in his fine bodily frame, he conducts into his garden all who come to visit him (even although he has never seen them before), and urgently presses them to strip to the doublet and try a turn with him at leaping.' Such actions, he notes,

can be practiced in public and in private, like dancing; and in this I think the Courtier ought to have a care, for when dancing in the presence of many and in a place full of people, it seems to me that he should preserve a certain dignity, albeit tempered with a lithe and airy grace of movement; and although he may feel himself to be very nimble and a master of time and measure.[15]

These are gardens that are experienced but that echo, of course, the dangers of the original garden, from which the proud and the boastful, the disobedient and the vain, were driven. Yet there is a haunting problem looming in such sentiment: 'with the growing moral rigidity of the seventeenth century, a sense of the possible contradictions between the goals aspired to was inevitable. Rectitude and an "elegant bearing" were felt by many Christian writers to be necessary to comply with the rules of civil behavior, yet to be dangerous to the child's conscience, which is liable to be trapped by vanity and "self love".'[16]

The Garden of Posture

The movement from the courts to the sitting rooms of the middle class takes place during the Enlightenment. Nowhere is this more manifest than in Jean-Jacques Rousseau's path-breaking account of childhood and education, *Émile; or, On Education*, published (and then publicly burned) in 1762. It is, of course, a fantasy, a tract that reads like the contemporary *Bildungsromane* (novels of education) and that places at its centre the corruption of our present state through its institutions. Education meant, for Rousseau, an acknowledgement of the natural state of children, not their fallen state into sin. It begins, of course, in a garden – but not the Garden of Eden.[17] Rousseau had showed a fascination with the garden in his novel *Julie, ou la Nouvelle Héloïse* (1761). He saw it as a reflection of his concern with his central 'theme, the natural goodness of man spoiled by culture and desiring to return to nature.'[18] But it is a very specific form of garden to which he turns: not the highly formed, ornamental gardens of Versailles but rather the English garden, structured and formed by the hand of man but appearing to be wild and natural. As the protagonist of this novel notes, 'Nature has done everything, but under my guidance.' And, as one commentator then remarks, 'freedom cannot be had unless cared for by education or arrangement. This garden is an image of man's reasoned endeavor, in which the results reflect by their sound proportions their relationship to man, the creator. The trees are of moderate height, since "a tree of twenty feet height puts him just as much under its shadow as one of sixty feet."'[19] It is a garden where biblical man would have felt at home.[20] But it is man's creation, not God's.

Rousseau begins *Émile* with a passage that framed both Immanuel Kant's metaphor and Johann Gottfried Herder's rebuttal of the idea of mankind as 'crooked wood':

God makes all things good; man meddles with them and they become evil. He forces one soil to yield the products of another, one tree to bear another's fruit . . . he will have nothing as nature made it, not even man himself, who must learn his paces like a saddle-horse, and be shaped to his master's taste like the trees in his garden. Yet things would be worse without this education . . . Prejudice, authority, necessity, example, all the social conditions into which we are plunged, would stifle nature in him and put nothing in her place. She would be like a sapling chance sown in the midst of the highway, bent hither and thither and soon crushed by the passers-by.[21]

Rousseau stressed the perfectibility of the human being as the central fact that differentiates him from the animal. Upright posture is a subordinate criterion for defining the human, a view that earlier Enlightenment thinkers read by Rousseau, such as the zoologist Buffon and the philosopher of law Montesquieu, supported. Thus posture takes a secondary role in defining humanness, but plays a role in educating the child for society:

let him learn to perform every exercise which encourages agility of body; let him learn to hold himself easily and steadily in any position, let him practise jumping and leaping, climbing trees and walls. Let him always find his balance, and let his every movement and gesture be regulated by the laws of weight, long before he learns to explain them by the science of statics. By the way his foot is planted on the ground, and his body supported on his leg, he ought to know if he is holding himself well or ill. An easy carriage is always graceful, and the steadiest positions are the most elegant.

Rousseau endorses a postural education that emphasizes the natural, rejecting the contrived positions of dance. He places himself in the position of an ideal, not a real, dance master, attuned to the nature of the child:

If I were a dancing master I would refuse to play the monkey tricks of Marcel, which are only fit for the stage where they are performed; but instead of keeping my pupil busy with fancy

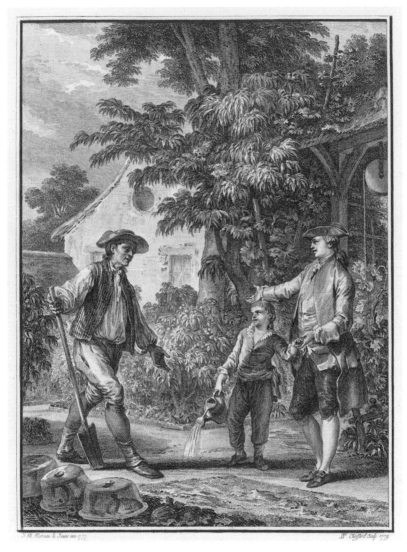

Pierre-Philippe Choffard, after Jean-Michel Moreau le jeune, 'Every One Respects Other People's Work So That His Own May Be Safe'. From *Collection complette des oeuvres de J. J. Rousseau* (London and Brussels, 1774).

steps, I would take him to the foot of a cliff. There I would show him how to hold himself, how to carry his body and head, how to place first a foot then a hand, to follow lightly the steep, toilsome, and rugged paths, to leap from point to point, either up or down. He should emulate the mountain-goat, not the ballet dancer.[22]

If we remember the lessons of the 'posture master', the artificial world of movement in dance and in military order, then Rousseau's admonition makes perfect sense. He goes on to argue also the contrary, that the movements of children, even in the stylized world of dance, reveal an underlying healthy posture:

> Now there is nothing commoner than to find nimble and skillful children whose limbs are as active as those of a man. They may be seen at any fair, swinging, walking on their hands, jumping, dancing on the tight rope . . . All Paris still recalls the little English girl of ten who did wonders on the harpsichord. I once saw a little fellow of eight, the son of a magistrate, who was set like a statuette on the table among the dishes, to play on a fiddle almost as big as himself, and even artists were surprised at his execution.[23]

Now the civilizing process damages human posture. But it also provides the conflicts that force the individual to grow and develop within societal norms.

If there is an answer to Rousseau's garden and its image of the controlled development of the individual, it comes in Kant's *Lectures on Pedagogy* (1803).[24] Advocating the need for a social structure, Kant evoked his older image of the tree and its 'crooked wood', maintaining that it is crooked wood that survives the real competition of social antagonism through a new, enlightened civic society.[25] The education of the prince, who is to shape society, is often isolated: 'in their youth no one resisted them. But a tree which stands alone in the field grows crooked and spreads its branches wide. By contrast, a tree, which stands in the middle of the forest grows straight towards the sun and air above it, because the trees next to it offer opposition. It is the same with princes.'[26] Kant's demand is that society provide a better alternative to Castiglione's courtier. Kant's text is written in support of the educational reforms of Johann Bernhard Basedow, whose experiments in education at his school, the Philanthropinum in Dessau, Germany, provided experiential training for his students' postures. Indeed, Johann Friedrich Simon, who taught gymnastics in 1774 at Basedow's Philanthropinum, is credited with being the first modern teacher of physical education. It is striking how Basedow's writing parallels Kant's own metaphoric language. When, in his *Elementarwerk* (1774), a compendium on education, Basedow talks about how we process the world, he observes that 'when you see a tree, that tree that you see through your senses is a perception, a representation in your soul, in yourself. It is not outside you but within you.'²⁷ Or, as he noted elsewhere about the very role of the educator: 'How can the tree be evil, if at the same moment its potential is known only to the master of the gardener?'²⁸ In Daniel Chodowiecki's famed illustrations for the *Elementarwerk*, the plate that illustrates the 'garden' has not only Rousseau's ideal garden laid out before us but a gardener trying to make a sapling stand tall.²⁹

Kant's is a reading of Rousseau that demands the ability in a conservative society for change in moral posture through the education of the leader, not merely in the physical training demanded by the military. Our discussion of Prussian military training, from Frederick Wilhelm I (the 'Soldier King') through Frederick II ('the Great') to Frederick Wilhelm III, king of Prussia when Kant was writing in 1803, stressed the rigid posture and code of the soldier. Kant's forest is the state; quite different from Rousseau's garden, but one in which social interaction as well as hierarchy are the forces that shape the citizen. Another of Chodowiecki's illustrations for Basedow's *Elementarwerks*

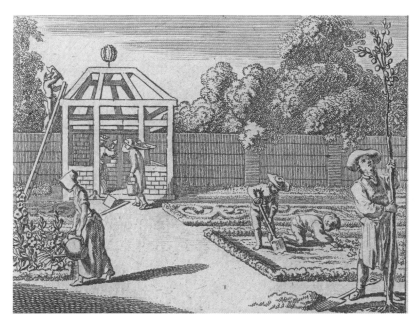

Daniel Chodowiecki, 'About Gardening, Building a Garden Shed'. From Johann Bernhard Basedow, *Des Elementarwerks* (Dessau and Leipzig, 1774).

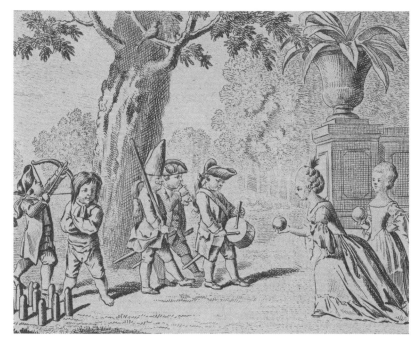

Daniel Chodowiecki, 'Playing at Soldiers. Shooting a Bow. Playing Bowls, Setting Up'. From Johann Bernhard Basedow, *Des Elementarwerks* (Dessau and Leipzig, 1774).

(plate 5a) represents the 'pleasures of the children'. The boys, of course, are playing at being soldiers with quite rigid posture (look at the boy drilling), while the girls try their hand at bowling.

Kant also tries to deal with the notion of what an education of the body implies. He evokes this in the notes to the published version of his lectures on anthropology offered to his students at Königsberg over two decades, and which appeared in print in 1798. In the margins of a discussion of the medical need for smallpox vaccinations, he wrote that 'the doctrine of happiness (*eudaemonism*) is the principle of gymnastics (negative: to sustain from or abstain) and the well (*salus*), *mens sana in corpore sano*, precedes moral teaching.'[30] He expands on this to the development of a moral philosophy where, citing Juvenal directly, he notes that this already demands a healthy rationality and a sound heart, the former created through experience and education.[31] This substantially echoes his lectures on pedagogy, where education is teaching, and teaching must incorporate the body, for – unlike in Herder's model – it forms and reforms human corporality in light of moral training. Given the association of such concepts within the realm of the state training of the body of the soldier (or those whose ideal is such a body), the healthy body houses the healthy mind of the new citizen.

The idea of education in mid-nineteenth-century Germany begins to absorb not only notions of moral training but German nationalism. We saw how Kant's successor at Königsberg, the right-wing Hegelian Karl Rosenkranz, began to describe the very nature of upright posture as a teleological measure of unequal human development, putting forward ugly posture as a sign of inferiority. In 1848 he published his widely used *Pedagogics as a System*, in which he subdivided education into classifications of physiology, pathology and therapeutics. This medical model dominates his understanding of the education of the young, but particularly their physical education. He sees modern education as a training that deforms, in the manner described by Rousseau, the 'natural' body. For him,

> the naive dignity of the happy savage, and the agreeable simplicity of country people, appear to very great advantage when contrasted on this side with the often unlimited narrowness of a special trade, and the endless curtailing of the wholeness of man by the pruning processes of city life. Thus the often abused savage has his hut, his family, his cocoa tree, his weapons, his passions; he fishes, hunts, plays, fights, adorns himself, and enjoys the consciousness that he is the centre of a whole, while a modern citizen is often only an abstract expression of culture.[32]

Natural man in his garden (with his cocoa tree) is far better off than the abstract, civilized man. For Rosenkranz the purpose of teaching is to restore balance, and the motto is that of the German advocates of gymnastics as a form of nation- (and body-) building:

> *Mens sana in corpore sano* is correct as a pedagogical maxim, but false in the judgment of individual cases; because it is possible, on the one hand, to have a healthy mind in an unhealthy body, and, on the other hand, an unhealthy mind in a healthy body. To strive after the harmony of soul and body is the material condition of all proper activity. The development of intelligence presupposes physical health. Here we are to speak of the science of the art of Teaching. This had its

condition on the side of nature, as was before seen, in physical Education, but in the sphere of mind it is related to Psychology and Logic. It unites, in Teaching, considerations on Psychology as well as a Logical method.[33]

While Rosenkranz rejected training in favour of an understanding of bodily education as part of the development of the self, he also saw the very nature of this education as part of the culture of the day. It is not merely the training of the nervous system or the formation of good habits.[34] The key to Rosenkranz's system is that the training of the body should reflect the military definition of physical competence. He notes that 'the system of gymnastic exercise of any nation corresponds always to its way of fighting . . . As soon as the far-reaching missiles projected from fire-arms become the centre of all the operations of war, the individual is lost in a body of men, . . . because of the resulting unimportance of personal bravery, modern Gymnastics can never be the same as it was in ancient times.'[35] Yet it is precisely within the modern system of pedagogy, the move to a healthy mind in a healthy body, that such posture training must take place.

To round out our account of the shaping of the body and the forming of the soul through education, we should turn to one visual commentator on posture, who references – if obliquely – the notion of the human as the 'crooked wood' that demands human attention. Of all the Romantics, none has a more strained relationship to science than the poet-artist-seer William Blake (think of his rejection of what he sees as Newton's mechanistic universe). Yet Blake seems to cite at least one rebuttal to that new science of postural restraint, the widely employed brace, so dominant in his age, in visual form. The frontispiece to Blake's *Songs of Innocence* (1789) sports not only a prominent tree with a vine entwined about it, but it is a very crooked tree. Growing in multiple directions, it is clearly not a tree that was ever braced by human hand. Set in a garden shaped by Milton's notion of the Garden of Eden in *Paradise Lost* (IX.186) that was 'nocent' – harmful because of the presence of the serpent – the entwined vine, the emblem of death, evokes the potential for that evil illustrated in Blake's parallel *Songs of Experience*.[36] Blake also contributed a plate to Erasmus Darwin's set of radical poems *The Botanic Garden* (1791), which provided arguments not only against slavery but for the new Linnaean science of plant classification. Such ideas are nowhere to be found in this image. Yet Blake's world of postural education is quite unlike most of the moral handbooks for children of the time, shaped by the urban world of the petit bourgeoisie, taking place as it does in a garden rather than in a nursery. Remember his abolitionist poem (in *Songs of Innocence*) 'The Little Black Boy', in which his black 'mother taught me underneath a tree'.[37]

Blake's image of moral instruction, too, is reversed from that of the moral handbooks of the time, such as Isaac Watts's *Divine Songs* (1715). For it is not the adult woman who is reading these poems to instruct the children at her knee, but the children themselves who read them and teach her in kind. Children, Rousseau noted, are themselves upright beings (in all senses), degraded only by the fashion of the day. Yet Blake imagines this moral universe as one in need of education by those uncorrupted by such fashion.[38] Thus his crooked wood is also that of 'the poison tree' in *Songs of Experience*, watered by fears 'Night and morning with my tears'.[39] When the friend sees the tree, he comes into the garden 'when the night had veiled the pole' and dies. Only moral insight – that of the uncorrupted child – can remedy this; not rationality, not fashion.

In an odd way, this trope of human posture as a growing sapling comes to a halt when the 24-year-old, newly minted professor of classics at the University of Basle, Friedrich Nietzsche, begins a series of five lectures on the nature of education at the Basle city museum in 1872. In the first, he bemoans the death of true education through the expansion of the new institutions that would give technical, scientific and humanistic education to the masses, thus robbing the elite of true culture. He echoes Matthew Arnold in *Culture and Anarchy* (1869), who condemns innovative educational practices, such as Ezra Cornell's new university, 'where any student could find education in any subject', that defile true cultural education. Nietzsche sets his lectures as a dialogue between an elderly professor and his young students, held on a 'rugged plateau' overlooking the Rhine, where there 'stood a long massive dead oak, silhouetted against the undulating hills and the open plains . . . a broad sharply pointed shadow reached out from our branchless tree trunk across the bare heath'.[40] Kant's crooked tree is quite dead by the time of the modern technologically orientated university, but still casts its shadow across education. Nietzsche sees the dead oak as a monument to the pernicious impact of society embodied in the rise of modern educational institutions that favour the earning of money

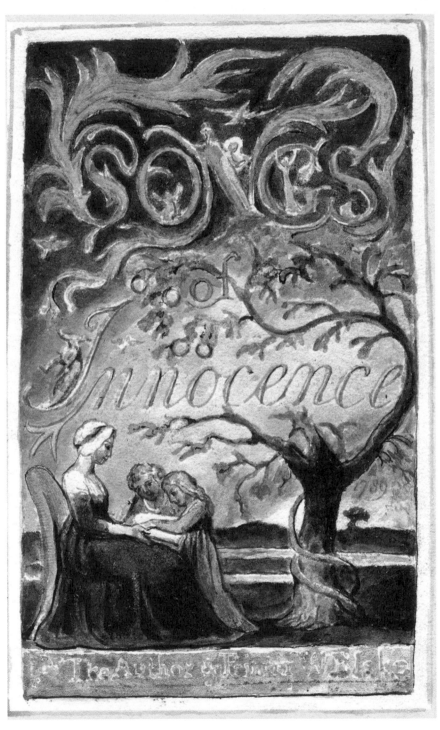

Frontispiece to William Blake's *Songs of Innocence* (1789).

over the improvement of the self. In his much-quoted account in *The Gay Science* (1882) about the death of God, he recounts the tale of the madman roaming the streets with his lantern during the bright morning hours, like Diogenes, shouting that he had searched for God and not found him. He had searched in all the churches, which turned out to be only the tombstones of God. It is society that has killed God, he preaches, and the churches and temples, much like the great dead oak, memorialize his loss. Nietzsche's tree, barren yet casting a long shadow, underlined the death of education through the modern university. Posture no longer matters.

Training for Correct Posture

Training the mind in the Enlightenment meant training the body in those arts (or skills) that provided access to the mind. Learning how to write – one of the signs of bourgeois Enlightenment attainment – was also a question of correct posture. It was further believed that girls had a natural proclivity for sewing as an art rather than for writing, which belonged to the world of little boys.[41] This is also the moment, as we saw with Daniel Paul Schreber's steel *Geradehalter*, that bad posture in the classroom could be ameliorated with braces and corsets. That there were handbooks of the time, such as that by Charles Paillasson, devoted to teaching girls to write with correct posture that did not 'deform the young lady's body', and that Rousseau simply seconds this notion of a gender-based posture, is part of the tale of posture and education.[42]

In Britain between the 1780s and the 1850s, middle- and upper-class girls, in particular, often had their posture mechanically corrected through the use of the posture board, also known as a back board. Placed across the back just above the waist, with the elbows tucked behind its ends, it forced the shoulders back, producing a rigidly upright posture. Those subjected to this regime were forced to remain aware of their posture or risk dropping the board. Educational reformers eventually concluded that this kind of method was too artificial, and that it led to vanity and self-consciousness.

The Anglo-Irish social commentator Maria Edgeworth described such a case in her *Moral Tales* (1801):

> Miss Fanshaw, an erect stiffened figure, made her entrée; and it was impossible not to perceive that her whole soul was intent

upon her manner of holding her head and placing her elbows, as she came into the room. Her person had undergone all the ordinary and extraordinary tortures of back-boards, collars, stocks, dumbbells, &c. She looked at Isabella and Matilda with some surprise and contempt during the first ten minutes after her entrance; for they were neither of them seated in the exact posture, for which she had been instructed to think the only position, in which a young lady should sit in company.[43]

Edgeworth, a follower of Rousseau, clearly reflected his sense of the artificiality of posture when it becomes merely body training. As a recent commentator observed, 'it is important [according to Edgeworth] not to choose a governess merely on the basis of her superficial

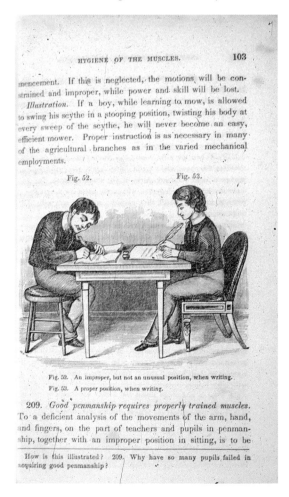

'Improper and Proper Posture when Writing'. From Calvin Cutter, *A Treatise on Anatomy, Physiology, and Hygiene Designed for Colleges, Academies, and Families* (Philadelphia, PA, 1849).

Posture board for a child,
English, *c.* 1820, elm wood.

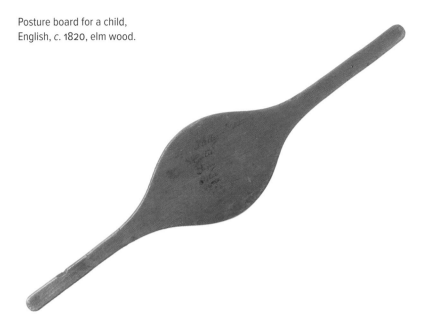

accomplishments. Rather, this person should be someone who has the wisdom to guide the young girl holistically in her development, not just in teaching her the correct dancing posture or a Parisian French accent.'[44] Erasmus Darwin, in his proposal for women's education, condemned the radically erect posture inflicted on young women: 'the stiff erect attitude, taught by some modern dancing masters, does not contribute to the grace of person, but rather militates against it; as is well seen in one of the prints in William Hogarth's analysis of beauty; and is exemplified by the easy grace of some of the ancient statues, as of the Venus de Medici.'[45] Darwin evokes Hogarth's rejection of the straight line in favour of the serpentine as the basis for an aesthetics of representation, but, like Hogarth, he extends such rules to the spheres of societal body training. The rejection of the social conventions of a rigid posture is part of the world of Jane Austen, who comments in *Sanditon* (1817) about

> just such young Ladies as may be met with, in at least one family out of three, throughout the Kingdom; they had tolerable complexions, shewey figures, an upright decided carriage & an assured Look; – they were very accomplished & very Ignorant, their time being divided between such pursuits as might attract admiration, & those Labours & Expedients

of dexterous Ingenuity, by which they could dress in a stile much beyond what they *ought* to have afforded; they were some of the first in every change of fashion – & the object of all, was to captivate some Man of much better fortune than their own.[46]

Their upright carriage marks their social climbing as much as their complete ignorance of the world.

Such training was condemned as unnatural from the mid-eighteenth century onwards. In his essay 'On Conversation' (1756), William Cowper complains about how this is taught and who teaches it: 'take notice of those buffoons in society the Attitudinarians and Face-makers. These accompany every word with a peculiar grimace or gesture: they assent with a shrug, and contradict with a twisting of the neck; are angry by a wry mouth, and pleased in a caper or a minuet step. They may be considered as speaking Harlequins; and their rules of eloquence are taken from the posture-master.'[47] It is our old friend the posture master who inculcates these artificial and unnatural postures.

It is not only in the world that framed Rousseau's anxiety about bodily training in the process of education that the posture master is feared. More than a century later, for Ralph Waldo Emerson, it is the family that serves to teach the infant, but in the false and destructive manner of the 'posture master', supplying the child with all the false gestures and postures that are filled with the cant of society:

> The babe meets such courting & flattery as only kings receive when adult, &, trying experiments every day, & at perfect leisure with these posture masters & flatterers, all day, – he throws himself into all the attitudes that correspond to theirs: are they humble? he is composed; are they eager? he is nonchalant; are they encroaching? he is dignified & inexorable. And this in humble as well as high houses; that is my point.[48]

This is the best of society made ludicrous and scabrous through posture training, which has percolated down all social ranks and has contaminated even the family.

In Germany the highest bourgeois goal of *Bildung* comes to be reconfigured following Rousseau and Herder in terms of posture. In

1776 Carl Friedrich Bahrdt understands 'by the *Bildung* of customs only the embellishment of decorum. It consists of walking, posture, gesture, facial expressions and tone – at the dining table, in society, and when distinguished persons are present.'[49] This is of course what Adolf Freiherr von Knigge observes when, in the first modern guide to manners, he notes that it is 'a breach of decorum to fit in an awkward posture at table'.[50] He continues that well-educated people know not to do such things; it is only the rising bourgeoisie who need to learn good posture (and the postures of dancing and morals and fencing . . .).

In *Makrobiotik oder die Kunst, das menschliche Leben zu verlängern* (Macrobiotics; or, The Art of Extending Life, 1796), one of the most widely read popular texts on health from the German Enlightenment, Christoph Wilhelm Hufeland (1762–1836) observed that

> if a child be obliged at an earlier age [than seven] to apply to learning, and be confined in a sitting posture, its body will be deprived of the noblest part of its powers, which must be now wasted by the business of thinking; and the consequences will be, a checking of the growth, imperfect formation of the limbs, muscular weakness, bad digestion, corrupt juices, the scrofula, and a preponderance of the nervous system in the whole machine which will become burdensome during life, by nervous affections, the hypocondrasis, and evils of the like kind.[51]

In other words, all adult problems come from early bad posture.

These idealized notions of posture come to shape (pun intended) educational policy towards posture training. Friedrich Fröbel, the inventor of the kindergarten, notes that: 'The progressive development of the senses is accompanied by the regular use of body and limbs in an order fixed by the nature of the body and the qualities of external objects . . . Thus is developed the use of the limbs for sitting or reclining, for grasping or seizing, for walking and jumping. Standing is the most perfect instance of the conjoint use of all the limbs and body; it demands the finding of the body's centre of gravity.'[52] Training makes the healthy body, and education becomes bodily training.

The High Victorian Lord Chesterfield frequently warned his son 'against those disagreeable tricks and awkwardnesses, which many people contract when they are young, . . . such as odd motions, strange postures, and ungenteel carriage.'[53] While this sounds like manners rather than medicine, it is also evident that Francis Galton, at least, saw the ability to perform at table with appropriate posture to be a quantifiable measure not only of the body but of human character. He suggested in 1884 that one could discern whether or not guests at a dinner party were attracted to one another by observing their bodily posture: 'When two persons have an "inclination" to one another, they visibly incline or slope together when sitting side by side, as at a dinner-table, and they then throw the stress of their weights on the near legs of their chairs.' This could be observed with the eye, but it could also be measured: 'It does not require much ingenuity to arrange a pressure gauge with an index and dial to indicate changes in stress, but it is difficult to devise an arrangement that shall fulfill the threefold condition of being effective, not attracting notice, and being applicable to ordinary furniture.'[54]

This became a mantra for education in the age of upward bourgeois mobility. 'PERFECT POSTURE, PERFECT POSTURE / Do not slump, do not slump' was the chorus that primary-school pupils were made to sing in unison.[55] Indeed, in the mid-nineteenth century the deportment chair, created by the surgeon and anatomist Sir Astley Paston Cooper, became a fixture of the Victorian classroom or nursery. Misbehave and you were sent to sit and correct your posture while you corrected your behaviour. It was a lesson well suited to the classroom, but also to the dining table. If we remember the discussion of the close relationship between postural training and dance, the image of a dance master, his students and both the posture board and the posture chair seems an obvious, if satirical, one. It is striking that the corrections are those of the nursery and the school – the posture board and the posture chair – but that there is also, as we saw in John Collett's satirical mezzotint of teaching grown men to dance, the corrective brace for the feet (see p. 151). The stance is forced so that you stand correctly and dance well.

Such views were true not only in the dining room but on the musical stage. In 1839 the French singer François Delsarte created a system of bodily training that quickly became the dominant manner of training the body in every aspect of the public sphere. Delsarte saw the emotions as natural, claiming that every emotion had an expression and posture. He defined the ideal posture as 'standing firm on both

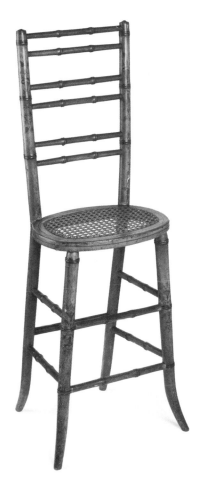

Astley Cooper deportment chair, English, c. 1835. The design of the chair forces children to sit on it 'correctly', that is, with a rigidly straight back and upright head.

legs'.[56] The Victorian singing teacher George Copland, addressing gifted amateurs, suggests that they 'stand up straight, and keep the shoulders well back, as this gives the lungs more room to properly expand . . . There need be no stiffness in the attitude'.[57] The singing master Francesco Lamperti illustrates as late as 1921 that 'the pupil should hold himself erect, with the chest expanded and the shoulders easy – in a word – in the position of a soldier'.[58] The line between health and posture seems clear; that between art and posture was equally evident at the time, since the aesthetic defines the human while the grotesque and deformed denies the very essence of humanness.

Education cured what education, to a certain extent, caused. In 1880 D. F. Lincoln argued following Rousseau that school itself was having 'injurious effects' on children's posture. 'A straight back may be said to be an element of beauty', he wrote, incorporating existing aesthetic standards; 'round shoulders and a twisted spine are an element of the opposite quality, beyond a doubt.' He argued that school experiences were causing between 83 and 92 per cent of all students to suffer deviation of the spinal cord.[59] Such views permeated every corner of childhood education. By the mid-twentieth century even that most radical opponent of rigid child training, Dr Benjamin Spock, commented in 1946 in his guide for parents on the need for some posture training, even though much of a child's posture was inherited.[60]

Education, Disease and Posture

Educational reformers remained obsessed with posture. The Italian reformer Maria Montessori created a wide range of classifications of postural pathologies in her *Pedagogical Anthropology* (1910).[61] Inspired by the forensic anthropology of Cesare Lombroso on degeneracy, she

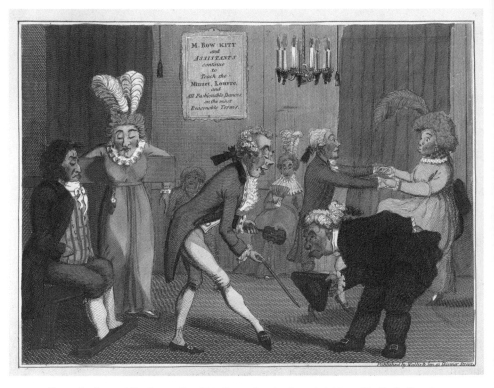

Grown Ladies and Gentlemen Taught to Dance, hand-coloured etching with stipple. Dancing is seen as a form of postural training in this satirical image from 1800–1810. To the left, two pupils are subjected to coercive technology to improve their posture. One sits on a deportment chair with a foot brace; the other uses the posture board.

sees some body types as having positive value: 'The macroplastic type is artistically more beautiful, but the europlastic type is physiologically more useful.'[62] But she also sees the rigidity of the formal classroom structure, with its fixed desks and hard chairs, as causing a wide range of illnesses because of postural deformities:

> It is not only the erect position that tends to reduce the stature, but the sitting posture as well. In fact, whether the pelvis is supported by the lower limbs or by a chair, the intervertebral disks are in either case compressed by the weight of the bust as a whole. If, for example, children are obliged, during the period of growth, to remain long at a time in a sitting posture, the limbs may freely lengthen, while the bust is impeded in its free growth, and the result may be an artificial tendency toward *macroscelia* [abnormal leg length or girth]. This is why children are more inclined than adults to throw themselves upon the ground, to lie down, to cut capers, in other words to restore the elasticity of their joints, and overcome the compression of bones and cartilages.[63]

Here Montessori echoes what is perhaps the most important modern text on education, John Dewey's lectures of 1899, published as *The School and Society*. Dewey's aim during his tenure from 1894 to 1904 at the laboratory school of the newly founded University of Chicago had been to rethink what the school actually did with children. He advocated for a school where the child would learn through an active environment that mirrored (and here he is close to Rousseau) his or her natural proclivities. It is a world where out

> of a spirit of social co-operation and community life, discipline must grow . . . and be relative to such an aim. There is little of one sort of order where things are in process of construction; there is a certain disorder in any busy workshop; there is not silence; persons are not engaged in maintaining certain fixed physical postures; their arms are not folded; they are not hold-ing their books thus and so.[64]

Posture for Dewey is associated with a stultifying of the natural impulses of the child for movement and interaction.

Montessori's emphasis on physical movement in the classroom is an answer to that force to which she attributes a variety of pathologies: being seated at school. She maintains that it predisposes children to tuberculosis:

> Now, the environment of school and the educative methods still in vogue in our schools, not only are not adapted to correct such a predisposition, but what is more, the school itself creates this predisposition! In fact, the sitting posture – or rather, that of stooping over the desk, to write – and the prolonged confinement in a closed environment, impede the normal development of the thorax and of all the physical powers in general. Many a work on pedagogic anthropology has already shown that the most studious scholars, the prize-winners, etc., have a wretched chest measure, and a muscular force so low as to threaten ruin to their constitutions.[65]

That tuberculosis is the result of bad posture was an assumption not only in the classroom but in the sweatshops. According to a report of the United States Public Health Service on workers' health in 1915, 'tuberculosis [was] undoubtedly the most serious disease prevalent among garment workers.' Its cause was seen in the 'inactivity of a sedentary occupation' and the resultant 'bad postural habits.'[66] Amelioration consisted of supplying seats with adjustable backs to improve posture. But other diseases, such as rickets, were defined by a worker's posture. Here, too, Montessori sees the dangers of the classroom in exacerbating such postural deficiencies:

> The treatment of rickets is medical and pedagogical combined. Children of this type should be removed from the public school, where the school routine might have a fatally aggravating effect upon the pathological condition of such children. In fact, gymnastics based upon marching and exercising in an erect position, together with a prolonged sitting posture, are likely to produce weaknesses of the skeleton and deformities, even where there are no symptoms of rickets![67]

The key to all these concerns is the fitness of the individual to reproduce. This becomes a central question during the course of the

Posture and Tuberculosis, one of a set of posters for a Modern Health Crusade exhibition that were available for purchase from the National Child Welfare Association.

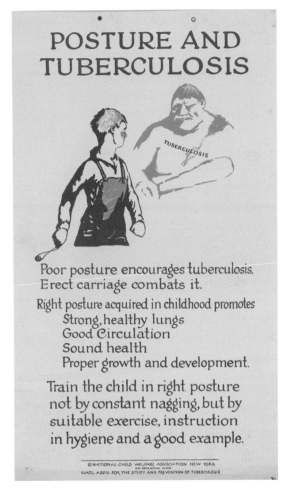

nineteenth century, when a heightened anxiety was articulated about whether the best and the healthiest were sufficiently reproducing or whether, indeed, the ability of inferior individuals (now protected by the new social network) to reproduce would undermine the vitality of the state.[68] Indeed, this eugenic fear paralleled a sense that the best races were not even reproducing at a rate to maintain themselves in the global struggle for domination. Thus Montessori ties feeble posture to poor childbearing:

A woman is not fitted for motherhood, even if physically developed, so long as her pelvis has not rotated normally. But if the rotation is exaggerated (due to prolonged sitting posture during years of growth), this is very unfavourable to normal childbirth. In rickets, associated with kyphosis, there is a form of exaggerated rotated pelvis (pubis high). The laborious 'modern' childbirth, and the dangerous childbirth in the case of women who have devoted much time to study, must be considered in connection with these artificial anomalies. Free movement and gymnastics have for this reason, in the case of women, an importance that extends from the individual to the species.[69]

And thus have an impact on the survival of the race.

Inheritance was also the key for such theories of posture within eugenics. The model for the nineteenth century was evolutionary biology with a Lamarckian assumption about the inheritance of acquired characteristics. These alterations in posture were read as positive (if they were seen to represent an increase in efficiency) or negative (if they were read as potentially a throwback to earlier, inefficient states of posture). The eugenicists thereafter 'probed participants' physical and mental health by measuring posture and strength, peering into eyes, ears, and throats'.[70] Doctors inspecting immigrants at Ellis Island at the same moment were convinced that 'a man's posture, a movement of his head or the appearance of his ears, requiring only a fraction of a second of the time of an observer to notice, may disclose more than could be detected by puttering around a man's chest with a stethoscope for a week'.[71] Examining older immigrants for physiognomic signs of degeneracy such as poor posture revealed moral as well as physical weaknesses that precluded them from entering America. A military notion of posture and the plumb line is inherent in this understanding of bodily perfection, but it could be acquired, at least in the young immigrant, through physical education.

The widely read Canadian physician and eugenicist Benjamin Grant Jefferis defined this perfect posture at the close of the nineteenth century as the antithesis of illness and moral decay: 'The following is said to be a correct posture for walking: Head erect: not too rigid; chin in, shoulders back. Permit no unnecessary motion about the thighs. Do not lean over to one side in walking, standing or sitting; the practice is not only ungraceful but deforming and therefore unhealthful.'[72]

The movement from eugenics to education and back continued well into the twentieth century. Arguments about the social causes of poor posture and the need for educational intervention haunted the pages of the *American Physical Education Review*, founded in 1898. In 1914 Jessie H. Bancroft formed the American Posture League, which dominated American discussions of posture well into the Depression. The league consisted of orthopaedic physicians, physical education specialists and efficiency engineers.[73] Posture became defined no longer solely in terms of scoliosis, as a malformation of the spine, but, as Robert Lovett argues in 1902, as a deviation from the military plumb line, measured from the mastoid process to the middle of the external

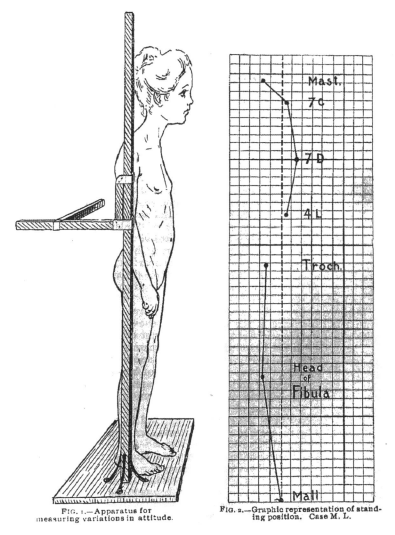

FIG. 1.—Apparatus for measuring variations in attitude.

FIG. 2.—Graphic representation of standing position. Case M. L.

The apparatus for measuring variations in attitude and their graphic representation. From Robert W. Lovett, MD, 'Round Shoulders and Faulty Attitude: A Method of Observation and Record, with Conclusions as to Treatment', *American Physical Education Review*, VII/4 (1902).

malleolus – that is, the military, rigid line that defined the 'normal' upright body from the sixteenth century to the twentieth.[74]

The range of fields engaged in the definition and institutionaliz-ation of postural reform was even more varied. It is important here that posture is not 'merely' physical, as we have seen with Alfred Adler, but rather must be acknowledged as a mental state: 'It does not seem enough that the patient acknowledge, semi-apologetically, that he stands poorly, possibly slumps or has a prominent "stomach": he should become aware, both of the insidious effects of poor posture . . . and of the definite details of his own faulty position that needs correction.'[75] Mind over matter matters.

Education, Posture and Race

By the 1930s and 1940s the study of posture had become all-consuming. Incoming freshmen (and women) at leading colleges in the United States were photographed nude to evaluate their posture, specifically to judge the impact of rickets, scoliosis and lordosis.[76] Such program-mes had their origin as early as the 1880s at Harvard. The notion that students were particularly at risk of poor posture has its roots at least in the Renaissance, as we can see with Erasmus. By the late nineteenth century, the poor posture of the student was thought to lead to a multitude of faults, including higher rejection rates from the armed services as well as various illnesses. Dudley Allen Sargent, professor of physical training at Harvard, observed in 1894: 'When we consider that a large amount of this sickness, suffering, and premature death is preventable, our responsibility in the matter is almost overwhelming.'[77] His remedy is clear: for the educated classes to do manual labour or at least mimic its action to preserve or improve posture:

No one can say that pulling chest weights is interesting, and yet the man who has sufficient character to use these develop-ing appliances regularly and systematically derives an immense amount of good from them. As a matter of fact, some of the most prominent athletes in our colleges and city gymnasiums laid the foundation for their strength and agility while doing farm work or engaging in industrial occupations or mechanical pursuits. It is the kind of efforts that one makes hundreds of times a day that affects the constitution most favorably or unfavorably, and not the spasmodic efforts that are made once or twice a week.[78]

Sargent taught both the German and the competing Swedish system of physical training, emphasizing the goals rather than simply the methods of both. It was vital for him that spinal health be maintained:

> There is no easier way of accomplishing this object than by repeatedly trying to straighten up and assume an erect attitude while sitting, standing, or walking . . . it may be well to mention that frequently drawing in full breaths and filling the lungs as completely as possible is one of the very best methods of straightening the spine and preserving the chest from deformities.[79]

Students most of all needed to keep fit, for their bodies defined their leadership role in a highly structured class society. One can note here that while the image that Sargent provides for his intemperate student is that of a man, this is the age of the introduction of physical education into the women's colleges, also with the intention of improving 'posture and carriage', so as to improve their reproductive faculties as well.[80] Sargent's Normal School of Physical Training in Cambridge, Massachusetts, founded in 1883, initially trained only women wanting to teach physical education in such settings. He stressed vigorous physical training for women as well as for men.

By the twentieth century class identity came to merge into race identity. The science behind this shift was most clearly articulated by William Herbert Sheldon, who is best known today for assessing and developing 'somatotypes', which he used to classify body physiques. Sheldon's taxonomy was part of an obsessive attempt, from the age of physiognomy in the Enlightenment, to reduce bodily form to a set of pseudo-Linnaean biological categories.[81] From Montessori in the field of education to Joel Goldthwait in that of medical science, Sheldon was building on a set of assumptions about the meanings ascribed to forms of posture. He was also involved in translating these concepts into what he called 'constitutional medicine', arguing that by examining a person's posture and physique one could assess temperament and intelligence. He claimed that somatotypes were 'unwavering determinants of character regardless of transitory weight change'.[82] All Sheldon's

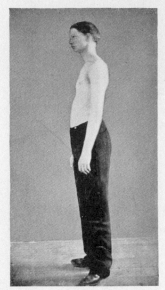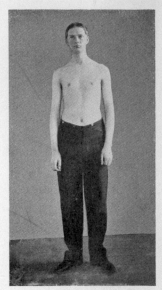

Typical figure, showing tendency of student life—stooping head, flat chest, and emaciated limbs.

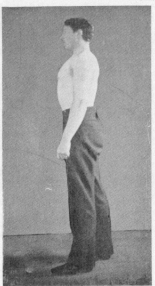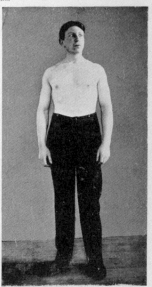

Typical figure, showing muscular development of chest and limbs, and large breathing capacity, produced by practice of gymnastics and athletics.

'Typical Figure, Showing Tendency of Student Life – Stooping Head, Flat Chest, and Emaciated Limbs', and the healthy body resulting from regular postural training. From D. A. Sargent, 'The Physical State of the American People', in *The United States of America: A Study of the American Commonwealth, its Natural Resources, People, Industries, Manufactures, Commerce, and its Work in Literature, Science, Education and Self-government*, ed. Nathaniel Southgate Shaler (London, 1894), p. 459.

body types, he claimed, correlated clearly with psychological profiles that reinforced existing notions of class and race. His somatotype system was an anthropometric technique of human classification, which measured body types, specifically the masculine physique. Using college students as his sample, he reduced all human variables to three body types, each of which had a different measurement of strength and character. He labelled these types endomorphs, mesomorphs and ectomorphs, and described their physical and psychological characteristics.

Sheldon's *Varieties of Human Physique* (1940), the classical statement of his 'constitutional psychology', had subdivided each of the three categories into 76 sub-classes and then into hundreds of mixed subtypes. Indeed, like the various classifications of race in 'race science', the fluid and often-contradictory nature of these categories led to ever more subtle subdivisions in order to process the clear contradictions inherent in such systems. Imagined categories, like dragons and unicorns, can have an infinite number of forms. Of the endomorphs, Sheldon argued in 1941, 'When well nourished . . . [they] tend towards softness and roundness throughout the body.'[83] Mesomorphs, in contrast, have good posture, an athletic shape, massive strength and muscular development because of the 'relative predominance of muscle, bone, and connective tissue.'[84] Yet in Sheldon's tripartite system, each of the primary categories can include aspects of the other two. Each individual is potentially made up of all the elements, with one predominating; therefore, even a primarily mesomorphic person could become fat if he also has high endomorphy.[85] However, mesomorphs with low endomorphy tend to be thin.

Posture seems to be a constant quality in Sheldon's classification. Ectomorphy is defined as the tendency to be flat and fragile throughout the body and stooped in posture. He explained: 'In the ectomorph there is relatively little bodily mass and relatively great surface area – therefore greater sensory exposure to the outside world.'[86] Ectomorphs also have the largest brain and central nervous system. It is telling that each of his subtypes is almost always defined, among other features, by its posture: thus, of subtype 127, 'The posture is straighter and the lumbar curve of the back is lower than in the 117.'[87] And of 434, 'one of the middle group of "normals"', he notes that 'The posture is erect and the general outline is inconspicuous, but a distinct tendency to roundness and softness pervades the body.'[88] Type 172, 'probably the masculine ideal', is 'the perfect serial action-thriller of the cinema', such as 'Tarzan,

Dick Tracy . . . and Superman . . . the lumbar curve of the back is low and sharp, since it involves the sharply defined, muscular buttocks.'[89] While all the types and subtypes have specific postures associated with them, each also has a specific character profile that reflects the meaning Sheldon reads into the posture. You are what your body says you are, he maintains.

When Sheldon developed his 'somatotypes' in the 1940s, he observed that Jews and 'Negroes' show an exaggeration in each of their body types. Thus endomorphic Jews (at least the three hundred Jewish students Sheldon examined) are somehow fatter than fat non-Jews, and have worse posture. They, like 'the 400 northern Negroes', tended towards the extremes of each type.[90] One should note that other such constitutional body-typing systems of the time, such as that of the psychiatrist Ernst Kretschmer at Marburg (1931), used similar divisions. Sheldon is clearly indebted to Kretschmer, and cites him. Kretschmer's types, the asthenic (weak), athletic and pyknic (fat), were used by Nazi eugenicists for racial typing, even though Kretschmer, himself badly politically compromised at the time, refused to acknowledge this use. Race science loved such seemingly objective classification. When Karl Landsteiner first began to unravel human blood types in Vienna in the first decade of the twentieth century, race science immediately tried to use these biological categories to distinguish among their invented racial groups. Unsuccessful, they turned to somatotyping for their evidence. To do so they needed what passed as empirical evidence, and they found it in the photograph.

In order to measure and document somatotypes, Sheldon assessed students and photographed them to illustrate the alignment of their body and certify that 'the picture as taken is for that subject the nearest approach to perfect bodily alignment [for somatotyping] that can be achieved.'[91] From observing these photographs, he noted that 'there appear to be nearly as many ectomorphs as mesomorphs', but there were 'appreciably fewer endomorphs'.[92]

Sheldon also concerned himself with the influences of both in-heritance and environment on a person's body type. He believed that one's somatotype was genetically determined and thus immutable over the lifetime, even though an individual's posture might change with fluctuations in his or her weight. The somatotype was thus a measure of his or her 'constitution' or hereditary biological endow-ment. Sheldon's reason for somatotyping was to 'provide a practicable,

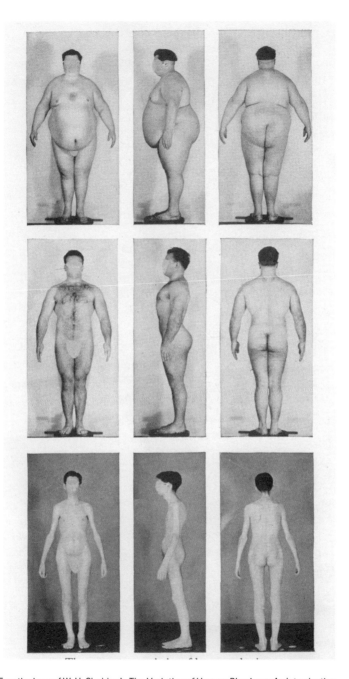

Frontispiece of W. H. Sheldon's *The Varieties of Human Physique: An Introduction to Constitutional Psychology* (New York and London, 1940). These are the exemplary cases. Note the rigid military posture of the mesomorph ('Tarzan or Superman'), the middle figure, and the very poor posture of the endomorph, above, and the ectomorph, below. For Sheldon, posture is character.

objective method for segregating and classifying the varieties of human physique.[93]

How such types and their concomitant postures correlated posture with mind can be seen in one of Sheldon's three types of constitutional psychology, the cerebrotonic form dominated by the 'higher functions' of the brain:

> Painful tenseness and restraint can be seen all over the body. All of the expressive movements are held in check, like horses under close rein. The body as a whole is carried stiffly, and there is the suggestion of a shrinking tendency . . . The favorite posture is a kyphotic, round-shouldered one, both in standing and in sitting . . . The walk suggests treading on eggs, or an attempt to move noiselessly in order not to attract attention. If a clinical examination is made, marked sphincter tension is noted.[94]

Here, too, race is a major factor. Sheldon observes that among Jews, 'The hands and feet are relatively small and weak-appearing for a physique which as a whole is mesomorphic, but this is a common characteristic among Jewish people. They are "centripetal", in the sense that their concentration of strength and mass tends to lie close to the center of the body.'[95] Sheldon sees 'inbreeding' as the cause of Jewish poor posture and bad character.[96] Education could do only so much to mitigate posture and as such to mitigate Jewish character.

Education, Class and Posture

Class as well as race is implicated in individuals with primitive posture, yet the idea that the lower classes are like more primitive animals never seems quite to vanish, as is clear from an essay in *The Lancet* in 1922: 'Some primitive races who have the squatting habit, and even many country people at home, keep knees and back bent and have a carriage and gait not much better than that of the higher apes. As a general rule, the more highly civilised the people the better is the carriage, but a perfectly erect carriage cannot be attained without drill.'[97] But 'drill' or postural training is not available to the lower orders, whether great apes or country folk. Stature and gait are already defined as biological predispositions of class, as the most important advocate of eugenics, Francis Galton, noted as early as his study *Hereditary Genius* (1869).

The medicalization of working-class and middle-class fashion affected posture, from the training of women to work more efficiently to the middle-class use of corseting:

> charwomen do not enjoy the 'all fours' position, for they do not adopt it but merely a pseudo-quadruped attitude – viz., on the hands and knees, principally the latter, so that the hands may be freer for work – and that is the source of most of their troubles, the pads which they should wear being either missing or insufficient. Otherwise their work is very healthy, and the source of the popular objection to it is rather the stress put upon the pride than upon the back. Young girls in cookery schools, too, are now so full of the pride of the erect posture and of that lofty atmosphere to which their emotions have raised them that who dare mention to them such a lowly attitude as the 'all fours' position, much less their adoption of it! Corsets, too, probably interfere.[98]

The anti-corseting literature, as we have seen with Rousseau, is full of comments on the poor posture that results from the wearing of the corset, repressing the fact that it was not merely a fashion item but was also a primary means of reforming the body of those suffering from poor posture, whether as a result of rickets or of poor education.[99] Indeed, in 1788 Samuel Thomas von Soemmerring argued that stays were the cause of 'tuberculosis, cancer, and scoliosis'.[100]

In 1888 the Rational Dress Society of London protested in an editorial note in the opening number of its *Gazette* 'against the introduction of any fashion in dress that either deforms the figure, impedes the movements of the body, or in any way tends to injure the health'.[101] Posture was natural; all corseting caused deformation of posture and gait. The medical literature against corseting was extensive and argued that corseting deformed posture, bracketing the fact that corsets were also a standard means of treatment for scoliosis and hernia. An exchange in 1909–10 between two British doctors in *The Lancet* about the dangers of corseting begins when the Wimpole Street physician Heather Bigg writes that 'women have found by centuries of accumulated experience that corsets are to them structurally indispensable, whilst modern science has also shown that they are physiologically beneficial'.[102] Cecil E. Fish responds, quickly condemning the very idea that

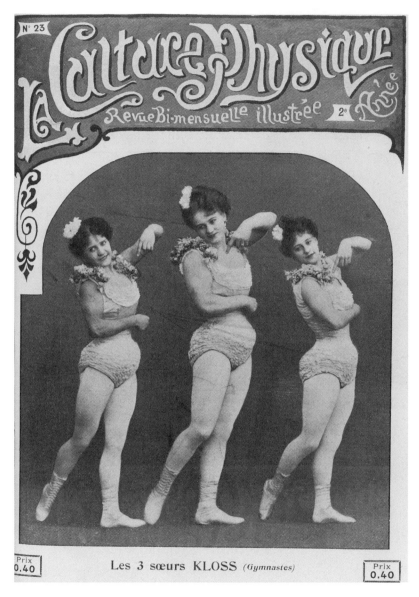

The Three Kloss Sisters (Gymnasts). The three Kloss sisters featured on the cover of the magazine *La Culture physique*, 23 (1905). Note the corsets and the extremely narrow waists. Gymnastics and corsets were not always seen as antithetical.

the corset may be beneficial for posture: 'If the erect posture demands it, then we should be wise to put our babies into stays as soon as they begin to toddle. God forbid it.'[103] Bigg's response to this is of interest since it argues that erect posture may indeed be the cause of a wide range of ailments. Evolutionary medicine in its first epoch (it returns at the close of the twentieth century) seems to be able to divine the essential nature of human posture – and it is not upright: 'man is built for a quadruped and not for an erect position . . . I advocated the use of corsets with the proper loin-band hold, because it appeared to me that they were in most instances positively necessary to combat the inherent structural disability under which mankind suffers when in the erect posture.'[104] The corset medically corrects a body damaged by its evolution to upright posture.

Corseting corrects the body that is ill – that is, if it is medical corseting. Corseting also reforms and beautifies the body if it is that of the middle class. Since both men and women corseted for both purposes, the confusion that existed in the meaning of reshaping the body's posture and form meant that health and beauty were elided, for good or for ill. To anyone opposed to corseting, the process deformed and made ill; to its proponents, it reformed and made healthy and beautiful. Such bodies were always on display, for posture was read immediately and seemingly without hesitation. It was in the age of photography that such bodies became, through the act of reproduction, part of the new science of posture, the world of movement frozen in time.

By the mid-twentieth century 'postural health' is defined as efficiency, illustrated by normative images of the healthy and unhealthy

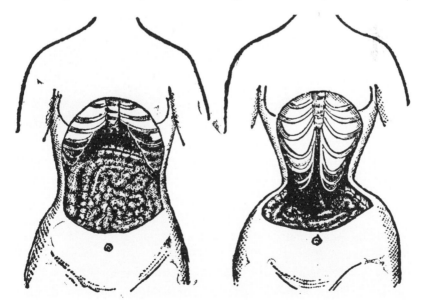

'Nature versus Corsets, Illustrated'. From John William Gibson, *Golden Thoughts on Chastity and Procreation* (Toronto, ON, and Naperville, IL, [1903]).

body within medicine. Seeing the body meant measuring, evaluating and diagnosing posture as healthy or pathological. Images of posture, both positive and negative, abound in public health advertisements, in etiquette books and in scientific journals of every possible medical and biological discipline. The science of seeing and evaluating, as with the race science of the time, also included a healthy dose of moral evaluation. Good posture is 'important for proper functioning of the body and contributes to good appearance. Proper alignment of the body parts promotes efficiency of movement and endurance. The person who has good posture and who moves gracefully projects poise, confidence, and dignity.'[105] It reflects character as well as health and beauty, since 'faulty posture' is 'unattractive'. Good posture demands a postural education and constant self-correction to stand up straight:

> Head is held erect, not turned or tilted to one side.
> Shoulders are level.
> Arms hang easily at the sides with the palms of the hands
>   toward the body.
> Hips are level, with the weight of the body borne equally by
>   both legs.
> Kneecaps face straight ahead.
> Feet point straight ahead or toe out slightly.
> . . . Good posture must be built from the feet up. If the feet
>   and knees are in good position, there is a better chance
>   that the rest of the body will line up properly.[106]

The 'disabled' body is thus seen as having poor posture that demands correction in order to be healthy. This has its roots in the Enlightenment notion of retraining or repairing bad posture. The idea of an efficient posture that is part of an evolutionary pattern that leads to an ideal military body demands correction of disabled bodies or, in terms of the model of evolutionary development that defines posture as the first principle, extinction. Disability is thus to be found, as we shall see, as defined by poor posture within a wide range of categories, including gender and race.[107]

By the twentieth century, functional definitions come to dominate the debate about posture, at least within medicine. Little attention is given to its origin. In 1947 the Posture Committee of the American Academy of Orthopaedic Surgeons defined posture as 'the relative arrangement of the parts of the body', making a distinction between 'good posture: the state of muscular and skeletal balance which protects the supporting structures of the body against injury or progressive deformity irrespective of the attitude in which these structures are working or resting' and poor posture as 'a faulty relationship of the various parts of the body which produce increased strain on the supporting structures and in which there is less efficient balance of the body over its base of support'.[108]

This is clearly the ideology that dominates Braune and Fischer's work on military posture in 1889 and becomes the officially accepted medical notion, so that a standard textbook of the late twentieth century can define posture as a 'position or attitude of the body; the relative arrangement of body parts for a specific activity; a characteristic manner of bearing one's body'.[109] The idea of the functional efficiency inherent in the military model never vanishes, but thinkers such as Moshé Feldenkrais at mid-century argue that such postural 'health' is not determined by an 'ideal' body. Even severely disabled bodies can achieve postural efficiency: 'Proper posture is such . . . that the movement is performed with the minimum of work, i.e., with the maximum of efficiency'.[110] Efficiency is a Fordist concept, which reflects the fascination in the 1920s with time and motion studies such as those by Frank B. and Lillian Gilbreth as well as Frederick Winslow Taylor; it is the appropriate effort expended in the realm of work to accomplish a task.[111] This defines good posture in the translation of a military concept to the industrial world.

Health and beauty can be found in the United States in the realm of posture well beyond the school classroom, and the counterpoint to the masculine history of posture is found in the history of modern feminine beauty. Such an attempt at public education came in the form of beauty contests judged on the basis of perfect posture. As a historian of posture noted, such contests

> had their beginning in the Most Perfect Spine Contest of the American Chiropractic Association (1922–1930) at its 1927 convention. At the 1935 NCA Convention in Hollywood, California, the winner of the two-hundred-contestant event was known as Miss Perfection. Life-sized, entire body x-rays were displayed along with a parade of finalists in bathing suits and evenings gowns with low backs.[112]

Local contests were held across the country, from Utah to Michigan: 'Barnard College held a posture contest for freshman every January, during which, according to Life magazine, "circling contestants walk[ed] for half an hour, rather like entrants in a live stock show." In Seattle there was a posture contest for preschoolers. The governors of Maryland, Minnesota, Arkansas, Kansas, and Kentucky all signed proclamations for Posture Week.'[113]

Such perfect posture contests, analogous to the beautiful baby and 'fitter families' contests of the same period, stress a eugenic model of the ideal body. While at the beginning of such contests, as with the beautiful baby contests, young men were also judged, this very quickly ceased. As a historian of these contests observed, 'they weren't as popular and didn't last very long,' adding, 'The guys always slouched.'[114]

Such contests claimed to place chiropractic in the same service to the healthy body as allopathic medicine in the public's eye. The winner received a scholarship for further study, placing the event squarely in the tradition of the beauty contests of the age, such as Miss America. But perfect posture, not only beauty or talent, was claimed to stand at the centre of the competition. The winner did not, by the end of interest in this tradition, sport a rigid, military body here any more than in more traditional beauty contests. The move was towards an idealized but eugenically perfect female body, orientated towards reproduction. In 1965 the contest took place in Salt Lake City and generated enough interest to be covered in the local newspaper. There the ideology of the world of chiropractic therapy intersected with that of the world of *mens sana in corpore sano*: 'Proper posture is essential to good health . . . Bad posture, say the experts, is due largely to a lazy or disorderly state of mind and to our soft way of living. The sharp-eyed judge who picks the violets from among the wild morning glories in these beauty bids, has been correcting defects for quite some time.' According to this judge: 'Straightening up like a tin soldier, chest out, shoulders back until they ache, isn't good posture. You must be relaxed . . . To hold your head properly, imagine you have a string tied back of each ear by which you are being dangled from the ceiling.'[115] Somehow, this latter image does rather bring us back to the quasi-military notion of a healthy, erect body. The final 'Posture Queen' contest took place in 1969. By then at least one goal of the contest had been achieved: chiropractic was licensed throughout the United States as a recognized postural therapy. By the 1960s, one can add, the white contestants

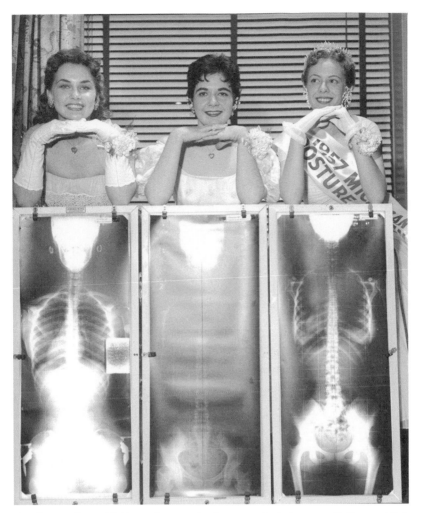

Miss Posture Queen Michigan of 1957 and unknown contestants pose with X-rays of their spines. The World Posture Contest was developed by Dr Clair O'Dell of the then Logan College of Chiropractic, and served as a way to promote chiropractic. It differed from a traditional beauty pageant in that a spinal X-ray was as important as the contestant herself. In fact, 50 per cent of judging was based on correct spinal posture and 50 per cent went towards evaluating the personality of the contestant.

would also have been confronted by the claims of civil rights for the inclusion of black contestants. Race mattered, even in evaluating the fittest posture.

Beauty (bathing suits), health (X-rays) and posture are not peculiarly American definitions of the healthy feminine physique – German and French sources of the nineteenth century point towards this as well – but the shift from the realm of the military to the realm of beauty represents the traditional universes of the masculine and feminine bodies defined here by posture. More importantly, one could see these bodies on the street: 'Take the apparently simple act of walking in the street . . . The dandy, "glorifying in his appearance", affected a slouching posture and "mincing" step. Meanwhile, the greenhorn loped along with a ludicrous "swinging gait", and the "impolite man of humble life" shuffled with downcast eyes.'[116] Educating the healthy body meant also displaying it in its correct posture. Such public competitions, as much as the debates within the schools and colleges, aimed for an idealized and objective notion of perfect posture, the perfect posture for the healthy citizen.

SEVEN

Anthropology Remakes Posture: Lamarck, Darwin and Beyond

W HEN I WAS AT UNIVERSITY in the early 1960s, we were
taught a number of characteristics that defined the uniqueness of human beings: language, the opposable thumb and
the use of tools, consciousness, morality, emotions and, last but not
least, upright posture. (Never mind Pliny the Elder's first-century
AD view in his *Natural History* that only man has ears that do not
move.[1]) 'Uprightness (or more prosaically bipedalism)', states Jonathan
Kingdon in his detailed survey of the question, is 'the central condition on which human evolution is predicated'.[2] For the discipline of
anthropology, this certainly became a truism. The British physician
James Alexander Lindsay stated the case in his Bradshaw Lecture on
Darwinism and Medicine in 1909:

> Man is a member of the animal series, and it is reasonable to
> expect that the ordinary laws of evolution would be exemplified
> in his structure and in his functions. This we find to be the
> case. The body of man is built upon the same lines – bone for
> bone, muscle for muscle, artery for artery – as that of the
> higher apes. The comparatively few distinguishing features of
> the human organism have relation to three points – viz., the
> assumption by man of the erect posture, his acquisition of
> special manual dexterities, and his higher cerebration.[3]

Over the past decades more and more of these qualities have (correctly
or not) been shown as shared with any number of animals, from the
primates to the anteater. Only upright posture has been maintained

as the quality that defines the human; indeed, it has come to be the defining attribute that draws the evolutionary line between the earliest human beings and their predecessors. A recent review of gait and posture states:

> Bipedality is commonly performed by a variety of primates and other mammals, even some artiodactyls. Human ancestors, however, adopted this odd gait as their exclusive form of locomotion, and so extensively modified their postcranium that every transport event, whether a simple stroll of a few yards or a desperate flight to avoid an attacking predator, became restricted to its use.[4]

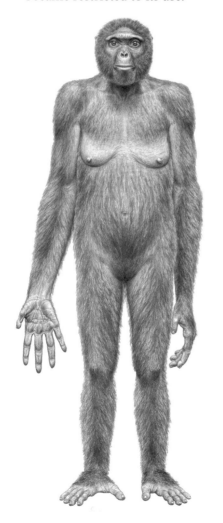

Jay Matternes, rendition of Ardi. From Ann Gibbons, 'Ardipithecus ramidus', Science, CCCXXVI/5960 (2009).

We are our posture.

The discovery in 2009 of *Ardipithecus ramidus* has our ancient ancestor defined as such because of 'upright walking': 'This remarkably rare skeleton is not the oldest putative hominin, but it is by far the most complete of the earliest specimens. It includes most of the skull and teeth, as well as the pelvis, hands, and feet – parts that the authors say reveal an "intermediate" form of upright walking, considered a hallmark of hominins.'[5] The representation of this 'ancestor' in the scholarly paper is of a hairy individual standing rigidly upright.

Not only bipedalism (walking on two feet and upright walking) but standing up straight defines human ancestry in an unspoken way. The reasons for this plumb-line upright posture have recently been found in the unique geography of where these ancestors lived: it is now claimed that they stood upright because *Ardipithecus ramidus* lived in 'a humid, cooler woodland' with small patches of forest high grass rather than moving from the trees to the savannah during the Pliocene. This earlier view argued that environmental changes had encouraged upright posture as she now had to stand erect to look over the grassy terrain.[6] This was quickly contradicted by a group of palaeontologists who argued that Ardi lived not in grassy woodlands but in a hot and dry bushy grassland.[7] Thus Ardi was living in a time of radical ecological transition from woodlands to savannah and could not be used to falsify the hypothesis that our ancestors began walking upright in grasslands rather than in the woods. Both of these variations countered Arthur Keith's view developed in the 1920s, summarizing Charles Darwin's perspective, that 'it was on the trees, not on the ground, that man came by the initial stages of his posture and carriage.'[8] To paraphrase Nietzsche, *Ardipithecus ramidus*'s posture was the result of what it ate, or at least where it ate it. Our earliest ancestors stand upright not reaching for the gods, but rather responding to radical environmental changes similar to those that haunt the nightmares of twenty-first-century humans.

Bipedalism is the Key to the Science of Posture

In this view of upright posture, modern anthropology inherits the mantle of the ancient world. Yet it is in the Enlightenment that the ideal manner of seeing the human being moves from the theological to the scientific. The science of the post-Enlightenment agreed with

Johann Gottfried Herder's sense that posture defined the human (now without citing the act of creation), rather than agreeing with Immanuel Kant's view of self-shaping. The human being is shaped rather than shapes himself, as Jean-Baptiste Lamarck claimed at the opening of the nineteenth century: 'Indeed, if any race of primates (quadrumanes) whatsoever . . . for a series of generations, be obliged to use their feet only in walking, and cease using their hands as feet; then there is no doubt . . . that these apes would finally be transformed into man (bimanes).'[9] For Lamarck, this posture is the result of human ancestors having left the trees for the open plain, analogous to his most often cited example of adaption: the lengthening of the giraffe's neck in order to eat leaves from the upper branches of trees.

Early evolutionary theory also sees such human development through adaptation in terms of race. Posture is one of the keys noted by the nineteenth-century ethnologist Karl Hermann Burmeister, who commented in 1855: 'Blacks and all those with flat feet are closest to the animals.'[10] This echoes Herder's Enlightenment distinction between the bestial and the human, with the uncivilized lying closer to the former. (He too drew an analogy between apes and pygmies.) Natural posture is primitive posture is bad posture; there is no plumb line. This is often contested, as in Frederick Arthur Hornibrook's early twentieth-

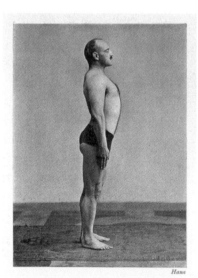
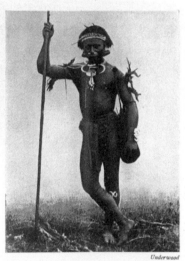

Hana

Underwood

FIG. 4. The military position at attention. Note the pouter pigeon chest and hollow back.

FIG. 5. Note the ease of attitude of the Polynesian native warrior shown here.

Civilized versus natural posture. From F. A. Hornibrook, *The Culture of the Abdomen* (London, 1927).

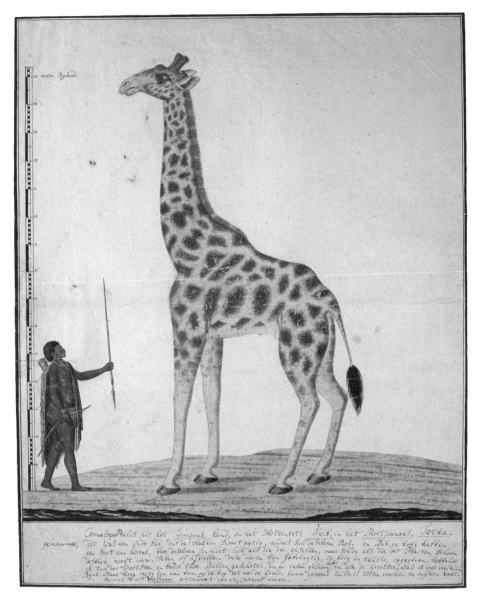

Robert Jacob Gordon, giraffe in Namaqualand, with a Khoi (Hottentot) at the left, 1779.

century account of the natural processes of digestion. The 'primitive' here has a healthier, more natural posture than the 'military position'.[11]

Thomas Huxley picked this up in his image of the 'natural' progression of the 'Skeletons of the Gibbon, Orang, Chimpanzee, Gorilla, Man' in *Man's Place in Nature* (1863).[12] This is one of the most often caricatured scientific images of evolutionary posture. For Huxley, upright posture is a given quality of man. He notes the intermediate stage of the gibbon, which 'readily takes to upright posture', and cites a source that describes the gibbon's ability to 'walk rather quick in the erect posture . . . When he walks in the erect posture, he turns the leg and foot outwards, which occasions him to have a waddling gait and to seem bow-legged.'[13] Likewise of the gorilla, 'when it assumes the walking posture, to which it is said to be much inclined, it balances its huge body by flexing its arms upward.'[14] Huxley sees that of the gorilla as closer to the upright gait of the human, at least *Homo sapiens sapiens*, than to that of the gibbon.[15] Thus the scale of evolution, with its teleological goal of the upright human being, is determined by the scale of posture.

Yet human beings on the evolutionary ladder after the great apes are also seen on a scale of upright posture, which meant that the poor 'Neanderthal Man' discovered in 1857 had (at least in the imagination of those who drew him) very poor posture – he was not quite human yet.[16] Huxley noted that Neanderthals represent 'the most savage primitive type of the human race, since [such] crania [also] exist among living savages, which . . . gives the skull somewhat the aspect of the large apes.'[17] Primitive indeed, but upright nevertheless, since he noted that the skeleton 'shows that the absolute height and relative proportions of the limbs were quite those of an European of middle stature. The bones are indeed stouter, but this and the great development of the muscular

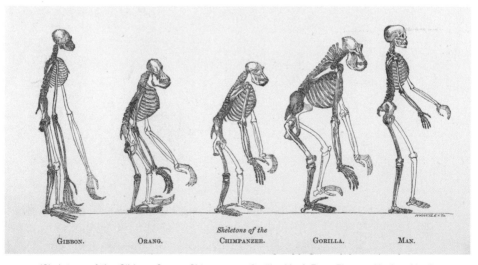

Skeletons of the
GIBBON.   ORANG.   CHIMPANZEE.   GORILLA.   MAN.

'Skeletons of the Gibbon, Orang, Chimpanzee, Gorilla, Man'. From Thomas Huxley, *Man's Place in Nature* (London, 1863).

ridges . . . are characters to be expected in savages.'[18] Indeed, there was an initial question about what actually was represented by the Neanderthal find. The great cellular biologist Rudolf Virchow was convinced that this was not a precursor of present-day humans. Rather, he thought it represented a very old human being, *Homo sapiens sapiens*, who had developed rickets as a child and died because he could not function well in an earlier hunter-gather society.[19] Not ancient, only diseased! Ironically, the rereading of some of the seemingly stooped remains of at least one Neanderthal in the twentieth century actually came to a similar conclusion. That particular example was stooped not because of his evolutionary position but because he was an elderly male Neanderthal suffering from osteoarthritis.[20]

With the discovery of further specimens in Europe, the definition of poor posture became more and more a defining means of differentiating older from newer bipeds, and 'the slumped posture of the Neanderthals' became a defining quality.[21] Indeed, it became the defining quality of virtually all the finds of early hominids, such as *Pithecanthropus erectus* (earlier Java Man), about whom was said 'with absolute certainty' in 1892 that he 'stood upright and moved like a human'.[22] This was based on the finding of a complete left femur. How human such specimens were remained in question. Indeed, the stooping posture of the Neanderthal came to define him as the 'missing link' between monkeys and modern man.[23] The finding of a hominid at La Chapelle-aux-Saints in central France seemed to document the poor posture of the Neanderthal.[24] Immediately thereupon, in 1908, Marcellin Boule of the Museum of Natural History in Paris wrote a review 'emphasizing the simian traits of the skeleton, even postulating that Neanderthal man had not carried himself entirely upright, but had had a rather stooping posture'.[25] This became a major story in both the French and the British illustrated newspapers of the day. The caption of the image reproduced in 1909 in the *Illustrated London News* (which also carried photogravures of the finds themselves) observed that this image was not fantasy, but, since it is 'not the artist's intention to depict merely a type of prehistoric man, but the actual man whose skull was found recently . . . Mr. Kupka has covered the bones with the muscles necessary to them: and still bound by the rules of anatomy, has given the face the expression it must have worn.' The description continues: 'The man must have been about fifty years old . . . and could not assume the upright position of the superior races,

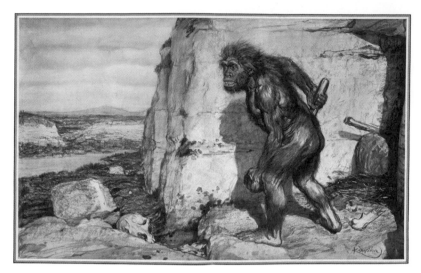

Franz Kupka, *An Ancestor: The Man of Twenty Thousand Years Ago*. From Anon., 'The Most Important Anthropological Discovery for Fifty Years', *Illustrated London News* (27 February 1909).

although his knee-pan[,] unlike that of the monkey, was in front, and he was more upright than the ape.'[26] A contemporary historian observes that

> This hairy creature, in a barren environment that seems to reflect its dull mind, is marked by an expressionless face, an uninventive club, bent knees, and a forward stoop of the upper body. His arms are long, his legs are short, and his chest is of incredible dimensions. In a large reproduction of the image, I can recognize the shape of an ape in his shadow. Obviously, he has not progressed far from such a stage.[27]

Marianne Sommers's meticulous analysis of the shift to a more benign image of the Neanderthal over the course of the middle part of the century shows that stooped posture remained as an index of their inherent difference.

Poor posture defined such early men even in the fiction of the day. Jules Verne imagines the discovery of such primitive men, the Waggdis, still existing in Africa in *The Village in the Treetops* (1901). They are defined by the fact that 'their posture, similar to that of man, showed that they were in the habit of walking upright.'[28] We still imagine 'Neanderthal Man' as a 'brutal, hunched, and hairy club-wielding humanoid' – not beautiful at all.[29] By the time of the discovery of *Pithecanthropus erectus*'s thighbone in 1891, there was no question that erect posture and assumed gait constituted the litmus test for evaluating the degree of 'humanness' of our earliest ancestors.

Why did erect posture evolve? To no one's surprise, Darwin's adaptation of Herbert Spencer's 'survival of the fittest' in his *Descent of Man* (1871) meant that posture was determinant in survival. For Spencer, fitness comes to be defined as physical well-being, and Darwin would echo this:

> If it be an advantage to man to stand firmly on his feet and to have his hands and arms free, of which, from his pre-eminent success in the battle of life there can be no doubt, then I can see no reason why it should not have been advantageous to the progenitors of man to have become more and more erect or bipedal. They would thus have been better able to defend themselves with stones or clubs, to attack their prey, or otherwise to obtain food.[30]

The 'battle for life', Spencer's notion, is a replacement for and extension of the very notion of a military posture developed in the seventeenth century. The plumb line defines the 'best built individuals'. Upright posture is the most efficient for this battle, and correct posture defines the process of civilization. For 'as the progenitors of man became more and more erect . . . endless other changes of structure would have become necessary. The pelvis would have to be broadened, the spine peculiarly curved, and the head fixed in an altered position, all which changes have been attained by man.'[31] All that is human is defined by the acquisition of upright posture.

When, late in his career, Darwin turns to the question of whether expressions are 'hardwired' in the psyche and the body, he concludes that expressions of anger, which he associates with aggression, would not have been possible because 'Our early progenitors, when indignant or moderately angry, would not have held their heads erect, opened their chests, squared their shoulders, and clenched their fists, until they had acquired the ordinary carriage and upright attitude of man, and had learnt to fight with their fists or clubs. Until this period had arrived the antithetical gesture of shrugging the shoulders, as a sign of impotence or of patience, would not have been developed.'[32] Even shrugging your shoulders, for Darwin a universal expressive gesture even found in the chimpanzee, is dependent on upright posture. But most of all, the sublimation of the idea of a military posture into the role of upright posture as a means of articulating aggression and therefore survival moves this from a cultural manifestation of the early modern period to a universal aspect of human development.

Subsequent rereadings of Darwin's claims were manifold. You will remember Kant's claim in the *Conjectural Beginning of Human History* of 1786 that being upright and having language were prerequisites of becoming fully human and having rationality. Such views come to hold rather a privileged place in the anthropological history of posture. In 1935 Joseph Shaw Bolton restated this in early twentieth-century terms: 'Connected with these physical changes [necessitated by upright posture], but always in advance of them, the new organ of mind, the cerebrum, gradually evolved in size and complexity.'[33] Upright posture did not give man rationality, only the pathway to human consciousness.

Rereading Darwin's Theory of Posture

One of the more engaged Darwinians was the creator of historical materialism, Friedrich Engels. A fragment dating from 1876 on the transition from ape to human stressed that upright posture was the first step in human development because it freed (following Darwin) the hands for work, and everything else resulted from this move to bipedalism. More radical than Darwin, Engels imagined that all aspects of human evolution began with the development of bipedalism, while Darwin assumed that cognitive ability (and brain size) developed before bipedalism and led to it. Engels imagines our ancestors as 'a particularly highly-developed race of anthropoid apes'.[34] They became human as a result of the specialization of the hands through work; 'these apes began to lose the habit of using their hands to walk and adopted a more and more erect posture.'[35] They began to 'stand up straight'; indeed, Engels states, 'this is the decisive step in becoming human.'

Unlike Darwin, Engels, in this essay on 'The Part Played by Labour in the Transition from Ape to Man' (1876), sees the impetus for upright posture in the need to maximize the value of the food gathered; that needed to be done using tools, for which upright posture was an absolute necessity: 'Labour begins with the making of tools. And the

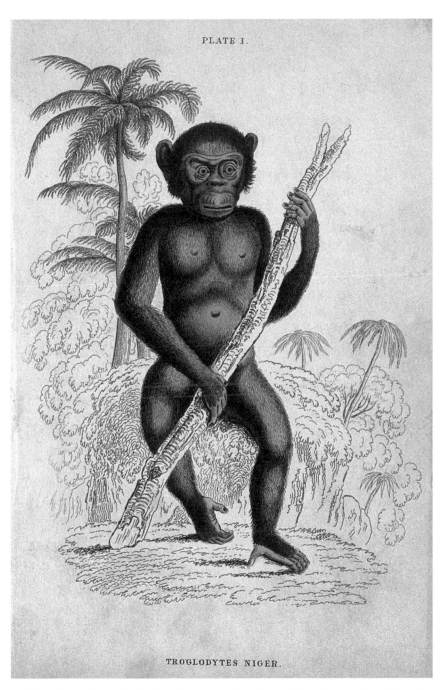

PLATE I.

TROGLODYTES NIGER.

William Home Lizars, *Troglodytes niger*, engraving after an illustration by James Stewart from Sir William Jardine's *Naturalist's Library* (Edinburgh, 1844). An ape of the species *Troglodytes niger* stands before a tropical scenery holding a large branch of a tree: the ape as a user of tools.

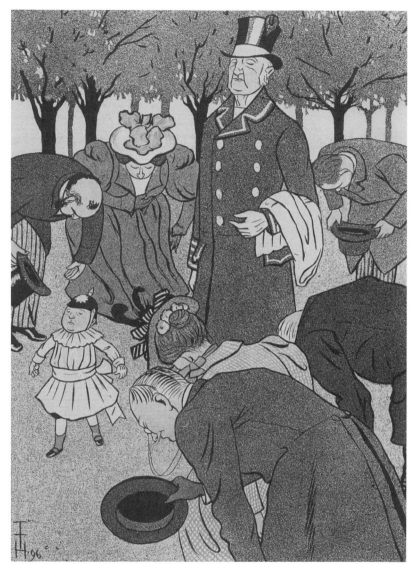

T. T. Heine, *Homo sapiens*. 'The Human Being (Homo Sapiens) Distinguishes Itself from Other Mammals by Its Upright Gait'. From *Simplicissimus*, I/14 (1896).

most ancient tools that we find . . . are hunting and fishing implements, the former at the same time serving as weapons.'[36] Tools precede weapons. 'Man the toolmaker', *Homo faber*, precedes 'man the warrior', *Homo necans*. This is the underlying rationale for the newest anthropological theories, from Herder to the present defining of the human being in terms of erect posture. Indeed, as late as the 1970s the eminent biologist Stephen J. Gould can mirror Engels's view, in an essay on the evolution of posture, that 'upright posture frees the hands from locomotion and for manipulation (literally, from *manus* = "hand"). For the first time, tools and weapons can be fashioned and used with ease. Increased intelligence is largely a response to the enormous potential inherent in free hands for manufacture – again literally.' Posture makes humans, even though it may well be the case that 'our early evolution did involve a more rapid change in posture than in brain size; complete freeing of our hands for using tools preceded most of the evolutionary enlargement of our brain.'[37]

There are those who take a contrarian view, noting that upright posture has led to all the cultural and physiological difficulties of modern human beings. For

> one of the penalties that the human being is forced to accept in his being the highest type of mammal, is that in locomotion, with the body used as an erect biped, gravity is constantly operating to drag the organs downward out of their normal position, as well as to draw the upper part of the body downward and forward into positions which must mean strain and weakness. This element, together with the anatomic form, seems many times sufficient to cause the conditions seen in chronic medicine.[38]

Among those conditions were 'unstable equilibrium, strategic weakness in direct physical attack or defense because the upright body forms a better target for missiles; vital and tender parts are more exposed than in quadruped position.'[39] As another writer puts it, 'Erect posture in man may still further impede the circulation of blood in the lower limbs. Hence we may explain the frequency with which gouty disposition in man first occurs.'[40] Or, indeed, 'imperfect motor paralysis of the upper and lower extremities' can be caused by 'obviously excessive coitus in a constrained (the erect) posture.'[41] Standing up straight can be very bad for your health. One can also add, based on the class system, that the constant debasement of *Homo erectus* into the perpetually bent subject as envisioned by the German satirist T. T. Heine at the turn of the century can be very bad for your sense of autonomy.[42]

Poor posture returns us to the very notion of what is human. At the close of the nineteenth century this question was very much up

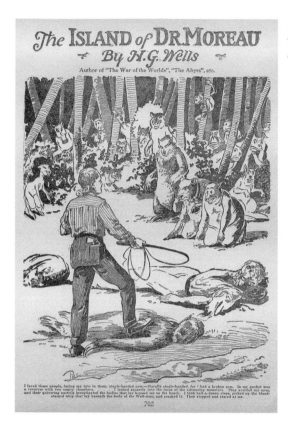

Frank R. Paul, illustration for H. G. Wells, *The Island of Dr Moreau*.

for grabs, following Darwin. 'We're all savages, more or less,' Higgins tells Eliza in George Bernard Shaw's *Pygmalion* of 1913.[43] This was nowhere better illustrated than in H. G. Wells's *The Island of Dr Moreau* (1896). Wells, in answer to the earlier moral arguments of such thinkers as Oliver Wendell Holmes, presents the horrors of Moreau's experiments to merge animals with humans in terms of the erect posture of the offspring: 'I could see the Thing rather more distinctly. It was no animal for it stood erect.'[44] Over time the hybrids become more primitive, 'and they walked erect with an increasing difficulty'.[45] Yet 'the dwindling shreds of the humanity still startled me every now and then, – a momentary recrudescence of speech perhaps, an unexpected dexterity of the fore-feet, a pitiful attempt to walk erect.'[46]

Wells's creatures are experimental throwbacks into the world before *Homo sapiens*, yet created by the very mind of the *Homo sapiens*. His critique relies on the illusion of human progress and the malleability of posture as well as character: 'a living being may . . . be regarded as raw material, as something plastic, something that may be

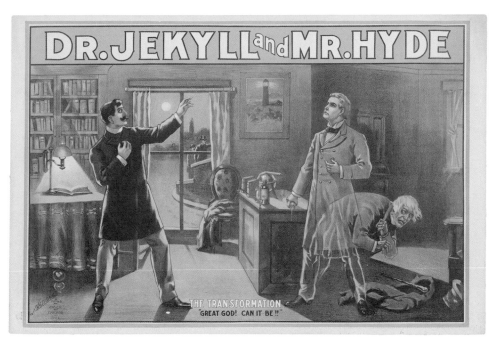

Dr Jekyll and Mr Hyde (The Transformation: 'Great God! Can it be!!'), *c.* 1880, colour lithograph.

shaped and altered . . . and the organism as a whole developed far beyond its apparent possibilities. We overlook this collateral factor, and so too much of our modern morality becomes mere subservience to natural selection.'[47] Posture may be changed, but there is always the anxiety of degeneration, of a 'morbid deviation from a primitive type' (to use B. A. Morel's classic formulation from mid-century), of being an upright, erect human and then devolving into someone or some 'Thing' that does not 'stand up straight'. Wells's 'Thing' is not quite human and therefore has not the erect posture that defines what is imagined to be the civilized being.

Without overstating the case, the model of 'deviant' posture as a form of 'throwback' to earlier evolutionary levels comes to have a strong resonance in the world of posture education. In 1923 Lillian Curtis Drew of the Central School of Physical Education in New York, writing in the authoritative *American Physical Education Review*, evokes, if not Wells, then his Victorian predecessor Robert Louis Stevenson's *Strange Case of Dr Jekyll and Mr Hyde* (1886). But what does Hyde look like? The theatrical representation of Mr Hyde is clearly that of the antithesis of the middle-class Dr Jekyll. How does one represent such difference? Stevenson provides a series of clues to Hyde's physiognomy. Mr Hyde is 'deformed somewhere'. He gives 'an impression of deformity although I couldn't specify the point'. Yet 'Mr Hyde was pale and dwarfish, he gave an impression of deformity without any nameable malformation.' There is overall 'the haunting sense of unexpressed deformity'. He is therefore 'a disgustful curiosity' and appears as 'something abnormal and misbegotten . . . something seizing, surprising and revolting'. He was primitive: 'the man seems hardly human! Something troglodytic.' Indeed, a troglodyte he was, like the Neanderthal find, 'ape-like', and his hand 'lean, corded, knuckly, of a dusky pallor and thickly shaded with a swart growth of hair'.[48] Primeval, deformed, unhealthy . . . Yet there is little specificity as to how this affect is triggered. Indeed, even Martha Stoddard Holmes in her *Fictions of Affliction* states that he is one of the characters with 'unspecified disabilities'.[49] On the stage it is clear: he is a hunchback, the mirror image of Jekyll's 'upright' character. And this is made explicit by his posture.

For Drew, good posture is simply an indicator of good character, and – in a New York teeming with immigrants from eastern and southern Europe, caricatured by bad posture – posture education meant creating moral citizens with 'mental and physical fitness':

> The objective is to establish in the individual such powers of motor control as will make the erect carriage a permanent habit, an integral part of the individual rather than a static position to be assumed in the gymnasium and associated only with this environment, or to be taken on admonition to 'stand up straight!' To be of any real value it must 'function in life'.[50]

Drew's reading of Stevenson, of course, misses the point of *both* characters being aspects of one personality, something that was not lost on the theatre audiences in the West End of London in 1888, when the dramatization of the story appeared simultaneously with the Jack the Ripper murders in the East End.

Class, Sexuality and Posture

Wealthy 'toffs' and working-class murderers were equally imagined in the press of the day as having an unhealthy posture. Toffs slouched, too, but very different meaning was attached to their posture. Formal posture, the posture of the posture boards and deportment chairs, gave way to an alternative 'life style', the slouch. At the close of the nineteenth century 'other Victorian staples, including norms of posture and definitions of ethereal love, began to be attacked or jettisoned as well.'[51] In one of the best-known satires of the aesthetic movement, the 'poor posture' of the aesthete is part of the image of the avant-garde. Here we have George du Maurier's response to the ultimate aesthete, Oscar Wilde, who remarked as a student that he found it 'harder and harder every day to live up to my blue china'. The position is one that reflects a number of contemporary photographs and caricatures of Wilde slouching. Wilde as a student 'let his hair grow; some said he altered his posture to match the languid sensibility prized by aesthetes. He couldn't – or wouldn't – keep his head upright.' One of his classmates observed: 'It fell side ways like a lily bloom too heavy for its stalk.'[52] The aesthete's posture was halfway between a stoop and a swoon, and was read as effeminate.[53] Indeed, the image of the slouching male as gay seems to be in answer to the more or less rigid posture ascribed to the bodies (and the morals) of Victorian bourgeois society.

This trope originates much earlier than the *fin de siècle*. For the Quaker preacher and moralist Joseph John Gurney in 1845, 'young people' must develop the habit

> of looking every man in the face[; it] is a matter of no trifling importance . . . It promotes mental vigour, a proper boldness of demeanour, and above all, openness and candour . . . Stooping must be regarded as a sort of auxiliary to indolence, bashfulness, and slyness . . . We might suppose that many robust young people in the present day, had been suddenly overtaken by the infirmities of extreme old age were we to form a judgment, from their perpetual inclination to an indolent posture of their bodies.[54]

Indeed, by the close of the nineteenth century 'certain tests had made it easier to ascertain if one were a true man: the duel, courage in war, and more generally, the possession of will power as well as the manly virtues of "quiet strength" and of an acceptable moral posture. Proper looks and comportment had provided proof of true manhood.'[55] This

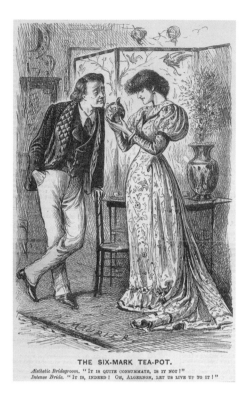

THE SIX-MARK TEA-POT.

Æsthetic Bridegroom. "IT IS QUITE CONSUMMATE, IS IT NOT?"
Intense Bride. "IT IS, INDEED! OH, ALGERNON, LET US LIVE UP TO IT!"

George du Maurier, *The Six-mark Teapot*. From *Punch* (30 October 1880).

posture became the goal of the elite young man in training. Slouch not, it reveals too much!

Drew's point, however, is that to transform the 'Hydes', the new immigrants who now populate the East Side of New York City, into young people of character, standing up straight had to become an essential part of their habituation. The link between the new city-dwellers and the new immigrants was implicit in his view, for 'Jews and homosexuals were not the only countertypes, but they were the most readily visible and frightening examples.'[56] Their transformation was possible through the training of the body. The alternative was not being of the avant-garde but being someone threatening to the new American context. Learning correct posture meant that they could overcome the inherited primitive nature of their background. The toffs already had, and through their posture threw the bourgeoisie into panic.

Darwin's legacy concerning posture is broad and deep in the culture. By the early twentieth century one arena in which it clearly had major impact is that of psychoanalysis. Sigmund Freud's account of the 'Rat Man', the pseudonym of the Viennese lawyer Ernst Lanzer

(1878–1914), who died in the First World War, centres on the idea of upright posture as the cause of neurosis. The Rat Man was ambivalent about a number of things, and especially fearful about his relationships with his fiancée and his father, and according to Freud it was these very contradictory ideas that caused his obsession, among other things, with being tortured by rats. In this case of obsessional neurosis from 1909 Freud observes his analysand's primitive fascination with smell: 'when he was a child he had recognized every one by their smell, like a dog; and even when he was grown up he was more susceptible to sensations of smell than most people . . . I have come to recognize that a tendency to taking pleasure in smell, which has become extinct since childhood, may play a part in the genesis of neurosis.' The Rat Man, according to Freud, was a *renifleur* or *osphresiolagniac*, which is to say that he both recognized everyone by their smell and was obsessed with the smells of his own body. This point is as ancient as Plato, who, as you will remember, in mapping the body finds symbolic significance in the head's position, after the human acquires upright posture, as being as far as possible from the organs of generation.

Freud postulates that the vestigial sense of smell in children and its repression may be the very cause of neurosis in modern man, asking

> whether the atrophy of the sense of smell (which was an inevitable result of man's assumption of an erect posture) and the consequent organic repression of his pleasure in smell may not have had a considerable share in the origin of his susceptibility to nervous disease. This would afford us some explanation of why, with the advance of civilization, it is precisely the sexual life that must fall a victim to repression. For we have long known the intimate connection in the animal organization between the sexual instinct and the function of the olfactory organ.[57]

We become less primitive by standing erect and therefore lose our sense of smell, a sense heightened in hunting animals.

Freud's fascination with the nose and smell, borrowed from his friend the otorhinologist Wilhelm Fliess, extended to imagining that smell was not only suppressed but shaped our conscious lives in complex ways.[58] He wrote to Fliess as early as 1897 about 'the abandonment of former sexual zones':

I was able to add that I had been pleased at coming across a similar idea in [the work of sexologist Albert] Moll. (Privately I concede priority in the idea to no one; in my case the notion was linked to the changed part played by sensations of smell: upright walking, nose raised from the ground, at the same time a number of formerly interesting sensations attached to the earth becoming repulsive – by a process still unknown to me.)[59]

Freud's insight here is for him a true 'aha!' moment. He has been, according to his own account, 'labouring' over this idea for weeks, and suddenly this major idea came to him. He even provides a footnote at this juncture: 'Only tall fellows for Sa Majesté le Roi de Prusse.'[60] What Freud means is that he has no little ideas, and this notion of uprightness and the origins of obsessive neurosis is a truly major one. Posture is never far from his mind at this moment. The reader will remember our discussion of Frederick Wilhelm I of Prussia's elite unit, known as the 'Giant Guard of Potsdam'. Not only upright Prussian military posture, but the posture of giants is Freud's analogy to the power of his understanding of the impact of human bipedalism on the psyche. Moll, whom he claims to have trumped with his gigantic idea, had in his *Untersuchungen über die Libido Sexualis* (Studies of Sexual Libido; 1897) stressed the phylogenic nature of fetishism, especially of those fetishes associated with smell.[61] Yet one can certainly observe that blaming upright posture for a wide range of human ills and states, both psychic and physiological, seems to have been a preoccupation of post-Darwinian medicine.

Freud's theory of the abandonment of erotogenic zones and their link to the notion of organic repression zones came, of course, well before the discovery of human pheromones and their role in sexual attraction. His emphasis is that those qualities captured by the lower senses are lost over time as the human begins to walk upright. Jacques Derrida notes Freud's parallel to Hegel's rejection of the 'lower senses' in his *Aesthetics*, since, as Hegel states, 'smell, cannot be an organ of artistic enjoyment either, because things are only available to smell in so far as they are in process and their aroma is dissipated through the air and its practical influence.'[62] Human aesthetic perception can be rooted only in the higher senses of sight and hearing, those that the human sharpens with upright posture. I must add here that the scale of higher (hearing and sight) and lower (smell, taste and touch) senses is a conceit of Renaissance aesthetics. The great debate in the nineteenth century is whether sight or hearing were more evolved, in that one or the other is more abstract or more concrete depending on which sense was favoured.[63]

For Freud and his contemporaries, posture – standing upright – compromised lower sensory functions and led to neurotic responses. Human evolution, with its alteration of posture, maintains in the unconscious traces of its pre-bipedal ancestry. It is the core of what makes the human civilized, as Freud stressed in *Civilization and its Discontents* (1930):

> With the assumption of an erect posture by man and with the depreciation of his sense of smell, it was not only his anal erotism which threatened to fall a victim to organic repression, but the whole of his sexuality; so that since this, the sexual function has been accompanied by a repugnance which cannot further be accounted for, and which prevents its complete satisfaction and forces it away from the sexual aim into sublimations and libidinal displacements . . . The genitals, too, give rise to strong sensations of smell which many people cannot tolerate and which spoil sexual intercourse for them. Thus we should find that the deepest root of the sexual repression which advances along with civilization is the organic defence of the new form of life achieved with man's erect gait against his earlier animal existence.[64]

Quoting St Augustine on the nature of becoming human in the material sense ('inter urinas et faeces nascimur' (we are born between urine and faeces)), Freud does not see the theological argument about upright posture as moving towards the divine as a possible corollary, even though he gestured towards it in the case of the Rat Man. Yet, for Freud, it is the residual qualities of our material existence before we acquired upright posture that are still manifested directly in the repression that resulted from upright posture shaping our civilizing process.

In the late nineteenth century evolutionary theory came to be read as political in the more limited sense. Lamarck and then Darwin postulated the acquisition of upright posture as one of the defining moments of becoming human. But the notion of military posture came quickly to be folded into this mix. At the opening of a military hospital in 1881 the great German physiologist Emil du Bois-Reymond declared, following Kant's view of human self-improvement, that the human was a 'self-perfecting optimizing machine' and the Prussians were truly 'self-made men' with their plumb-line posture.[65]

Even though the popular view is that organized religion disavowed Darwin (or better, the various varieties of Darwinism that quickly sprang up), the religious response was in no way uniform. The Philadelphia reformer Rabbi Joseph Krauskopf, in a series of books and essays at the end of the nineteenth century, saw Darwin's model as divinely ordained, and posture as a defining quality of the human who is able 'to seize and combine and utilize its laws like a God, and like a God to attain to the highest discernment of good and evil. From the horizontal movement of his primordial ancestor he has elevated himself to the upright posture.'[66] The theological notion of upright posture defining the moment when human beings became human is not new, as we have seen. But the theological adaptation of Darwin's explanation stressed an acceptance of the notion of 'how' the human became upright, but not 'why', and this came to be the bone of contention within most organized religion and some of the science of the succeeding epochs.

Posture from Anthropology to Philosophy and Back

In 1952 the phenomenological neurologist Erwin Straus published his groundbreaking paper 'The Upright Posture'.[67] Straus's view synthesized Darwin, Freud and Martin Heidegger. His approach seems to be one that was deeply embedded in mid-twentieth-century thought but that also provided much material for a rethinking of posture as an essential human quality grounded in notions of stability.

As do many of our commentators on posture, Straus sees human posture as 'the civilizing force that created the human being'.[68] Thus he defines the development of posture in terms of a version of ontogeny recapitulating phylogeny: 'Whereas animals move in the direction of their digestive axis, sight precedes the locomotion of the upright human organism . . . Sight penetrates depth, sight becomes insight.'[69] Following Freud, Straus sees uprightness as changing the emphasis of the senses, and this moves the human being from an olfactory to a visual animal:

'Upright posture has lifted eye and ear from the ground. In the family of the senses, smell has lost the right of the first-born. Seeing and hearing have assumed dominion . . . Bite becomes subordinate to sight.'[70]

The human infant is thus in an intermediate state, 'uprightness in waiting': 'Upright posture characterizes the human species. Nevertheless, each individual has to struggle in order to make it really his own. Man has to become what he is.'[71] Yet in becoming mobile while standing erect, 'the precarious equilibrium reached in standing has to be risked again.'[72] Straus's important distinction between static and mobile posture provides a means of imagining a new instability, one that is inherent in uprightness itself. 'The space that surrounds me is not a piece of neutral, extended manifold, determined by a Cartesian system of co-ordinates. Experienced space is action-space; it is my space of action. To it, I am related through my body, my limbs, my hands. The experience of the body as mine is the origin of possessive experience.'[73] Posture and gait enable us to experience the world around us, and that experience becomes a quality of who we feel we are.

G. H. Estabrooks, a psychologist at Colgate University in upstate New York in the mid-twentieth century, was clearly anti-Darwinian when it came to the course of human development. He was convinced that the human began to deteriorate from the moment he adopted upright posture, arguing that the plague of bad sinuses in modern man is the result of his uprightness.[74] Becoming human means losing a connection to the 'natural' body, he maintained. This counter-argument becomes a means of glorifying the 'primitive' as being closer to the ideal, or at least closer to nature. Science is in a dynamic relationship with politics in which each serves as a resource for the other. Science may serve as a 'cognitive, rhetorical or institutional resource', transforming its very content or practice in a political context.[75] In this manner, posture can serve as a litmus test for such transformation: anti-Darwinian views are also political positions.

Posture thus takes on the coloration of the political ideology of the moment. Indeed, in the 1970s, with a very different notion of the history of human development, the left-wing theorist Klaus Theweleit questioned any positive meaning to be associated with upright (now read as military) posture in his examination of the notion of a relationship between fascist fantasies of the plumb-line posture and masculinity.[76] In evoking 'posture', he pointed to its extensive use in the racial science of the early twentieth century, in which 'good' or plumb-line posture was denied to the weaker, corrupt 'Eastern' races.[77] By the 1990s upright posture is part of a philosophical fantasy of the right-wing German writer Peter Sloterdijk, who suggests that the very act of awakening and sleepily swinging one's legs out of bed is our morning 'ontogeny recapitulating phylogeny', of daily moving to bipedalism, upright posture and transcendent intelligence:

> Nobody has to tell me that the aim of the exercise is to achieve the vertical, even on this morning there is something in me ready to meet the generic fate that moved us to risk being on two legs and having free hands – head now available for considered perspective now placed at the highest point. No one can say that I have not followed the call of human dignity this morning. The improbable – it now takes place, walking upright, it is the event. My standing here now on no more than two legs is an accomplished fact. From now on it will be easy to traverse the path of humanity to consciousness.[78]

Are we our posture, or are they *their* posture? This strikes me as the central question that reverberates through the history of posture.

Yet many scientists today continue to spin their notion of what makes the human 'human' around the development of upright posture, and thus reveal the biases about what actually defines the essential nature of the human being. Thus the controversy surrounding the American anthropologist C. Owen Lovejoy's claim in 1981 in his monogamy-provisioning hypothesis, which imagined that among the earliest 'Miocene hominoids' the proto-human male stood upright in order to improve the efficiency of his foraging for his home-bound mate. Lovejoy claimed that there would be 'a strong selection for bi-pedality, which would allow provisions to be carried "by hand" [and that] would thus accompany provisioning behavior . . . The need to carry significant amounts of food was a strong selection factor in favor of primitive material culture.'[79] All other evolutionary developments depart from this increase in efficiency. Lovejoy somewhat later defines upright posture in a way that seems to be functional:

> Our upright posture, in contrast, places our center of mass almost directly over the foot. If we stand erect and lengthen

our legs by straightening the knee and rotating the ankle, the ground reaction is directed vertically and we end up on tiptoe. In order to propel our upright trunk we must reposition our center of mass ahead of one leg. The trailing limb is lengthened to produce a ground reaction while the other leg is swung forward to keep the trunk from falling. The strength of the ground reaction is limited, because much of it is still directed vertically and also because the trailing limb is already near its limit of extension owing to our upright posture: the hip joint is fully extended and the knee joint nearly so.[80]

The image of human posture contrasts the way the pelvis and leg of the chimpanzee and human 'reflect the differing demands of quadrupedal and bipedal locomotion'.[81] It is as radical a representation as was Huxley's of the difference between pre-human and human, with the latter defined quite clearly by the plumb-line representation of upright posture. This view of evolutionary efficiency caused uproar in the first age of feminist science studies, not because of its argument about the efficient human body, but because of its claim of the primacy of *male* evolution and monogamy.[82] To bring us full circle, C. Owen Lovejoy was one of the primary figures in the public debates about *Ardpithecus ramidus* and the origins of human bipedalism in 2009. To no one's surprise, no mention of the 'monogamy hypothesis' litters that debate.

EIGHT

'Natural Posture': Posture and Race

I S POSTURE *MERELY* a question of human biology? If posture is a quality of the body, whether static or in motion, the answer is, of course it is! 'Certain postures may occur in all cultures without exception, and may form a part of our basic hominid heritage. The upright stance with arms at the sides, or with hands clasped in the midline over the lower abdomen, certainly belongs in this category.'[1] Yet as the very notion of a 'biological' definition of the body changes radically over time, so do the meanings attributed to seemingly identical postures depending on their context. 'Good' or 'natural' posture and the plumb line seem to separate 'primitive' from 'advanced' peoples as well as the 'ill' from the 'healthy' and even the 'human' from the 'pre-human'. When we turn to the debates within the arena of race theory and the 'science of race', we find that posture defines race and refutes racial assumptions simultaneously.[2] Just as our assumed boundary between nature and nurture – like that between science and culture – is specious, as each shapes the findings of the other, posture is used on both sides of the debates about race as evidence for each position. The line of demarcation, to use the Austrian-British philosopher Karl Popper's term from 1935, is an artefact of how we need to see each as autonomous of the other, rather than the sort of absolute that Popper desired to see between 'science' and 'pseudo-science'.[3] There is no clearer case than the function of posture within the discourse of racial science.

In this chapter we will examine the rise (and transmutation) of the notion of the racial body and the function that posture had (and has) in defining it. We must remember that race, meaning the biologically pre-programmed nature of specific, clearly defined groups, was inherent to all the 'sciences of man' from the late eighteenth century to the mid-twentieth (and perhaps even beyond). This was the world in which all the human sciences, from medicine to anthropology to education (indeed, every arena of Western thought that classified human beings), were informed by racial science.[4] Such disciplinary boundaries drew powerfully on the idea of pathological predispositions of the 'inferior' races. The false assumption of the equivalence of all such races, however defined in whatever system evoked, created symmetry among the pathology ascribed to such groups. What categories were used and how race functioned in these categories varied widely. When we turn to posture as a marker of race, what we see is the odd collapsing of the boundaries between the various disciplines that used such classifications. Perhaps the most egregious cases are those of races whose inferiority is defined by biology but whose struggle against such labels demanded alternative understandings of what posture implies.

Racial Difference and Posture

We have already seen that race, as the marker of biological predisposition to bad or good posture, is interlaced with notions of medicine and education in the first age of biology, which runs from the Enlightenment through to the mid-twentieth century.[5] Posture, gait and race are connected too, through models of education. When Native American children were compelled into boarding schools, they were also forced to wear formal school shoes in order to 'correct physical posture, [and encourage] proper ways of moving and of exercising and correct details of dress'.[6] Racial difference is assumed, for good or ill, to be a biological marker, and posture is one of its indicators.

But the notion that posture defines our social body rather than our biological one is as old as the idea of the racial body. As early as the English physician John Bulwer's *Anthropometamorphosis: Man Transform'd* (1650), national bodies were seen as being based on cultural assumptions of appearance.[7] Bulwer's work examines the widest range of body modifications, from tattooing to circumcision. His focus is an attack on fashion and change with clear political overtones: the French seem inherently different from the Scots, and the English different from everyone else, 'Almost every Nation having a particular whimzey as touching corporall fashions of their own invention'.[8] Only transitory fashion and cosmetic appearance make them so. Bulwer condemns practices that, he charges, disfigure the human body, and his intent is to guide the reader towards keeping that body created by God. Thus, for Bulwer, certain nations exhibited acceptable posture; others had idiosyncratic posture, which was to be condemned or corrected. It is striking that his comments on fashion overlap with other categories of examining posture as normative or deviant. Thus, in commenting on how the Irish stand, Bulwer notes that the 'Irish are good footmen' because of the shape of their calves. But he explains this as:

> many times Children about the second yeare of their age, when they begin to go are wont to vari and go wide and straddling with their feet, their Knees inkling to each other. About this feared deformity, their mothers, being solicitous, crave help of Chirurgions, who for the most part endeavor with divers Machins to erect and keep straight their Legs and Thighs, but in vaine, because of themselves, and the just accord of Nature, for the most part about the time they are three or four yeares old, their Legs and Muscles grow more firm and strong, and the parts return to their natural state.[9]

Here, being 'knock-kneed' (*genu valgum*) is seen as the natural state of the Irish, a sign of their innate difference, unchangeable even through the good offices of physicians and their braces. The Irish are thus unlike the English, who have inherently 'normative' posture unless it is deformed by fashion. One can note here that 'for the English the group that was first to be shunted into this discursive derogation [of inferior other] and thereafter invoked as almost a paradigm of inferiority was not the black "race" – but the Irish "race."'[10] Irishness and the deformity of posture maps well on to later notions of a black postural inferiority inherent in the debates about slavery. But the bad posture of the Irish is also attributed to a disease process.

We discussed earlier the function that diseases such as rickets had in shaping the notion of postural disability. Rickets, rather than being Irish, is a common cause of being knock-kneed, something early physicians recognized. Rickets and other nutritional diseases were endemic to Ireland after Cromwell in the 1650s and the suppression of the island's population by the English. By the early eighteenth century

Bulwer's image of the 'knock-kneed' Irish and their posture. From John Bulwer, *Anthropometamorphosis: Man Transform'd* (London, 1653).

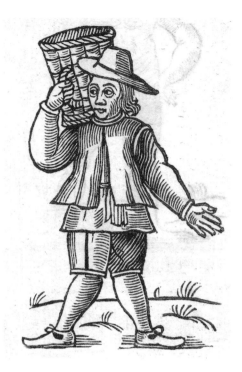

it can be noted that 'in Ireland this disease [rickets] is wonderful rife now, but that nothing near been so long known there as in England.' It is read as 'a disease peculiar to young children.'[11] Rickets and other postural deformations caused by malnutrition were the immediate result of the politics of the day, yet Bulwer sees them as the natural state of the Irish body. Rickets comes to be seen in the United States, even as late as the twentieth century, as a particularly Irish-American disease, and such bodily deformity is read as a sign of the Irish body.[12] Reforming the Irish body is a question, then, of creating a normal body through the refashioning of Irish posture. Here the physician who attempts to correct posture is placed in the same position in Bulwer's account as the purveyors of other fashions. Good as well as poor posture and gait is fixed, unalterable by mere human intervention. It defines the very nature of difference.

Africans, Slaves and Posture

In the United States race maps almost exclusively on to skin colour and African descent, and it is here that the idea of black posture, as a marker, becomes a means of validating slavery. When posture is evoked, Enlightenment debates about polygenetic theory – whether there was one human race or many arranged in a hierarchy of values – come to define the overlap between biological, indeed evolutionary, science and theology. Such debates spanned the world between science and theology in the age when theology was giving way, at least in part, to science. The so-called pre-Adamite views argued that before the biblical Adam, who was created by God to stand upright, the human slouched. At least, commentators on Genesis claimed this, since they viewed human posture as an index of hierarchical difference. These views defined, for theologically orientated racism, the difference between the white, post-Adamite man, and the black, a relic of the pre-Adamite age. The historian John Haller notes in his classic study of the science of race that the belief that

> there were major anatomical differences between the Negro and the white was commonly accepted . . . [Scientific texts of the day argued that] the evolution of races . . . showed the development of an upright posture which led to corresponding changes in the thorax, pelvis, and lumbar vertebrae . . . the posture 'shifted the weight of the abdominal viscera from the thorax to the pelvis . . . and also the last lumbar vertebra tended to fuse with the sacrum, thus tilting up still further the pelvis'.[13]

It is central here that the black body was defined as the body of the slave, predisposed to his inferior status.[14]

The poor posture of the slave has an ancient pedigree as 'physical differences are invoked, between the crouching posture natural to a slave and the upright posture of a free man. This is archaic aristocratic material, going back, for instance to Theognis: "A slave's head is never upright, but always bent, and he has a slanting neck."'[15] For Aristotle, 'the posture of the natural slave is less erect than that of the natural master, so that the former is better suited to performing tasks involving stooping (manual crafts and agriculture), whereas the latter was intended by nature to practice the *politikos bios*, the life of a citizen.' Aristotle recognizes that 'very often natural free men . . . stoop and so have (ser)vile bodies.'[16] Striking in Aristotle's treatise *Physiognomics* is the fact that this dichotomy mirrors his definition of masculinity: 'The characteristics of the brave man are stiff hair, an erect carriage of body, bones, sides and extremities of the body strong and large, broad and flat belly . . . The signs of the coward . . . not eager but supine and nervous.'[17] Moral value, not merely social status, is reflected in posture.

Yet Aristotle has difficulty with this claim of an absolute relationship between the slave's occupations and the slave's appearance. Given the Platonic definition of the good citizen as ἀγαθὸς καὶ σοφὸς, 'wisdom and nobility', defined by inner character and values rather than by any outward manifestation of the body, Aristotle must hedge his position.[18] He writes in the *Politics* that

> The intention of nature therefore is to make the bodies also of freemen and of slaves different – the latter strong for necessary service, the former erect and unserviceable for such occupations, but serviceable for a life of citizenship . . . ; though as a matter of fact often the very opposite comes about – slaves have the bodies of freemen and freemen the souls only; since this is certainly clear, that if freemen were born as distinguished in body as are the statues of the gods, everyone would say that those who were inferior deserved to be these men's slaves.[19]

For Aristotle, the real difference is the presence of rationality (*logos*) in the freedman but not the slave. Different they are; the only question is what is the measure by which we recognize this difference.

When translated into the language of racial biology in nineteenth-century America, the black body is defined as the body of the slave, but the slave is also thought to be a more primitive form of human being. The link between the primitive and the inferior body (and soul) is an example of Johannes Fabian's theory of the 'denial of coevalness', which construes 'the savage, the primitive, the Other', different racial, criminal or mentally ill types, as not only pathological and inferior, but temporally Other, belonging to an earlier, more primitive time.[20]

Thus in 1861 the New York physician John H. Van Evrie defended black slavery by claiming that 'The negro is incapable of an erect or direct perpendicular posture . . . the *tout ensemble* of the anatomical formation, forbids an erect position. But while the whole structure is thus adapted to a slightly stooping posture, the head would seem to be the most important agency, for with any other head or the head of any other race, it would be impossible to retain an upright posture.'[21] Rather, his argument goes, mirroring the pre-Adamite view that the

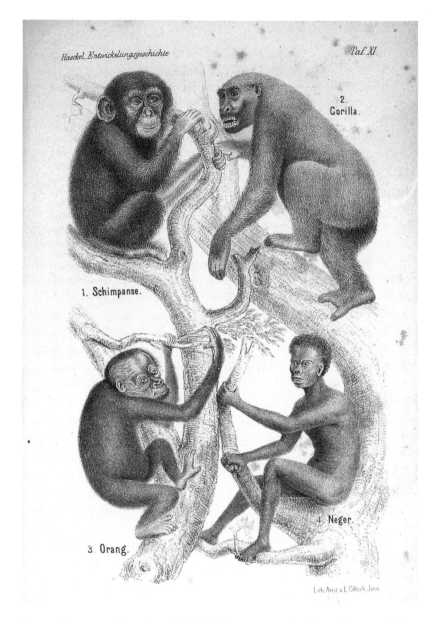

Comparative posture. From Ernst Haeckel, *Anthropogenie, oder, Entwickelungsgeschichte des menschen Keimes- und Stammesgeschichte* (Leipzig, 1874).

black slaves' ancestors were quadrupeds that survived on Noah's ark: 'The negro, from the structure of his limbs, his head, etc., has a decided inclination to the quadruped posture, while the ourang-outang has an equal tendency to the upright human form.'[22] In contrast, 'the Caucasian can be confounded with no other . . . the flowing beard, oval features, erect posture and lordly presence, stamp him the master man wherever found.'[23] White posture is lordly; black posture is servile.

Slaves 'slouch', as Mrs A. C. Carmichael noted in her work on Jamaica in 1833, describing a slave 'walking some paces, holding down his head, and with a slouching gait'.[24] Or, in Thomas Dixon's infamous *The Clansman: A Historical Romance of the Klu Klux Klan* (1905), on which D. W. Griffith based his notorious film *Birth of the Nation* (1915): 'The negro drew himself up, pulling his blue uniform into position as his body stretched out of its habitual slouch'.[25] The slave's posture was simultaneously the key 'to judge moral character, intelligence, and social tendencies'.[26] His posture as well as his mental state predisposed him to slavery, since the character of the black is written on his slouching body. The only question that remained was the classic debate about whether what Jean-Jacques Rousseau in 1754 puzzled over as 'national character' is fixed, as David Hume stated in his essay 'Of National Characters' (1748) specifically about blacks, or malleable, as Montesquieu states in *De l'Esprit des lois* (1748).[27] Could their character as well as their posture be reformed?

Such dehumanizing views echo earlier arguments about the divine origin of upright posture well past the abolition of slavery into the Jim Crow era, when, in 1900, Charles Carroll wrote a book entitled *The Negro a Beast; or, In the Image of God*. In it, Carroll concludes that Negroes are pre-Adamite creatures and could not possibly have been made in God's image and likeness because they are beastlike, immoral and ugly. It is the fallacy of evolutionary theory, rather than biblical teaching, that has made the black human: 'Under the influence of The Theory of Natural Development, the Negro has been taken into the family of man.'[28] But his argument is not merely of race but of the biblical admonition that upright posture is a true sign of the human before the Fall:

We observe that the first curses which God visited upon the serpent were directed solely at his posture. Had the tempter of Eve been a snake, God's sentence, 'Upon thy belly shalt thou go,' would have been of no effect . . . But when we come to understand that the tempter of Eve was a beast – a negro – this whole subject appears in a very different light. The habitual posture of the negro is the erect. Hence, God's sentence, 'Upon

thy belly shalt thou go,' wrought the most radical change in
this negro's posture, and was a most terrible punishment.[29]

The following year the American theologian William Gallio Schell
commented on this passage that 'when we change men into beasts and
snakes into men, we are confronted with ridiculous and conflicting
ideas.'[30] At best.

These examples paralleled a clearly theological perspective defending Jim Crow laws that relegated the black to second-class citizenship
and continued a theological argument that has been powerful in the
defence of slavery, the argument about the sons of Ham. They were a
commonplace of the time. But they are also found in the more serious
eugenic literature of the day. The theology of race morphs quite easily
into the comparative arguments about racial eugenics by the 1920s, as
Haller indicated. At the Second International Congress of Eugenics in
1921, held at the American Museum of Natural History in New York
(one of three held between 1912 and 1932), some 53 scientific papers
were presented, most by Americans, and Alexander Graham Bell
served as honorary president. One of the most often cited is the paper
of the eugenicist Robert Bennett Bean of the School of Medicine at the
University of Virginia on the differences in posture of the various races. Bean had been head of the anatomical laboratory at the University
of Manila from 1907 to 1910, where he had published on the racial
types of the Philippines. He returned to the United States, to Tulane
and eventually Virginia, where he became one of the leading eugenicists working on the physical anthropology of race, mirroring his initial work at the University of Michigan in 1905–7 on the 'brains of the
Negro . . . with [anthropometric] measurements taken on Ann Arbor
students.'[31] This combination, as we shall see, links race science and the
obsessive measurement of elite posture.

In 1921 Bean returned to his fascination with exotic posture. He
stressed his clinical as well as anthropological expertise, since he had
'observed for many years the sinuosities of the vertebral column in the
negro . . . in the dissecting room . . . The back cannot be straightened
and the thorax and buttocks project backward and the head and
abdomen forward when the negro is standing.' He found that 'the great
muscular development of the trunk in the negro may be explained in
part by . . . the attempt on the part of the negro to maintain the erect
posture.' 'Natural posture' for the black was some form of quadrupedia:

blacks walked upright as a force of will in emulation of whites, and not as their natural capacity, given that 'the pelvis is tilted forward to bring the body to the center of gravity.'[32] Bean accompanies his argument with a series of three photographs of semi-clad figures showing the poor posture of the 'negrito' from the Andaman Islands.

Such views of black posture reflect what Erving Goffman labels 'canting posture' in modern advertising art. 'The level of the head is lowered relative to that of others, including, indirectly, the viewer of the picture. The resulting configurations can be read as an acceptance of subordination, an expression of ingratiation, submissiveness, and appeasement.'[33] Bean's images, in common with much of the anthropological images of non-Western posture of the day, gesture at such a

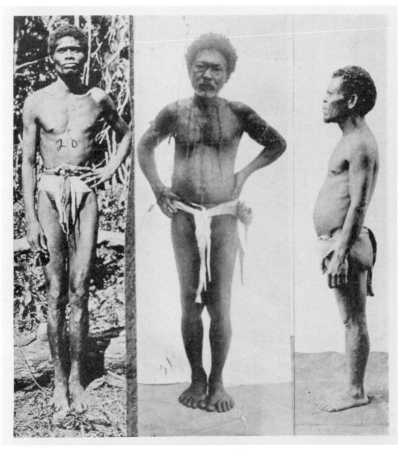

The posture of the 'negrito' from the Andaman Islands. From Robert Bennett Bean, 'Notes on the Body Form of Man', *Scientific Papers of the Second International Congress of Eugenics, September 22–28, 1921* (Baltimore, MD, 1923).

subservient stance as part of the 'documentary nature' of the image as evidence of inferiority.[34] While Goffman's illustrations are mainly of women, such images of passive posture have older analogies in the image of the black slave, male or female. These are images of a submissive posture as 'the black figure is . . . trapped in an everlasting posture of debasement, as the freed slaves are in the manumission imagery'.[35] But the bent posture has other meanings with regard to the black. We can apply Goffman's notion of stigma here, for the black is 'reduced in our minds', as he writes, 'from a whole and usual person to a tainted, discounted one'.[36]

If posture degrades the black into the subhuman, anti-slavery campaigners argue that it is slavery that marks the destruction of the black's humanity by destroying their posture. Accounts of the slave ship and the Middle Passage often commented on the cramped conditions of the ships and its impact on the slaves' constitution:

> The height between the floor and ceiling was about twenty-two inches. The agony of the position of the crouching slaves can much easier be imagined than described, especially that of the men, whose heads and necks are bent down by the boarding above them. Once so fixed, relief by motion or change of posture is unattainable. The body frequently stiffens in a permanent curve; and in the streets of Freetown I have seen liberated slaves in every conceivable state of distortion. One I remember who trailed along his body, with his back to the ground, by means of his hands and ankles. Many can never resume the upright posture.[37]

Such images haunt the abolitionist literature of the time. In 1823 a broadside of the slave ship the *Vigilante* by John Hawksworth, printed by Harvey, Darton & Co. in London, circulated in Great Britain. The caption reads:

> The representation of the brig *Vigilante* from Nantes, a vessel employed in the slave trade, which was captured by Lieutenant Mildmay, in the River Bonny, on the coast of Africa, on the 15th of April 1822. She was 240 tons burden & had on board, at the time she was taken 345 slaves. The slaves were found lying on their backs on the lower deck, as represented below, those

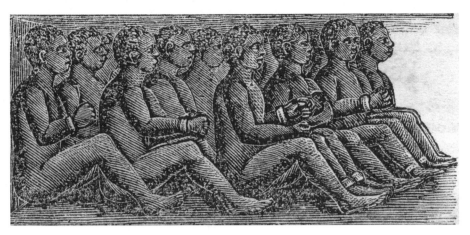

'Interior of a Slave Ship', woodcut illustration. From John Warner Barber, ed., *A History of the Amistad Captives* (New Haven, CT, 1840).

> in the centre were sitting some in the posture in which they are
> shown & others with their legs bent under them, resting upon
> the soles of their feet.

Anti-slavery campaigners used this print to remind the public of how extraordinarily cramped conditions were on slave ships. The image also shows how men and women were segregated on board. The men are shown restrained in pairs with handcuffs and leg irons. The image of the bent and tortured posture of the slaves had by this point become part of the visual charge against the Atlantic slave trade.

In 1840, during the trial in the United States District Court for the District of Connecticut of the Africans who had seized the Cuban slave ship *La Amistad* in 1839, the horrors of confinement were stressed by the defence, which had one of the defendants, Grabeau, testify that

> they were fastened together in couples by the wrist and legs,
> and kept in that situation day and night . . . By day it was no
> better. The space between decks was so small, – according to
> their account not exceeding four feet, – that they were obliged,
> if they attempted to stand, to keep a crouching posture. The
> decks, fore and aft, were crowded to overflowing.[38]

The nature of the postural restraints became an inherent part of the image of the horrors of slavery. The court held in favour of the

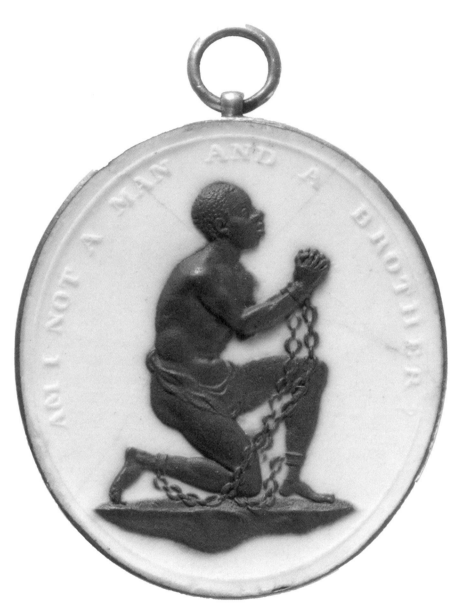

William Hackwood (modeller) and Wedgwood (maker), *Am I Not a Man and a Brother?*, c. 1787, oval medallion of white jasper with a black relief set in a gilt metal hoop. The medallions were not sold commercially, and were never listed in the Wedgwood catalogues. Instead, Wedgwood probably bore the cost of their production and distribution. Others of similar size sold at three guineas each, which gives an indication of the considerable sums involved. They were probably distributed through the Society for the Abolition of Slavery. Certainly, Wedgwood is known to have sent consignments to both the American statesman Benjamin Franklin, who was then president of the Philadelphia Society for the Abolition of Slavery, and Thomas Clarkson, a leading abolitionist and author of *A Summary View of the Slave Trade*.

Africans, who were thus not required to be turned over to the slave traders in Cuba, and mandated the federal government to return them to Africa, from where they had been kidnapped.

Perhaps the best-known image of the anti-slavery crusade is the kneeling, supplicant slave asking the question 'Am I not a man and a brother?' Josiah Wedgwood produced William Hackwood's design for the Society for Effecting the Abolition of the Slave Trade in 1787, and it came to be the reigning visual image of the posture of the slave, often reproduced in many media. Thomas Clarkson, the leader of the London abolitionists, wrote of the immense popularity of the icon: 'Of the ladies, several wore them in bracelets, and others had them fitted up in an ornamental manner as pins for their hair . . . At length the taste for wearing them became general, and thus a fashion . . . was seen for once in the honourable office of promoting the cause of justice, humanity and freedom.'[39]

In William Lloyd Garrison and Isaac Knapp's abolitionist newspaper *The Liberator* in 1834, Garrison wrote: 'In order to keep my sympathies from flagging, and to nourish my detestation of slavery by a tangible though imperfect representation of it, I have placed on my mantel-piece the figure of a slave (made of plaster) kneeling in a suppliant *posture*, and chained by the ankles and wrists.' The piece was presented to him in London by an esteemed friend, and elicited the following:

My heart is sad as I contemplate thee,
Thou fettered victim of despotic sway;
Driven like a senseless brute from day to day,
Though equal born, and as thy tyrant free.
With hands together clasped imploringly,
And face upturned to heaven, (heaven shall repay!)
For liberty and justice thou dost pray,
In piteous accents and on bended knee.
That exclamation, 'AM I NOT A MAN?
A BROTHER?' thrills my soul. I answer – YES!
Though placed beneath a universal ban,
That thou art both, all shall at last confess:
To rescue thee incessantly I'll plan,
And toil and plead thy injuries to redress.[40]

Thus it also appears in 1837 on the broadside publication of John Greenleaf Whittier's anti-slavery poem 'Our Countrymen in Chains', which gave words to the image:

> And shall the SLAVE, beneath our eye,
> Clank o'er *our* fields his hateful chain?
> And toss his fettered arm on high,
> And groan for freedom's gift, in vain?[41]

As has been cogently observed about this icon of the slave among abolitionists, 'though this black has been given his freedom and has had his chains physically removed, he is still imprisoned within the posture and gestures that the abolitionists invented and that white society considered the most acceptable official icon of the Atlantic slave'.[42] What is striking, however, is that it is not only the supplicant posture with the upraised hands but the physical deformity of the spine that defines the slave's body. Ultimately, the slave's body in modernity is understood as having poor posture owing to malformation of the body, whether because of the nature of his race or because of the oppressive nature of slavery itself.

Such questions about the slave's posture re-emerged in a complex way in the United States immediately after the Civil War. On 14 April 1876 the President, Ulysses S. Grant, dedicated the Emancipation Memorial in Washington, DC, sometimes called the Freedman's Memorial and designed by Thomas Ball. Depicting Abraham Lincoln holding the Emancipation Proclamation standing before a kneeling freed male African-American slave, it was decried by contemporaries such as the leading African-American abolitionist Frederick Douglass. Douglass, who spoke at the unveiling, departed from his written text to state that the kneeling image 'showed the Negro on his knees when a more manly attitude would have been indicative of freedom'.[43] This according to the Howard University historian John Cromwell, who was at the dedication. In 1916 Freeman Henry Morris Murray, one of the first black art historians, saw the 'kneeling – or is it crouching? – figure' as a version of the conventional image of Jesus and Mary Magdalene, coming 'perilously near making Mr. Lincoln saying, "Go, and sin no more" or, "Thy sins be forgiven"'.[44] Indeed, as recently as 1997 the figure was condemned as 'a monument entrenched in and perpetuating racist ideology' because of the posture of the black figure.[45]

The sculptor had initially conceived the figure as an allegory of freedom, with a crouching black slave wearing a 'liberty cap'. (A maquette of this initial figure is in the collection of the University of Michigan Museum of Art. It is very similar to a plaster maquette of Randolph Rogers's proposed Emancipation monument for Philadelphia created shortly after Lincoln's assassination in 1865, also in the Michigan collection.) Ball's initial figure seemed too passive to the St Louis-based Western Sanitary Commission that had ordered it and paid for it with contributions from African Americans. It 'was re-thought as a muscular former slave with shackles freshly broken'.[46] It was completed with the new figure bearing a likeness of the freed slave Archer Alexander, the hero of a popular contemporary biography by William Greenleaf Eliot. Yet,

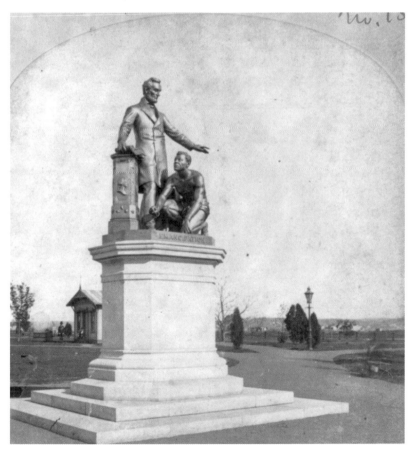

Half of a contemporary stereographic slide of Thomas Ball's *Emancipation Monument* (1876), Lincoln Park, Washington, DC.

compared to the original design, in which Lincoln's hand seems to awaken the slave to his new freedom and to the realization that his shackles are gone, the current memorial is more of an amalgamation of approaches. It is no longer allegorical but realistic. In fact, Lincoln never met Archer Alexander, so it is historically inaccurate. While the original design poses a question – will this slave become a man? – the revision erases that query and instead implies a relationship between two men who never actually knew each other.[47]

At the same moment, at the Centennial Exposition in Philadelphia in 1876, the Italian artist Francesco Pezzicar's statue *The Freed Slave* was first exhibited. This artist's interpretation of emancipation – a lone black male clutching Lincoln's Emancipation Proclamation and rising from the earth, breaking his chains – stood in dramatic contrast to the memorials of Rogers and Ball. The great interest in Pezzicar's statue on the part of African-American visitors was captured in the fact that it was reproduced by Fernando Miranda as an illustration for *Frank Leslie's Historical Register of the Centennial Exposition*. But, unlike that of Ball and Rogers, Pezzicar's statue went unsold, only to be shipped back to Italy at the close of the exhibition.

Yet the subliminal question of this and other critiques is whether the posture of the freed slave was an indicator of his former or present status. The masculinity of the slave, in the revised version that was eventually cast, points to the status of freedom. Yet even the hint of submission in his posture raises the spectre of inferior status. Is the freed slave in motion, standing upright, in order to be recognized as 'a man and a brother', or is he frozen in the posture of submission? Viewers then and now seem unable to judge. Ambiguity in reading posture meant that it was impossible to distinguish between the various meanings present.

The mutilation of race through oppression remains a trope well into the middle of the twentieth century, yet with interesting shifts based on how the disabled body presents itself in the culture of the time. Coming out of the Second World War, Frantz Fanon, in *Black Skin, White Masks* (1952), refers to a scene from the film *Home of the Brave* (1949; dir. Mark Robson), which, he argues, makes the mutilated arm of Mingo, a white solder, parallel to the race of Ross, the black soldier. Is race mutilation? Fanon responds: 'with all my being, I refuse to accept this amputation. I feel my soul as vast as the world, truly a soul as deep as the deepest of rivers; my chest has the power to expand to infinity. I was made to give and they prescribe for me the humility of the cripple.'[48] It is the rejection of the idea of race as an absence, not as deformation, that haunts Fanon's world. Indeed, his image is of the psychologically deformed, not physically mutilated, colonial subject suffering from identification with the aggressor:

> I recommend the following experiment to those who are unconvinced: Attend showings of a Tarzan film in the Antilles and in Europe. In the Antilles, the young Negro identifies him-self *de facto* with Tarzan against the Negroes. This is much more difficult for him in a European theater, for the rest of the audi-ence, which is white, automatically identifies him with the savages on the screen.[49]

If there is an imaginary film playing in the heads of Fanon's black colonial subjects it is Tarzan, and that is the body with which they identify. It is a strong, masculine body, neither mutilated nor scorned.

The legacy of the black slave's posture continues well after the be-ginning of the renewed struggle for American civil rights in the 1950s. The black nationalist Malcolm X commented on posture in a talk in 1964, reflecting that when he visited Africa, he noted the 'sense of poise and balance that [Africans] over there have', and lamenting that Ameri-can blacks have lost their natural posture and need to be taught it:

> They have a tendency to be other than with dignity, unless they're trained. When their little girls go up to these, you know, hi-falutin' schools, and they want to teach them how to walk, they put a book on their head. Isn't that what they do? They teach them how to walk like you. That's what they're learning how to walk like, like you. But you were almost born with a book on your head. You can throw it up there and run with it.

He argued that blacks must 're-adopt' erect posture to 'walk with dig-nity' and as a proud reflection of their African heritage.[50] This has re-cently been echoed by the African American sociologist Michael Eric Dyson, who argued that 'black nationalism's psychology of race insist-ed on the upright posture of black manhood. Given the context of the times, this was meant to signify the entire race, but its references to the restored egos of black *men* is unmistakable.'[51] The gendering of posture is neither new nor specific to this moment. It is, however, striking that Malcolm X evokes 'little girls' who attend American schools to learn what he considers to be the lost, natural posture of the African.

On the other side of the civil rights divide, Martin Luther King, Jr, does not evoke posture but folds it into the need for higher standards in the black community. On 6 September 1960, in a speech before the National Urban League that stated 'the Negro must make a vigorous effort to improve his personal standards,' he argues that 'our lagging standards exist because of the legacy of slavery and segregation, inferior schools, slums, and second-class citizenship, and not because of an inherent inferiority.'[52] Quite aware of the judgemental aspects of white society, he demands that blacks adopt better personal standards as a form of transformation to reify their social as well as political potential, 'to develop a positive program through which these standards can be improved'. Rather than stressing, as did Malcolm X, the inherent qualities of the black as the baseline for black culture, King notes that 'the Negro who seeks to be merely a good Negro, whatever he is, has already flunked his matriculation examination for entrance into the university of integration.'[53]

Such arguments echo through works reflecting the question of an appropriate black posture into the twenty-first century. Garnett S. Huguley writes in his self-published autobiography about the 'Sambo behavior' that is reflected in the posture of the black, 'who grinned or trembled frequently, who typically shuffled or stuttered in front of whites'. The only 'alternative to this behavior or legacy is to teach our children to walk with an upright posture, heads held high, chins up, shoulders back and straight backs. This change in posture appears more rational, beneficial and I believe it will promote a positive legacy and a new image and attitude for African Americans, demonstrating to others, culture pride and confidence.'[54] Upright posture comes to define identity in the twentieth century, for African Americans as well as all others.

Posture and the Jews

By the seventeenth century national characteristics of posture had come to be understood as biological realities defining group differences, a fact that is nowhere better illustrated than in Robert Burton's *Anatomy of Melancholy* (1621), which echoes such contemporary views and specifically cites the Jews in terms of their poor posture. Burton writes of the 'pace' of the Jews, as well as 'their voice . . . gesture, [and] looks', signs of 'their conditions and infirmities'.[55] The German Orientalist Johann Jakob Schudt commented in 1718 on the 'crooked feet' of the Jews, among other indicators of their physical inferiority.[56] Difference in posture and gait defines the Jew, but this difference may or may not be racial in origin. Indeed, to paraphrase Burton, it may be the result of their oppressive lives and the illnesses that result from them.

What is folkloric (and Burton is not quite medical science) in the seventeenth century becomes part of the science of race in the nineteenth. By the early nineteenth century, as we have seen, representations of the philosopher Moses Mendelssohn in Germany did not shy away from stressing his postural deformity (he was a hunchback).[57] As early as 1804, in Joseph Rohrer's study of the Jews in the Austrian monarchy, the weak constitution of the Jew and its public sign, 'weak feet', were cited as 'the reason that the majority of Jews called into military service were released, because the majority of Jewish soldiers spent more time in the military hospitals than in military service'.[58] This linking of the weak feet of the Jews and their inability to be full citizens (at a time when citizenship was being extended piecemeal to them) was for Rohrer merely one further sign of the inherent, intrinsic difference of the Jews. Thus Balduin Groller could claim that the overwhelming evidence is that 'the physical composition' of both Eastern and Western Jews 'is not normal'.[59] Groller cites the statistical records of a Russian military doctor on the prevalence of Jewish degeneracy: the average size of an adult Jew is 162.7 centimetres versus 165–70 centimetres for a non-Jew; Jews have less developed chest bones and musculature, including a 60 per cent smaller chest size than the norm; Jews suffer from bad posture as well as a greater susceptibility to tuberculosis, skin disease, eye infections, myopia and nervous and psychological disorders; finally, they have a greater incidence of hernia.[60]

Joseph Pennell, the Victorian illustrator and friend of James Abbott McNeill Whistler, in a small book on *The Jew at Home* (serialized in the *London Illustrated News* at the same time), states more or less the same problem among Russian Jews for a popular audience:

Much sentiment has been wasted over the poverty-stricken appearance of the Russian Jew, his consumptive, hollow-chested look, and his shambling walk . . . The Jew naturally is not physically weaker than the peasant. As a soldier, when he is made to stand up straight, he is as fine a man as any other Russian, with the exception that he cannot march as well, but becomes quickly footsore. This is because he never takes any exercise; he never walks, he never uses his hands or his legs if he can help it.[61]

Every view of the Jew's body has bad posture at its core, reflecting in one way or another the character of the Jew.

The American novelist and social commentator Jack London, in London for the coronation of Edward VII in 1902, spent months in the city's overcrowded East End. His account of urban poverty at the turn of the century, that of the displaced Eastern European Jews in the ghettos of the East End of London, as in other American and European cities, notes that 'when . . . segregated in the Ghetto, they cannot escape the consequent degradation. A short and stunted people is created, – a breed strikingly different from their masters' breed, a pavement folk, as it were, lacking in stamina and strength. The men become caricatures of what physical men ought to be, and their women and children are pale and anemic, with eyes ringed darkly, who stoop and slouch, and are early twisted out of all shapeliness and beauty.'[62] For London, the posture of the slums is not only a sign of the impact of the ghetto but the result of eugenics. The best and most powerful men (his word) had long abandoned such places, leaving the poorest specimens, 'a deteriorated stock', behind to reproduce.

It is of little surprise that among the earliest medical specialists in the rather new field of orthopaedics dealing with posture are two mid-nineteenth-century Jewish orthopaedists in Berlin, Moritz Michael Eulenburg and Heimann Wolff Berend. The latter was the first to use anaesthesia for surgery in Berlin, and he also made early use of patient photographs to document and publicize their treatment.[63] Berend and Eulenburg were heavily influenced by the Swedish system of medical gymnastics developed by Pehr Henrik Ling with the intention of reforming posture and restoring health through directed exercises. Bodies, even those of the Jews, were deemed infinitely adaptable, at least through medical intervention.

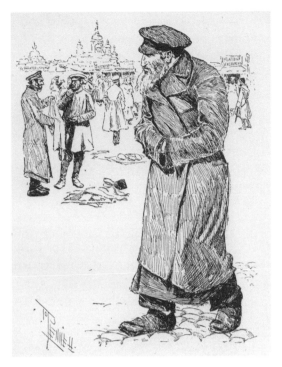

Joseph Pennell, *The Jew at Home: Impressions of a Summer and Autumn Spent with Him* (New York, 1891).

By the turn of the twentieth century Jews too had accepted the notion of their bad posture as a sign of Jewish maladaptation to the modern world. In his opening speech at the Second Zionist Congress in Basle on 28 August 1898, Max Nordau, the most important figure in early Zionism after Theodor Herzl, invented one of Zionism's most famous, most fraught and most challenging ideals: the 'muscle Jew'. His essay on '*Muskeljudentum*' (often translated as 'A Jewry of Muscle'), which he originally gave in 1903 as a dedicatory speech for the opening of yet another Jewish gymnastic club, condemned the 'degenerate modernity' that he had earlier seen as defining the modern world: 'Unreal, too, are the studied postures, by assuming which the inmates are enabled to reproduce on their faces the light effects of Rembrandt or Schalcken. Everything in these houses aims at exciting the nerves and dazzling the senses.'[64] The answer to Jewish degeneracy indeed became a range of sports clubs, mirroring the anti-Semitic *Turnvereine*. Perhaps the most famous in the pre-war period was the Makkabi Deutschland, the Jewish sporting club founded in 1903 after Jews were substantially excluded from the *Turnvereine*. When the Jewish philosopher and educator Franz Rosenzweig visited one of the Makkabi clubs, he noted that while there were signs in Hebrew on the wall stating *mens sana in corpore sano*, the young men seemed to know nothing about religious practice or belief.[65] A strong mind in a strong body meant postural training. During the First World War the 'new Jew' on the front, trained now for physical fitness, 'exposed as lies the fairy tale of the bent and crooked Jews, as our youth grows to maturity in good health and with straight bodies'.[66] Bodily training undertaken to refute the calumnies of the postural deficiencies of the Jew has become a leitmotif of Jewish reaction to anti-Semitism. It is not sufficient merely to reject such arguments; the Jewish body must have perfect posture to rebut such claims.

The red line that connected early Zionism and other forms of bodily reform, such as 'Muscular Christianity', was the resurgence of interest in classical Greece fomented by the Greek Revolution against the Ottoman Empire in the early 1820s. Not only did it show Jews that older ideas of nationalism could be reclaimed, but it was closely associated with notions of bodily reform and politics. (Think of the sporty though disabled Lord Byron, dying at Missolonghi in 1824, as the ideal hero of the Greek rebellion.) Inherent in this was the staggering importance of Greek sculpture in providing models for the ideal national posture, but it also led to the resuscitation (or invention) of models for bodily reform such as the modern Olympic movement, which has its earliest modern form in the 1830s among the Greeks, then in Great Britain in the 1850s, and finally in Athens under the leadership of Pierre de Coubertin in 1896. This renewed tradition, as part of a modern nationalist bodily reform, was particularly important for early Zionism since 'Jewish nationalists largely rejected rabbinic spirituality, non-belligerence and the disdain for athleticism which dominated Jewish life after Rome destroyed the Jewish state in 70 CE.'[67] Here the Jews overcame specific ideas of bodily reform and embraced the more widely held understanding of postural reform as part of the new nationalistic body.

As Nordau noted, by the early twentieth century bad posture had become a central maladaptation of the Jews: 'The Jews' terrible posture does not come from any natural trait. It is but the result of a lack of physical education. In this way, there is not really a difference between Jew and Aryan.'[68] He stated in 1903:

> I said: 'We must once again think of creating a Jewry of muscle'
> . . . Once again! For history is our witness that such a Jewry

once existed. There is no shame to admitting this need: Our new muscle Jews [*Muskeljuden*] have not yet regained the heroism of their forefathers . . . But morally speaking, we are better off today than yesterday, for the old Jewish circus performers of yore were ashamed of their Judaism and sought, by way of a surgical pinch, to hide the sign of their religious affiliation . . . while today, the members of Bar Kochba proudly and freely proclaim their Jewishness.[69]

The warrior Simon Bar Kochba led the Jews in their failed revolt against the Romans in AD 132, but his martial spirit gave the name to the Jewish sports club in Berlin in 1902. For Nordau and his contemporaries, Jews and non-Jews, the Jews were the sick *men* of Europe:

The Zionist societies use every effort that the members and the Jewish masses in general may know the history of their nation . . . They care, in the measure of their strength, for the amelioration of the hygiene of the Jewish proletariat, for its economic improvement by means of association and solidarity, for well-directed education of children, and for the instruction of the women . . . They preach the duty of leading a faultless, spiritual life, the rejection of a crude materialism, into which the assimilation Jews, on account of the want of a worthy ideal, are only too apt to sink, and strict self-control in word and deed. They found athletic societies in order to promote the long neglected physical development of the rising generation.[70]

In speaking about the newly established Jewish National Fund during the Fifth Zionist Congress in Basle in 1901, Nordau argued:

The physical elevation of the Jewish people is a money question. If the [majority] of Jews were in a good position it would not be necessary to waste words on their physical improvement . . . look at the Jewish families who for the past three generations have been men of wealth! Compare these stately horsemen, these first rate fighters, these stylish dancers, these prize-winning gymnasts and swimmers, compare their robust bodies with the emaciated and cough-racked frames of the Eastern ghettos. Then you will immediately form an idea of the means required for the physical amelioration of the Jewish race . . . The mass has neither the time nor the means for gymnastics and sports. If we offer them any hygienic suggestions it must be such that cost nothing.[71]

Such views came to be commonplace. The image of Jewish postural transformation is at the core of the image of the Jew in the work of non-Jewish (and certainly non-Zionist) thinkers of the day. In his essay 'Die Lösung der Judenfrage' (Solving the Jewish Question; 1907), the future Nobel Prize-winner Thomas Mann saw the 'Jewish question' as 'purely psychological' because the Jew is 'always recognized as a stranger, feeling the pathos of being excluded, he is an extraordinary form of life'.[72] Mann's views paralleled the discussion of the deformed Jewish body as a central trope of the debates of the time, including those among the other contributors to the special issue of the German newspaper the *Münchner Neuesten Nachrichten* on 14 September 1907, in which Mann's essay appeared. The progress of German culture, not Zionism, Mann argued, permitted – indeed, demanded – the spiritual integration of the Jews into Europe, and that resulted in the transformation of the Jewish body. Mann's fantasy of the Jews imagines them primarily as crippled and malformed inhabitants of the ghettos of Eastern Europe. Their movement into European culture in Germany is not mere social acculturation but physical transformation.[73] Mann sees this movement as the replacement of the ghetto Jew, with his 'hump back, crooked legs and red, gesticulating hands', by 'young people who have grown up with English sports and all the advantages without denying their type and with a degree of physical improvement'.[74] We must remember here that Mann's very first successful attempt at the writing of fiction was his short story 'Little Mr Friedemann' of 1896, the tale of the disabled aesthete, 'with his pigeon chest, his steeply humped back and his disproportionately long skinny arms'.[75] After a life of self-imposed asceticism because of a youthful rejection, he falls in love with Frau Gerda von Rinnlingen, the homely wife of the military commander of the town in which he lives. She mocks him when he declares his love for her and his only recourse is to commit suicide. Physical imperfection (even, indeed, the evocation of Friedemann's Jewish-sounding name) gestures towards the psychological self-doubt of those with imperfect posture. For Mann, this malformation and its potential for transformation are part and parcel of the 'general cultural

'In the Dreyfus Affair, the more that is exposed, the more Judah is embarrassed.' From the Viennese anti-Semitic journal *Kikeriki*, XXXIX (23 April 1899).

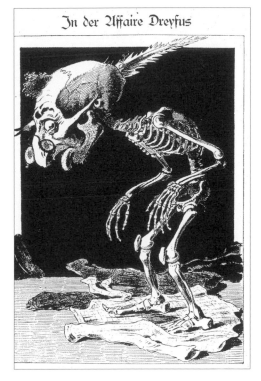

In der Affaire Dreyfus

development' of Europe – of the new cosmopolitanism of healthy bodies as opposed to degenerate ones.

This biological notion of the regeneration of good posture is in line with Herzl's views on adaption and maladaptation: 'Education can be achieved only through shock treatment. Darwin's theory of imitation [*Darwinsche Mimikry*] will be validated. The Jews will adapt. They are like seals that have been thrown back into the water by an accident of nature . . . if they return to dry land and manage to stay there for a few generations, their fins will change back into legs.'[76] And, one can add, they will 'stand up straight.' As Paul Higate puts it, 'only by providing a "previously emasculated Central European Jewry with an honorable and manly posture" did Theodor Herzl believe the goal of the regeneration of a Jewish state could be achieved.'[77] But this was not only an ideal. The self-consciously Jewish strongman Siegmund (né Zishe) Breitbart (1883–1925) became the image of the 'new muscle Jew' in Herzl's Vienna and beyond:

A human being of supernatural powers. Breitbart. He bends steel as if it were soft rubber, bites through chains as though

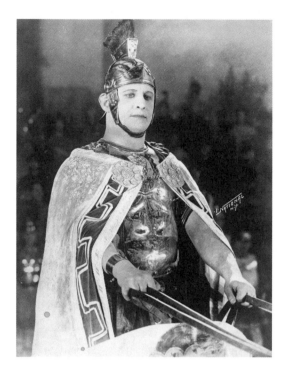

Siegmund Breitbart's most featured stage entrance and his signature persona as a Roman centurion. From *Das Programm, Artistisches Fachblatt*, 1,187 (4 January 1925).

they were tender meat, drives nails into thick wood with his bare fist . . . A bridge loaded with hundreds of kilograms of concrete block is lowered onto his gigantic body, and the blocks are pounded with hammers.[78]

Costuming himself as Bar Kochba or a Roman centurion (no matter how contradictory those two personae were), he came to represent the new muscle Jew as pseudo-military figure. Sport becomes the means, as it was in the nineteenth-century German national movement, of regenerating not only a healthy body but a healthy mind. Through such twentieth-century transformations the Jew regains a pride in being Jewish through the newly revitalized Jewish body.[79]

In 1908 the German-Jewish eugenicist Dr Elias Auerbach of Berlin undertook to produce a medical rebuttal of the claims of Jewish postural inferiority, contesting the 'fact' of the predisposition of the Jew to certain disabilities that precluded him from military service in an essay entitled 'The Military Qualifications of the Jew'.[80] Auerbach begins by attempting to 'correct' the statistics, which claimed that for every 1,000 Christians in the population there were 11.61 soldiers, but for 1,000 Jews there were only 4.92 soldiers. His correction (based on the greater proportion of Jews entering the military as volunteers and who, therefore, did not appear in the statistics) still finds that a significant portion of Jewish soldiers were unfit for service (according to his revised statistics, of every 1,000 Christians there were 10.66 soldiers and of 1,000 Jews, 7.76). He accepts the physical differences of the Jew as a given, but questions whether there is a substantive reason that these anomalies should prevent the Jew from serving in the military. He advocates the only true solution that will give Jews equal value as citizens: the introduction of 'sport' and the resulting reshaping of the Jewish body, even though this will not necessarily make them better qualified to be soldiers. In 1909 Max Zirker argued in the *Jewish Gymnastics Journal* that the Jewish people must develop a 'class of farmers' who can till the ground, something that will counterbalance their 'mostly intellectual work'. As such, they will develop the bones, musculature and posture necessary for serving in the military and becoming national citizens able to defend a future homeland, while also honing their intellectual prowess and 'mental hygiene'.[81]

These disruptions of the healthy mental map of the body came to be seen as forms of mental illness, as the Italian psychiatrist Enrico Morselli observed when he coined the diagnostic category of 'dysmorphophobia' in 1891. Dysmorphophobia is, according to Morselli, the fact that patients stress their own fixed physiognomy as the source of their unhappiness. He described the patients' fixation on specific qualities of that body: the low and mashed forehead, the absurd nose and the bandy legs. Bad posture and badly formed bodies, then, are the origin of mental illness.

This view of the pathological meaning of poor posture is found throughout such defences of the Jews with the rise of racial anti-Semitism at the close of the nineteenth century. In his 'defence' of the Jews in 1893, the French historian Anatole Leroy-Beaulieu notes that the Jews are characterized by the predominance of the nervous system over the muscular system: 'too little muscles; too much nerves, *il est tout nerfs* [he is all nerves]'. The Jew is all nerves because of his 'oriental origin' and his sedentary life.[82] At the same moment, the anti-Semites are making the same argument and drawing the same connections. In 1893 the German physician and writer Oskar Panizza, in his depiction of the Jewish body, observed that the Jew's body language was clearly marked:

When he walked, Itzig always raised both thighs almost to his mid-rift so that he bore some resemblance to a stork. At the same time he lowered his head deeply into his breast-plated tie and stared at the ground. – Similar disturbances can be noted in people with spinal diseases. However, Itzig did not have a spinal disease, for he was young and in good condition.[83]

The Jew looks as if he is diseased, but it is not the stigmata of degeneracy that the observer is seeing but rather the Jew's natural stance. Panizza's Itzig undertakes massive corrective surgery, including having his bowlegs broken and reset. Itzig then appears 'somewhat taller and resembled a respectable human being', standing 'straight and tall like a pine tree'.[84] At the conclusion of the tale, after he has tried to pass as a German, Itzig's body returns to its 'natural' posture, revealing his immutable Jewish character. Yet with the rising tide of Zionism (and indeed a general sense of distaste at the notion of a degenerate Jewish body), especially among intellectuals in the United States, a counter-image arose of the ancient Israelites as warriors possessing perfect posture.

For Jews in Germany, some of whom had 'nose jobs' beginning in the 1890s to be able to 'pass' more easily, postural anomalies revealed too much. Alexander Granach, one of the most popular film and stage actors in Weimar Germany, was a Jew from Austrian Galicia who came to Berlin as a teenager before the First World War. He starred in a series of important films, from the silent *Nosferatu* (1922) – in which he played Knock, the mad, hunchbacked estate agent – to one of the first 'talkies', *Kamaradschaft* (1931). In one of his most memorable stage performances, in Munich in 1920, he even played Shylock. A major star, he emigrated to the United States and continued his film career until his untimely death in 1945. In his autobiography, *There Goes an Actor* of that year, Granach explains how he transformed himself from an Eastern European Jew into a German by having both of his legs broken to correct his 'crooked knock-knees'.[85] (It is unpleasantly reminiscent of Panizza's anti-Semitic caricature.) Granach's self-consciousness about this was to no little degree because it was seen as a sign of Jewish posture, or at least Eastern European Jewish posture. Studiously, his friends 'said they had never noticed that my legs were crooked'.[86] He saw this postural deficiency as a sign of something other

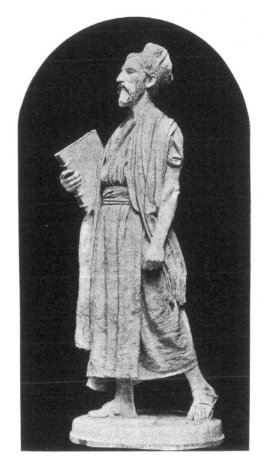

Katharine M. Cohen, *The Israelite*, 1896, marble. In 1887 Cohen, a Jewish American sculptor, went to Paris to study. While there, she was elected an honorary member of the American Art Association. The academic jury chose her life-size sculpture *The Israelite* for the Paris Salon in 1896, a definitive sign of her arrival as an artist. This image, with its upright, hyper-correct posture, defined the biblical Jew in its day. Widely reproduced, it came to represent the potential for Jewish postural transformation.

than race, attributing his 'crooked baker's-legs' to his hard work in his father's bakery, rather than to malnourishment or to race.[87]

Immigration policy in the United States at the time Mann was writing was shaped to no little extent by the posture of Jewish immigrants from Eastern and Central Europe who flooded into New York City at the close of the nineteenth century. The medical examination at Ellis Island begun after the federal government took control of the borders with the Immigration Act of 1891 was constituted to identify 'irregularities in movement', among a wide range of other disabilities. Immigrants were watched as they carried their luggage to observe if 'the exertion would reveal deformities and defective posture'. One inspector wrote: 'It is no more difficult to detect poorly built, defective or broken down human beings than to recognize a cheap or defective automobile . . . The wise man who really wants to find out all he can about an automobile or an immigrant, will want to see both in action, performing as well as

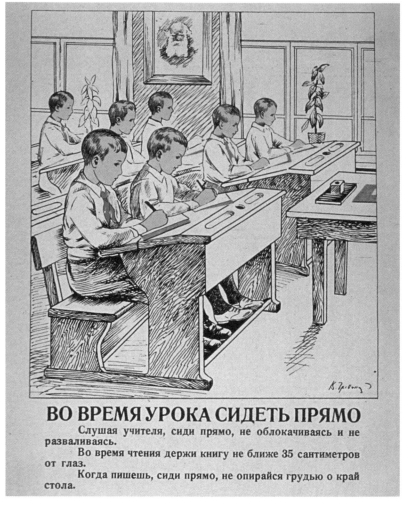

ВО ВРЕМЯ УРОКА СИДЕТЬ ПРЯМО

Слушая учителя, сиди прямо, не облокачиваясь и не разваливаясь.

Во время чтения держи книгу не ближе 35 сантиметров от глаз.

Когда пишешь, сиди прямо, не опирайся грудью о край стола.

'During the lesson you must sit up straight.' The new Soviet man is shaped through posture education. One of the public health posters from 1944 published in Moscow by the Institute for Health Education in a series of rules for schoolchildren. Lithograph.

at rest.'[88] Those with 'defective' posture quickly had an 'L' chalked on their backs. They were then ordered to the shipping companies for transportation back to Europe. If they were admitted to the United States, that is, if they were judged to be healthy and of good posture, they were still seen as deformed. At the turn of the twentieth century the distinguished Boston physician Richard C. Cabot, sitting opposite such an immigrant in an examining room, saw 'not Abraham Cohen, but a Jew; not the sharp clear outlines of this unique sufferer, but the vague, misty composite photograph of all the hundreds of Jews who in the past ten years have shuffled up to me with bent back and deprecating eyes, and taken their seats upon this stool to tell their story'.[89] Reality, Cabot recognized, was masked by assumptions about the Jewish body. By 1931 the historian James Truslow Adams had coined the phrase 'the American Dream' in his *Epic of America*, to describe the imagined goals of the new immigrants. Adams defines it as 'a dream of social order in which each man and each woman shall be able to attain to the fullest stature of which they are innately capable . . . regardless of the fortuitous circumstances of their birth'. A liberal understanding of the resiliency of human posture shapes his notion of human stature.[90]

Such demands for bodily transformation in the 1930s are not limited to the United States. Scholars of body politics of Stalinist Russia in the 1930s have pointed out that the cultural and public discourse of the time was marked by the rhetoric of reforging (*perekovka*) human beings. In spite of this culture's Marxist emphasis on the supremacy of the economic and social environment for human formation, the concept of reforging was paradoxically linked to the notion of biological change within an organism. Various Jewish writers, such as the Soviet children's author Lev Kassil, made attempts to demonstrate the success of such a reforging of the body and soul as exhibited in many of the Russian and Jewish literary characters in the writing of the 1930s. The human body's biological essence was viewed as a product of the forces of nature, against which remedies had to be found. As Mikhail Zoshchenko's diaries attest, Nordau's turn-of-the-century concept of degeneration continued to be influential among the generation of the 1930s, who were concerned with how to overcome it.[91] Learning to stand up straight was a key to this in shaping the new Soviet Man (as well as the new Fascist Man and the new Zionist Man), as the historian of sexuality George Mosse argued about the varieties of masculine identity that dominated these disparate political directions.[92]

Such views penetrate Marxist ideology in the 1930s beyond the Soviet Union, and merge with assumptions about race science and posture. The utopian Marxist philosopher Ernst Bloch 'saw the upright gait as a moral orthopedics of human dignity, as strengthening the backbone against humiliation, dependency, and subjugation'.[93] Bloch reads upright gait as a political act and sees it as standing behind Marx's demand 'to overthrow all relations in which man is a degraded, enslaved, abandoned, or despised being'. He observes that 'the claim to the upright gait was within all rebellions; otherwise there would not be uprisings. The very word uprising means that one makes one's way out of one's horizontal, dejected, or kneeling position into an upright one.'[94]

Bloch's greatest work, *The Principle of Hope*, was written in exile from the Nazis between 1938 and 1947, but published only in the 1950s. In it he places posture as a key to his understanding of the altered physiognomy of the body under capitalism. He notes that

> genuine athletic postures are very different from cosmetic postures in front of the mirror, from makeup that is wiped off a woman's face again at night, or from other rebuilding which is dismantled when we take off our clothes again. The body should not be concealed at all but rather shed the distortions and disfigurements which an alienating society based on the division of labour has inflicted on it too.[95]

Capitalism may seem to encourage healthy posture, but it masks the need for money to maintain it: 'Of course there are people who breathe correctly, who combine a pleasant self-assurance with well-ventilated lungs and an upright torso, which is flexible to a ripe old age. But it remains a prerequisite that these people have money; which is more beneficial for a stooped posture than the art of breathing.'[96] This is Immanuel Kant's note that all humans are 'crooked wood' now translated into the world of capitalistic exploitation. It reappears in the guise of the world of the poverty-stricken and the simple struggle for food, not in Rousseau's garden but in the brutal world of fascism:

> Many things would be easier if we could eat grass. In this respect the poor man, kept as a brute animal in other ways, does not have it as good as that animal. Only the air is readily available, but the soil first has to be tilled, over and over again. In a stooping, painful posture, not as one grows choice fruit upright against the wall. The days of collecting berries and fruit, and of free hunting have long been a thing of the past, a few rich people live off a lot of poor people. Constant hunger runs through life, it alone compels us to drudgery, only then does the whip compel us.[97]

But Bloch, in American exile as a Jew, also rejects any notion that such postural differences are the result of race: 'Thus even the chances of nobility do not stem from breeding; it is rather that social hygiene, a society in which an upright posture is not suppressed any more, in which no mean trick pays off any more, reveals noble behaviour anyway, indeed it is truly revealed by that society alone. Only here does the "breeding" of geniuses really succeed, of these true and solely desirable "blood minorities".[98] Very different in its rhetoric, this evokes Nordau's view that only a true reform of society can enable the corrupted posture of the Jew to be reformed. For Bloch it is clear that capitalist society takes over the role of anti-Semitism as the force deforming the social body, echoing the Frankfurt School's view, articulated by Max Horkheimer in the 1930s, that anti-Semitism was merely a secondary phenomenon of late capitalism. It is the world of capital that for Bloch trumps the claims of race. He had been forced to flee Germany in 1934 as a Jew, eventually settling in the United States where he wrote his magnum opus before returning to the German Democratic Republic after the war. There he became a major critic of the repressive communist state. Whether he felt that German communism provided better posture for its citizens is doubtful, but this ceased to be an obsession for him.

Locating the unhealthy Jew and separating those Jews from potentially healthy citizens permeated the ideology of Zionism at virtually the same moment. This comes to be rooted in 'the idea of "productive" labor' in early Zionism in Palestine:

> Physical labor became part of a Jewish body politics with regard to the Zionist citizen-to-be. The target group those Zionists addressed with their call for productive, physical labor was not so much non-Jewish society and even less the anti-Semites, but rather the religious Jews who stuck to their books and religious practices. In a quite condescending manner, they used to call them 'ghetto-Jews' in contrast to the new 'Halutz' (pioneer) who had yet to be trained.[99]

The question was whether posture was remediable, and for whom. Posture came to be the means of distinguishing permanent factors that disqualified the Jew from those imposed bodily deficits that could be remedied by a new ideology of the body.

Let us be clear: this image of the hunchbacked Jew does not vanish with the establishment of the state of Israel and its creation of a new Muscle Jew. It continues well into the twenty-first century. The Jewish-

Russian-American novelist Gary Shteyngart, who emigrated to New York City from the USSR in 1978, when he was six, turned his 'American Jewish' experience into his first novel, *The Russian Debutante's Handbook* (2002). His account stresses the impossibility of integration, a theme well known in the American as well as the Soviet discourse of the time. His protagonist, the Soviet Jew Vladimir Girshkin, is employed by the Emma Lazarus Immigrant Absorption Society, a position that his middle-class professional parents find well below his potential. Yet he remains too Russian (and therefore too Jewish) for a cosmopolitan America, made up of Jews who stand up straight. His mother had noted that, unlike American Jews, his difference is written on his body: "'Look at how your feet are spread apart. Look how you walk from side to side. Like an old Jew from the shtetl . . . How can a woman love a man who walks like a Jew?'"[100] His mother endeavours to walk like a 'normal' American, and urges:

> *You, too, could walk like a gentile.* You had to keep your chin
> in the air. The spine straight.
> Then the feet would follow.[101]

But Vladimir never quite learns this lesson and remains posturally (and thus identifiably) Russian Jewish, his body unreformed into the sporty American physique that stood up straight. In other words, stand up straight and walk upright like a real American (read: Gentile) if you want to survive American white nationalism enveloped in neo-liberal capitalism. Michael Chabon, in his novel *Moonglow* (2016), gestures at this when he has his Jewish-American protagonist alter his posture as he walks from his Jewish neighbourhood in Philadelphia through the Italian one abutting it: 'you studied the nuances of people's ways of . . . carrying themselves . . . if you hoped to avoid a beating on Christian Street, you could alter your gait and the cant of your head.'[102] This is what Bloch had gestured at in the 1940s as the orthopaedia of the upright carriage translated into claims for human dignity. As we have seen, the use of posture to demarcate the Jewish body race merges into theories of national identity and the corrected posture of the Jews. This has rather a long reach today.

NINE

'Political Posturing': Posture Defines the Good Citizen

H OW WE STAND DEFINES who we are in the eye of the beholder, but also reflects our internalization of cultural norms about posture. These become our own bodily sense. Among the various uses to which posture has been put and which quickly became part of the body map of modernity is as a litmus test for the healthy modern body of the perfect citizen.

The political theorist Benedict Anderson argued in his widely cited *Imagined Communities: Reflections on the Origin and Spread of Nationalism* (1983) that the image of the modern nation-state is 'fully, flatly, and evenly operative over each square centimetre of a legally demarcated territory. But in the older imagining, where states were defined by centres, borders were porous and indistinct, and sovereignties faded imperceptibly into one another.'[1] Anderson's now classic formulation holds that the very concept of the nation 'was born in an age in which Enlightenment and Revolution were destroying the legitimacy of the divinely-ordained, hierarchical dynastic realm . . . nations dream of being free, and, if under God, directly so. The gage and emblem of this freedom is the sovereign state.'[2] Religious identity, as with the power of religion in general, gives way beginning with the Enlightenment to other indicators of power. In such new symbolic orders, the terms of belonging to the new nation become naturalized. Anderson writes, 'in everything "natural" there is always something unchosen. In this way, nation-ness is assimilated to skin-colour, gender, parentage and birth-era – all those things one cannot help. And in these "natural ties" one senses what one might call "the beauty of *gemeinschaft*". To put it another way, precisely because such ties are not chosen, they have

about them a halo of disinterestedness.'[3] Posture is also one of these
variables that seem natural to the citizen, especially the citizen-soldier
of the nineteenth century liberal nation-state. While the 'Prussian'
body (if we can so summarize the development of military posture in
the eighteenth and nineteenth centuries throughout the world – from
a unified Germany to Meiji Japan, from an expansionist United States
to colonial India) stressed the development of the professional soldier
in the modern nation-state, the idea of the citizen-soldier, shaped by
the French Revolution and by the failed Revolutions of 1848, comes to
redefine the national project.

The body of the new citizen, like that of the professional recruit,
can be shaped and improved. This might take the form of 'whitening'
(as in Argentina) or of the constant improvement of aspects of the
body, including posture. The nation thus has a symbolic body that
is always engaged in the process of meaningful alteration, as the
philosopher Ernest Gellner asked provocatively in his article 'Do
Nations Have Navels?'[4] They have origins, they have traditions,
but they also have postures. What was a simpler world structure
rooted in kinship has become, even by the time of the Greek city-
state, a nascent nation where cultural norms become the new con-
stitutive principle. Gellner comments elsewhere that 'the hold of a
shared literate culture ("nationality") over modern man springs from
the erosion of the old structures, which had once provided each man
with his identity, dignity and material security, whereas he now depends on education for these things.'[5] We might amend this to note
that education is but one of the disciplines through which this task
is undertaken.

Through these disciplines lines are drawn between those bodies
that cannot be improved, where education as a citizen will not change
the body markedly, and those healthier bodies that can be reshaped.
In the shaping of modern national identity, religion as a reflection of
kinship systems gives way to the symbolic language of the new state,
a central symbol of which is the reformed body of the citizen. Work
on this new symbol runs parallel to the development of the military
stress on posture, but it is embedded into a new symbolic vocabulary,
that of the new bourgeoisie, as Anderson notes.[6]

Posture has symbolic value in defining citizenship as well as 'national identity'. This symbolic identification between the citizen's body and
that of the nation arises from 'that paradigm condition in which a mass

of people have made the same identification with the national symbols
– have internalized the symbols of the nation – so that they may act
as one psychological group.[7] Posture can and does become a symbol of
the healthy citizen. This national symbolic language is not necessarily
one of affirmation, since 'the nation-state into which the infant is born
as citizen is in a state of permanent competition with its international
environment. Other countries are competitors in the great international game.'[8] But such citizens, to paraphrase George Herbert Mead,
are inherently symbol-generating animals, understanding themselves
as both subject and object, both self-aware and aware that they are
self-aware. Such individuals, Mead claimed, make the 'distinction
between body and self, between physique and consciousness.'[9] But
they also have the ability to see in their own bodies, in the posture that
defines them, the symbolic representation of the nation.

Indeed, the philosopher Charles Taylor has noted that in the end
we are all 'self-interpreting animals', each of us constituted in part by
an ongoing and open-ended process of collective self-interpretation.[10]
Our bodies are part of this process, and it can be seen clearly in the
development of 'national' bodies with a 'national consciousness'. Jürgen
Habermas has argued that this process of self-interpretation is not
merely limited to questions of our performance of identity and our
various roles in society, but rather incorporates questions about what
it actually means to be human.[11] For Taylor and Habermas, the image
of the 'symbolic game' demands a new image of the players' bodies,
defined to no little degree by their posture as citizens.

German Nationalism and Posture

The idea of a political posture is, in the nineteenth century, more closely
associated with German nationalism than with British eugenics, the
creation of Francis Galton. Rooted in the German Enlightenment definition of the nation – inherently abstract, since there were more than
two hundred German free cities, principalities and bishoprics – ideas
of education and posture as advocated by such reformers as the theologian Johann Gottfried Herder came to define the transcendental
German national body. Herder, in his *Ideas of Philosophy of the History
of Mankind*, stated that education, *Bildung*, meant mimicking the *imago
Dei* realized on the sixth day of Creation in the making of upright
Adam.[12] As we have seen, the initial, indeed primary, definition of this

divine body is the upright stature of mankind. Herder argued that we could achieve reason only through language, and for him language comes to define membership of the nation-state; the nation is 'a group of people having a common origin and common institutions, including language'. The nation-state represents the union of the individual with the national community; each people is unique, and indeed polyglot entities, such as Switzerland (or the Tower of Babel), were 'absurd monsters contrary to nature'.[13] But Herder's understanding of the divine form of nature is also part of his construction of the nation. For the citizen's body is defined divinely: by the upright posture given to mankind by God. Such a view dominated Enlightenment medicine. Christoph Wilhelm Hufeland noted in his widely read *Makrobiotik*, drawing on Hippocratic practices of exercise and moderation, that the healthy bourgeois body with an upright and solid posture is the key to health and long life. The practical resolution of this is found in the elaboration of ideas of *Bildung* as defining the new middle-class citizen by thinkers such as Carl Friedrich Bahrdt as early as 1776. Bahrdt's core idea of *Bildung* included 'walking, posture, gestures, facial expressions and tone'.[14] But it was in the turn to a new national politics that posture would assume a central role.

How such a philosophy of national identity came be converted into the '"tribal" gymnastics' that define the body in the Third Reich is a tale of the world following the Napoleonic wars.[15] Friedrich Ludwig 'Turnvater' Jahn (1778–1852) did more than any other individual to make bodily discipline a formal constituent of German national identity.

Jahn was a minor, rural Prussian patriot without a university education or much real military experience (he had held a minor rank in a volunteer brigade during the Napoleonic Wars), who used his own enthusiasm for gymnastics as a building block for a new German nationalism, clearly linked to racism: 'While elements of racism antedated the rise of nationalism, the nation-state is a necessary precondition for the entrenchment of racism, for the former establishes the utility of large-scale forms of collective identity and encourages the collective ideology of identity that sustains racism.'[16] This was nowhere more evident than in the fragmented, multiple German states in the eighteenth century as they responded to the claims of an overarching identity as 'German' after the Peace of Westphalia (1648).

After absorbing the teachings of physicians such as Karl Basedow, the grandson of Johann Bernhard Basedow, and the educator Johann

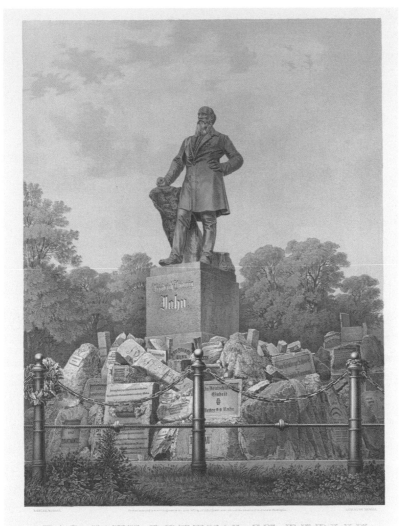

Edward Mendel, *The Jahn Memorial in Berlin* by Erdmann Encke (1872), lithograph. This lithograph was printed in Chicago, and illustrated the Berlin monument, with its dedications and contributions from gymnastic societies across the world. Note Jahn's rigid, plumb-line posture, defining him as a good citizen.

Christoph Friedrich Guts Muths (1759–1839), Jahn took popular gymnastics a step further, making it the cornerstone of an organic German nationalism that included mind, body and politics. For Guts Muths, gymnastics created a new sense of masculinity: 'The balanced proportions and the harmony of all parts of the body, as well as the proper posture[,] are important, for "who would not be impressed by the letter of recommendation beauty provides?'"[17] But the notion of what comes to be cross-training remains large in Guts Muths's understanding of bodily training. His handbooks certainly stressed masculine undertakings such as gymnastics as well as military drill, but he also saw dancing as a danger of postural training:

> The art of dancing may contribute greatly to a graceful demeanour; but if its measured steps and regular carriage be adopted in our habitual movements and attitudes, we shall announce more pedantry than taste. An easy display of strength and suppleness in all our gestures, without the least appearance of art or constraint, is most to be admired . . . These, however, are not so completely within the sphere of the dancing master, as is generally supposed, but depend in great measure on the early management of children.[18]

Rousseau's warning about freedom versus training is never far from the eye of the German nationalists. Its Romantic notion of a human freed from constraint, postural and partisan, and moving towards a 'natural' political solution is key. Notions of appropriate masculinity haunt the world of German nationalism from its inception, in terms of the physicality of the new citizens.

In 1809 Jahn began to reshape physical education as a particularly German form of activity, in which 'German' was meant to have both a national and a racial component. He advocated what we would today call 'field sports', from running to the javelin, as well as gymnastics, such as the vaulting horse. Indeed, he developed a range of equipment that mirrored various bits of military body training, from the pommel horse, the parallel and horizontal bars and the vaulting blocks, to postural training aids such as dumbbells and Indian clubs.[19] He saw all these as preparing the German citizen for an active role as a citizen-soldier. He excluded dance from physical education and was lukewarm about the inclusion of fencing, since he saw both as elite rather than bourgeois activities.

For Jahn in 1816, gymnastics was a discipline that could re-establish 'the lost harmony of humanity'.[20] The notion of a unified German spirit and body, a body that was clearly defined as bourgeois, was that of the true German citizen. He (and the citizen was always male) would be part of a healthy, landed middle class that would form the political core of Jahn's imagined German parliamentary monarchy. One of his contemporaries noted in 1818 that the lower classes were interested only in tightrope-walking and strongmen; the upper classes had 'a distaste for the very essence of Jahn's gymnastics, community and camaraderie. In the middle class there are fewer indifferent opinions, more foes and more friends, especially the former.'²¹ The movement to create a German middle class across the boundaries, both geographic and religious, that fragmented the German-speaking world into multiple competing states was one of the agendas of the Enlightenment; it also became one of the core ideas of German nationalism.

Jahn's *Deutsche Turnkunst* (1816), written with Ernst Eiselen, became the bible of German gymnastics just as his *Deutsche Volksthum* of 1810 had heralded his turn to nationalism. *Deutsche Turnkunst* began by evoking a definition of posture that echoed established images of the military body: 'Posture: Feet and knees must always be as close as possible. Body erect, belly inwards, breast outwards. Particular care must be taken to maintain the posture of the upper part of the body. In this way the back can be drawn in, the shoulders recede, and a firm and noble posture of the body be effected.'²² For Jahn, such posture and the very collegial structures of the gymnastics society come to represent a new political turning, a reoccupation of the Prussian body he had experienced in the volunteer Prussian Lützow Free Corp, fighting Napoleon in 1813, with a new notion of the German. It was not the parochial Prussian but a new German – in the terms of the time a liberal, if not democratic, German. Imprisoned by the Prussians for sedition, Jahn was exiled but continued to encourage the use of gymnastics to build the body of the citizen of this imagined new state.

But if the Germans (a mental construct that has its roots in the eighteenth century) were to have a new body, it had to be in contrast to other bodies: those of the French, the Poles, the priests, the aristocrats and especially the Jews, whose postural anomalies were stressed in the popular as well as the scientific literature of the day. Jahn had argued as early as 1810 that the abstract Germany of the Enlightenment needed a national space, for 'a nation without a state is a dead, floating chimera like the nomadic Gypsies and Jews. A state and *Volk* together create a *Reich* but it is the power of the *Volksthum* that preserves it.'²³ Nomads cannot have any sense of national identity; they are zombies because 'they have died and yet are not dead, they continue in this corpse life like a madman's horrific double' damned to eternal wandering.[24] And their wandering bodies were marked by their posture, among a wide range of other observable qualities.

Out of Jahn's ideological demand for institutions that supported the idea of a German spirit in a German body arose the *Turnvereine*, the gymnastics societies, the motto of which was *mens sana in corpore sano*. That phrase, which as we have noted comes from Juvenal, takes on a new and rather specific German coloration in the period of growing nationalism. By Goethe's time it had taken on a quite modern meaning, referencing health, gymnastics and bodily hygiene.[25]

For these *Turner* (members of the *Turnvereine*) in the early nineteenth century, the sense that the German states had not only abandoned a German identity but bankrupted the German body was central. The movement, often with the ideological baggage of German nationalism or at least civic reform, spread quickly worldwide as people flooded out of the German states after the economic collapse that was quickly followed by the failed Revolutions of 1848. Friedrich Hecker, who had helped to lead the unsuccessful Baden Revolution in 1848, came to America, where he turned abolitionist and then became a Union colonel during the Civil War. He founded the first American *Turnverein*, in Cincinnati in 1848. The ideology of the *Turnvereine* was clear: it encouraged the 'cultivation of rational training, both intellectual and physical for the express purpose of strengthening the national power and of fostering true patriotism'.[26] By 1860 there were more than 160 *Turnvereine* across the globe. Even those who distanced themselves from Jahn's political and religious views saw body training as essential to the goal of a new German. Thus the physician Carl Ignatius Lorinser (a follower of Hufeland) bemoaned in an essay published in 1836 the abandonment of training in the schools for mental strength, 'a harmony and unity which needed to follow the healthy precepts of Juvenal's notion of *mens sana in corpore sano*'.[27] One must stress that education in the gymnasiums was open only to males of a certain class. For women, such training was seen as inappropriate. The American physician and educator Edmund Hammond Clark wrote in his *Sex in Education* (1874): 'Identical education . . . defies the Roman maxim, which physiology has fully justified, *mens sana in corpore sano*. The sustained regimen, regular recitation, erect posture, daily walk, persistent exercise, and unintermitted labor that toughens a boy, and makes a man of him, can only be partially applied to a girl.'[28] Virtually always in the nineteenth century, we are speaking of male posture and male identity.

The exception – and it is not a minor one, as we can see from Clark's comments – is when the question of reproduction arises. One of the mass fantasies driving late nineteenth-century European nationalism is the sense that the nation (whether the English, the German, the French or, indeed, the Jewish) is not reproducing at a rate that would enable the maintenance of national identity. Thus, in a handbook on sex facts for young American women produced by the American Bureau of Social Hygiene, preceding any discussion of reproduction is the admonition that 'proper erect posture is always beneficial and attractive, inspiring grace and ease.'[29] Or, as the educator William D. Lewis writes in an essay on 'The High School and the Girl' in the *Saturday Evening Post*, 'The first thing that society wants of our girl is good health . . . The future of the race so far as she represents it, depends on her health . . . It pays no attention to the curvature of the spine developed by the exclusively sit-at-a-desk-and-study-a-book type of education.'[30] The 'monotonous posture' of factory work, too, deforms the female, as the sexologist Havelock Ellis remarks during the First World War, and makes reproduction difficult: 'After leaving the work for matrimony the deformities caused by the work become apparent . . . Miscarriages occur oftener among factory wives than in the general population.'[31] Good posture makes good citizens, or at least enables them to be conceived.

The question of the healthy body becomes a leitmotif not only of German nationalism but of the very definition of the healthy German male. In his 23rd lecture on politics, held at the University in Berlin over decades and published posthumously in 1897–8, the historian Heinrich von Treitschke defined the role of the army:

> For it is an advantage to a nation when it has a strong and well-organized army, not only because the army is intended to serve as an instrument for foreign policy, but because a noble nation with a glorious history can employ the army for a very long time as a dormant weapon, and because it forms a school for the peculiarly manly virtues of the people, which so easily become lost in an age of profit and enjoyment . . . It is a defect of English civilization that it does not know universal military service.[32]

What was for Jahn a relatively vague and unencumbered concept of military posture comes to be, by the end of the nineteenth century, the very definition of masculinity and nationalism. It is the antithesis of the imagined body of the Jew. Treitschke's highly strung antithesis to the military were the 'Jews who are nothing more than German-speaking Orientals' with their slouching, weak posture.[33] He had recognized the 'complicated historical causes which gave all too easy an explanation of the unmilitarist sentiments of the Jews' in the Prussian state.[34] In his new and united Germany, they constituted a foreign body that could not be assimilated into the new German nation.

Jahn became one of the central figures of the German national pantheon, for good or for ill.[35] Treitschke dismissed him as a 'crank . . . whose buffooneries had sufficed to make him a person of note', yet he was appropriated for a wide range of German national causes.[36] In 1928, in the Weimar Republic, his bust became one of the immortals enshrined in Ludwig I of Bavaria's 'Valhalla' hall of great Germans.[37] But by 1930 he was already being praised as a 'famed National Socialist'.[38] In 1933 Adolf Hitler, following the beginning of the integration of the gymnastics movement into German youth sports activity, spoke publicly about Jahn's role in creating a German national model for education.[39] Posture had clearly become politics. As a rising political force in the early 1920s, Hitler refined his sense of the leader's posture

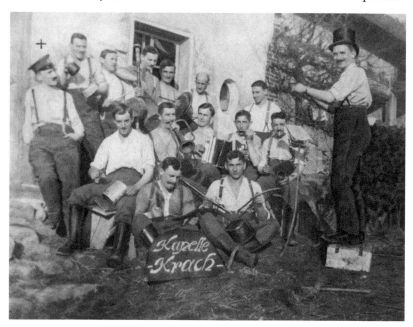

Adolf Hitler slouching in a group portrait of his unit's pop-up band, the 'Noisy Band'. From *Hitler wie Ihn keiner kennt*, ed. Heinrich Hoffmann and Baldur von Schirach (Berlin, [1940]).

by undertaking speaking exercises in front of Heinrich Hoffmann's camera. It is no wonder, since he had been labelled as having 'lazy posture' by Fritz Wiedemann, one of his superiors during the First World War.[40] A leader could not have poor posture.

Jahn's notion of a German nationalism, rooted in the soil of the fatherland and by definition anti-Semitic, was appropriated easily by the National Socialist state, especially by the semi-official state philosopher Alfred Baeumler, who saw in Jahn the shaping of the German body that presaged the theories of the Nazis.[41] Baeumler writes that gymnastics demanded a political orientation, because 'Gymnastic tradition underlies the notion that physical education and sport are not performed by the individual for individual fun, relaxation or prestige, but rather as a national duty in the service of the nation state.'[42] He denies the middle-class origins of gymnastics, since 'German physical activities could not be created from the needs and habits of the bourgeois society. They developed as a result of the political movements of the time of the struggles for liberation and they will be renewed by the political movement of our day.'[43] Only physical education could lend itself to the revival of national unity: 'The principle of physical activities is not a life of beauty, not the wish to keep oneself "healthy and slender", but the fresh happy life in the community of the Volk.'[44]

The opposite was also true. The police, using a model from Imperial Germany, collected specific data about those accused of a crime. During the Nazi period these crimes included violation of the so-called racial laws. The data ranged from specifics of the accused's 'legs and feet; identifying marks; visible ailments; tattoos; build; presence; posture.'[45] The anthropologist Hans F. K. Günther, known at the time as *Rassen Günther* (Race Günther), had published pictures of characteristic Jewish posture in the Weimar Republic. He was one of the scientists who popularized *Rassenkunde* (race science) and the idea of Nordic supremacy, and he was one of the few race scientists to have been a member of the Nazi Party before 1933. He contributed to the new Nazi undertaking of identifying Jews by describing a pathological but 'typical Jewish posture.'[46]

Günther used posture as a sign of racial difference, and he 'believed that the virtues of the Nordic race were expressed in its male body type, with its straight posture, pronounced chest, and small abdomen. This posture (chest out and belly in) was alien to the Eastern man, whose appearance was a negation of the beauty ideal of the Occident.'[47]

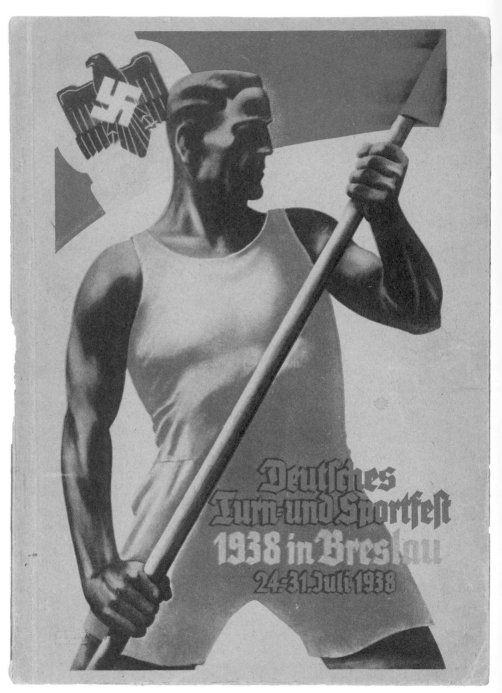

Poster for the National Track and Field Competition in Breslau, 24–31 July 1938. The poster promotes 'Aryan' physical ideals through its depiction of blond, athletic German men.

The military plumb line becomes the standard of male racial beauty. This view became the touchstone for Nazi racial politics in a pragmatic manner. When Heinrich Himmler's 'race office' developed criteria to sort 'racially acceptable' from 'unacceptable' individuals among the occupied nations of Europe after 1941 for inclusion as Aryans, 'erect bearing' trumped all other criteria. As Peter Longreich noted in his biography of Himmler, Himmler would not have been defined as 'racially acceptable', given his poor posture.[48]

Focusing on the centrality of posture in modern nationalist thought in terms of bodily reform, earlier Western claims about posture as defining the quality of the healthy citizen generated a demand to define

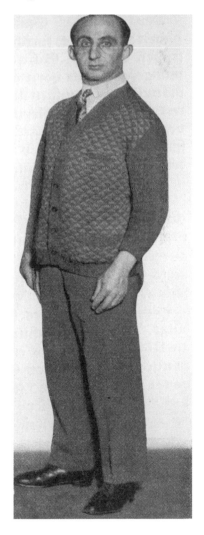

Announcer of a Jewish Wrestling Troup. His Posture Reveals Something Unmistakably 'Jewish'. From Hans Günther, *Rassenkunde des jüdischen Volkes* (Munich, 1930).

and then reform unhealthy posture. If healthy posture could not be inculcated (as in the case of the Jews), then the bright lines defining the national body excluded those with poor posture. The use of military definitions of posture to reinforce retrograde nation-states following the crushing defeat of the 1848 Revolutions in Europe and the Congress of Vienna came to define new revolutionary movements, such as those at the beginning of the twentieth century in Asia.

Chinese Nationalism and Posture

In Asia, 'bad' posture was 'good' posture, since 'Chinese posture also reflects social relationships: rounded shoulders characterize the bow, which is an expression of humility before superiors, and in the case of athletes, also before audiences.'[49] As Western medicine came into China during the nineteenth century, this notion of posture defined the 'sick man of Asia'.[50] Such views had been a staple of Western images of China since the Enlightenment. Kant, Montesquieu and Herder – even the putative advocate of China, Gottfried Wilhelm Leibniz – viewed the 'yellow' race as dangerous, if not backward and corrupt.[51] By 1895, when the notion of the 'Yellow Peril' (*gelbe Gefahr*) was coined in Imperial Germany, evoking the cholera epidemic that decimated Hamburg as well as the racial politics of the global movement of peoples from Asia, the link between China and the risk of disease seemed overdetermined.[52] But being 'sick' in the late nineteenth century was also seen as a reflex of the degenerate culture of late Imperial China: 'Few nations make use of so many compliments as the Chinese. Bowing, kneeling, and prostrating themselves are the different grades of the respect they show towards each other.'[53]

Such social posture quickly came to be a sign of the degeneracy of Chinese culture in the creation of sick bodies:

> The myriads of beggars also go in for voluntary deformation crawling on their knees till they cannot assume an upright posture; welcoming and encouraging an ulcer or a skin disease or a blind eye until the utmost possible deformity and condition of filth are attained. When no better result can be accomplished, something may always be done with paint and plasters, and a very good imitation of the real thing produced.[54]

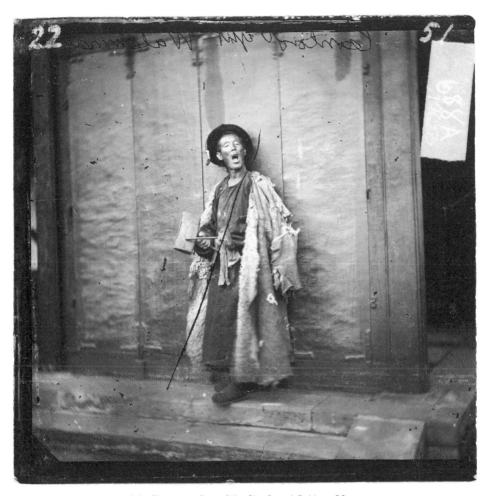

John Thomson, *One of the City Guard, Peking*, 1869.

Degeneracy was the key.[55] Yet it was a socially created degeneracy, and was seen that way at least by the most radical writer of the time, Lu Xun, who wrote in 1918: "'The world is going to the dogs. Men are growing more degenerate every day. The country is faced with ruin!" such laments have been heard in China since time immemorial. But "degeneracy" varies from age to age. It used to mean one thing, now it means another.'[56] What it means is clearly coloured by Western fantasies of disease and posture, which Lu Xun knew exceptionally well, since his major literary work, *A Madman's Diary* (1918), is a fictive case study of madness read through Western medical models. The answer was bodily reform, and that meant the importation of Western, specifically German, forms of postural training. The motto of the China Gymnastic

School in the 1920s was 'Build up the physical strength of the Chinese nation. Wipe away the humiliation of the Sick Man of Asia.'[57]

The notion of the Chinese having defective posture becomes part of the Western clinical portrait of 'mongolism', Down's syndrome, well into the twentieth century. In his monograph of 1924, Francis Graham Crookshank writes of the 'Mongols expatriate':

> we see around us many men and women, not easily or greatly distinguished from their fellows, who would justly resent the epithet of Mongol, and yet do display, in head form, in feature, in proportion, in expression, in posture, or in the morphology of this or that organ or member, some one or more of the *indicia* of racial Mongolism . . . they have certain tendencies to disease, which are best appreciated when the racial tendencies are understood.[58]

The stigmatizing fantasy was that individuals with Down's syndrome were evolutionary throwbacks and represented a 'lower' level of humanity, and that this could be seen in their 'Oriental' posture.

Posture remained tied to the question of pride and confidence, so to 'lift one's head' is not only what the Chinese nation should do metaphorically on the global stage but also what the Chinese people must do literally to march into 'modernity'. Confidence, as with Max Nordau and the Zionists, is tied to notions of pride in a new Chinese body. Being 'spineless' and 'slouching' is not only a problem of the Chinese nation on the political stage, but a problem of the people's bodies. There are scattered references to this kind of argument in journals and magazines of the 1920s (especially in etiquette manuals telling one how to dress, eat, meet and greet, and walk – complete with illustrations – which carry this nationalist rhetoric to varying degrees). Even Zhang Jingsheng, the Shanghai commentator known as 'Dr Sex', touches on the question of sitting/standing up straight in his 'aesthetic utopia'; according to him there is one universal, 'aesthetic' way of sitting or standing that must be adopted by all.[59] There is a counter-discourse to this in the 'modernist' loafer such as Lin Yutang, who observes in his *Importance of Living* (1937) that there is nothing wrong with loafing, lying around – that all this talk of how people should sit, stand and walk is oppressive, enforcing conformity and turning everyone into efficient soldiers and machines with no individual character.[60]

It is hardly surprising that, just as the Jews were reforming their bodies as part of a new national ideology of Jewish identity, revolutionary China came to the same conclusion: reform posture and you reform the system. Social Darwinism entered the country with modernization. Yan Fu was one of the principal figures to introduce Darwin's 'natural selection' to China in the late nineteenth century.[61] Central to this was the notion of adaptability, and posture is fundamental to that idea. Chen Duxiu, the co-founder in 1921 of the Chinese Communist Party, made this idea part of the ideology of Chinese communism, especially in his periodical *New Youth*. In 1915 he complained that

> Whenever I look at our educated youth, I see that they have not the strength to catch a chicken, nor mentally the courage of an ordinary man. With pale faces and slender waists, seductive as young ladies, timorous of cold and chary of heat, weak as invalids – if the people of our country are as feeble as this in body and mind how will they be able to shoulder burdens and go far?[62]

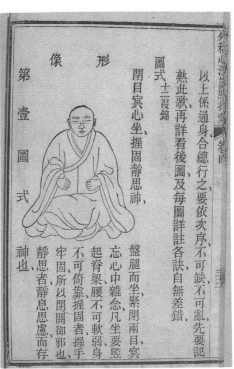

Woodcut from *Waike xinfa zhenyan zhinan* (Guide to Tried and True Methods at the Heart of External Medicine; 1887). It shows the first posture in the practice of the Twelve Brocades of Cultivation, to be performed at the beginning of the session. One must sit cross-legged and straight-backed, without leaning against anything or slouching, with both hands closed into fists and both eyes firmly shut, letting go of distracting thoughts and allowing one's mind to become calm and still.

The noted historian of modern China Frank Dikötter describes how

> A strict upright posture was prescribed to youngsters under the Guomindang's New Life Movement in the 1930s, and today it is still the characteristic way in which young party members are portrayed in communist propaganda . . . After 1900 there was an emphasis on physical training and martial vigour, and this ranged from Luo Zhenyu's recommendation to turn Confucian temples into physical training centres to [Mao Tse-Tung's] writings on physical exercise.[63]

While Mao Tse-Tung's youthful work on combating the degeneracy of Chinese society and the body was at the time truly marginal, it can serve as a model for the arguments about reforming posture that paralleled the Zionist case.[64] His essay 'A Study of Physical Education' (*Tiyu zhi yonjiu*), which appeared under the pseudonym 'Twenty-eight Stroke Student' (*Ershibahua Sheng*), was published in April 1917 (in *Hsin ching-nein*). In it Mao argues, in the model of 'Turnvater' Jahn, that sick minds inhabit sick bodies: 'Those whose bodies are small and frail are flippant in their behaviour. Those whose skin is flabby are soft and dull in will. Thus does the body influence the mind.'[65] And the ill mind of the Chinese is reflected in their politics. Later Mao said to Edgar Snow: 'my mind was a curious mixture of ideas of liberalism, democratic reformism and utopian socialism. I had somewhat vague passions, about "nineteenth century democracy", utopianism and old-fashioned liberalism, and I was definitely anti-militarist and anti-imperialist.'[66] But this was also his practice at the time. He needed to re-create his own body as a revolutionary: 'In the winter holidays, we tramped through the fields, up and down mountains, along city walls, and across the streams and rivers . . . All this went on under the title of "body training".'[67] This essay from 1917 reveals Mao as a Chinese modernizer following the Xinhai Revolution of 1911 that ousted the Qing dynasty and established the Republic of China. That was before his turn to communism as a member of the Marxist study society at Beijing University in 1918.

Yet Mao's argument is very much that of social Darwinism:

> Because man is an animal, movement is most important for him. And because he is a rational animal, his movements must

have a reason. But why is movement deserving of esteem? Why is rational movement deserving of esteem? To say that movement helps in earning a living is trivial. To say that movement protects the nation is lofty. Yet neither is the basic reason. The object of movement is simply to preserve our life and gladden our hearts . . . Physical education not only strengthens the body but also enhances our knowledge. There is a saying: Civilize the mind and make savage the body . . . When the body is perfect, then knowledge is also perfect.[68]

The result is the creation of the upright posture advocated for the military from the seventeenth century onwards: 'Our nation is wanting in strength . . . If our bodies are not strong we will be afraid as soon as we see enemy soldiers, and then how can we attain our goals and make ourselves respected? Strength depends on drill, and drill depends on self-awareness.'[69] The military model is Darwinian but also revolutionary.

The link to the West is made clearly in Mao's text: 'East and West differ in their interpretations of it. Chuang Tzu followed the example of the cook, Confucius drew on the lesson of the archer and the charioteer. In Germany, Physical Education has gained the greatest popularity. Fencing has spread all over the country.'[70] This link has been overlooked because it seems such an offhand remark. Fencing as a popular sport? Rather duelling! And it is duelling that is historically the litmus test in late nineteenth-century Germany for answering the question of Jewish masculinity and identity in bourgeois society. During the nineteenth century Jewish students were automatically admitted to the general fraternity systems in Germany, which were duelling societies. There one learned the rules of social behaviour and physical deportment. Sabre fencing had its own specific posture. Many acculturated Jews, such as Theodor Herzl, 'relished the test and adventure of the duel, the so-called *Mensur*, which was considered manly and edifying'.[71] Students challenged one another to duels as a matter of course, without any real need for insults to be exchanged; being challenged was a process of social selection. 'Without exclusivity – no corporation' was the code of the fraternities as late as 1912.[72] By then, Jews had been expelled from the general fraternity system, and Jewish duelling fraternities sprang up. Being *satisfaktionsfähig* (worthy of satisfaction) meant that members of these fraternities were seen as honourable equals and thus could be challenged to a duel. Marked on the duellist's scarred face and erect posture was his integration into German culture. This was the context in which the Jewish fraternities (most of which did not duel) sought to reconfigure the sickly Jewish body into what Nordau called the 'new muscle Jew'. The Jewish fraternity organization stated in 1902 that 'it desires the physical education of its members in order to collaborate in the physical regeneration of the Jewish people'.[73] For some Jews, a duel and the resulting scars marked the socially healthy individual. Much of this ideology of the body comes to be integrated into the creation of the ideal citizen of the state of Israel. As Oz Almog notes, the ideology of the Sabra has deep roots in a rejection of the image of the Jew in the Diaspora. Some figures, such as the Israeli general Moshe Dayan, become representative of the ideology of the muscle Jew, down to the meaning of his upright posture.[74]

Chinese nationalism was as much in thrall to the waves of postural reform as was political Zionism. Mao, in his essay on physical education, actually cites three sources for the Western as well as Eastern relationship between physical education and the training of the new Chinese body. In a letter to Li Jinxi on 9 December 1916 he wrote, as he would later in his 'Study of Physical Education', that Roosevelt, Sandow and Kano 'have developed mighty bodies out of frail ones'.[75] 'Roosevelt' is clearly Theodore Roosevelt, the apostle of the 'strenuous life' as well as muscular Christianity. For the Chinese he was also the figure whose mediation in the Russo-Japanese war put him on the side of the modernizing revolutionaries. Roosevelt knew that such an approach to the moral and physical education of Americans builds good soldiers. In August 1903 he spoke to the Society of the Holy Name at Oyster Bay, Long Island:

> I should hope to see each man who is a member of this society, from his membership in it become all the fitter to do the rough work of the world; all the fitter to work in time of peace; and if, which may Heaven forfend, war should come, all the fitter to fight in time of war. I desire to see in this country the decent men strong and the strong men decent, and until we get that combination in pretty good shape we are not going to be by any means as successful as we should be.[76]

'Kano' is Kanō Jigorō, the founder of Judo both as a sport and as an ideology. Like Roosevelt, he was a believer in 'Mutual Welfare and Benefit' (自他共栄 *jita kyōei*, the moral training inherent in the practice of sport). It is in Meiji Japan that the German military posture is introduced, including the goose step, but it is also the world in which Nagai Michiakira introduces the '*kiotsuke*' moment, when the teacher enters the classroom and all the students stand at attention with rigid posture.

The third of Mao's sources is the German bodybuilder Eugen Sandow (1867–1925). Sandow was not only a pioneer of modern bodybuilding as a form of the avant-garde *Lebensreform* (reforming life) movement, but as such was an advocate of *mens sana in corpore sano*: 'Yes; you can all become strong if you have the will and use it in the right direction. But, in the first place, you must learn to exercise your mind.'[77] Sandow was early a follower of his fellow Prussian Jahn, training at the *Turnhalle* in Königsberg (Kant's old university town). He credited Jahn as the inspiration for his work.[78] Sandow was one of the first global celebrities in this age of the origin of modern celebrity advertising, and he also employed this new advocacy of bodybuilding within a growing sense of the national body. Yet his aesthetics tended towards the neoclassical. As it had done for Hegel and for William Hogarth before him, the world of classical sculpture, such as the Farnese *Hercules*, gave him a model for a healthy posture (and provided moral cover for his beefcake poses, which were widely enjoyed by Victorian men and women).

For Sandow, who moved to England in the 1890s, it became a force in shaping the British body, especially in the colonial setting. The physician and writer Sir Arthur Conan Doyle, the creator of Sherlock Holmes (perhaps not the best example of a healthy mind in a healthy body), introduced one of Sandow's massive volumes on body training in 1907 by noting,

> The strength of a nation is measured by the sum total of the strength of all the units which form it. It is a truism that anything that raises any portion of a man, his body, his character, his intelligence, increases to that extent the strength of the country to which he belongs. Therefore, since the State is so interested in these matters, it has every reason to examine them and to regulate them.

He then cites the Education Act of 1870, which, according to Conan Doyle, stated that 'we must *force* you to keep yourself in better order.' We now need, he notes, an inspector of bodies, who can accost 'the obvious offender . . . saying to him: "Your back, sir, is too rounded, your chest is too cramped, your knees are too bent. You are not an efficient physical unit of the State."'[79] Posture remains the litmus test by which the good citizen is judged, even at first glance, and is defined as that quality in need of reform.

By 1894 Sandow had starred in a series of bodybuilding films made by the pioneering Edison Studio. Indeed, it has recently been argued that modern yoga practice, so deeply associated with the Indian sub-continent and older Ayurvedic traditions in the West, is the direct result of Sandow's extensive travels and network in British India.[80] Indeed, according to this reading, much of Gandhi's own obsession with bodily reform at the time comes out of this mix. In 1904 Sandow extended his travels into China and Japan, where his work was wide-ly read and very favourably received.[81] His periodical *Physical Culture* reached even wider audiences.

The Chinese had been exposed since the middle of the nineteenth century both to German gymnastics on the model of the *Turnvereine*, using implements such as vaulting horses that mimicked military training, and to Pehr Henrik Ling's system of Swedish gymnastics and body training, modelled on martial arts as well as on military drill.[82]

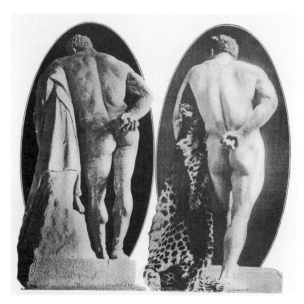

(Left) 'The original Farnese Hercules, to whom the Author has been compared. (Right) The Author in a similar pose. Many say that the Author's proportions are the more symmetrical of the two.' From Eugen Sandow, *Life is Movement; The Physical Reconstruction and Regeneration of the People (A Diseaseless World)* (London, [192?]).

Both systems were present in the Chinese army. In 1879 the Imperial Army under Li Hongzhang had sent seven Chinese officers to the new Germany, where they learned the rudimentary forms of German gymnastics; this was only a precursor to the important role that such systems had in the lead-up to the Revolution of 1911 and the founding of the Republic of China.[83]

But in Sandow, Mao, shortly thereafter, found a system that also argued against the vices of civilization as it then existed.[84] Civilization had not only deformed the natural body but led to rampant immorality, and only rigorous postural training could restore both the healthy body and morality. Sandow wrote:

> All 'Varsity men' will know from their own experience that the moral degenerates among the undergraduates are not to be found among the athletes, and when the subsequent life of the athlete is followed up, it is very rare indeed that he is found among the 'legion of the damned', that ignoble crowd of men, who starting apparently with every advantage, have 'gone under'.[85]

Uprightness in both the spiritual and postural senses of the word defines morality for Sandow: 'We speak of the "upright" man, and the expression can be made to bear a double interpretation, and the erect attitude of the body taken as an illustration of the righteous mind.'[86] The abandonment of morality through civilization is a violation of the 'natural' order, and the only recourse civilized humans have is to postural training:

> The children and savages whom I have used, by way of illustration, have no scientific system of physical exercise, and yet they represent a state of health to which two-thirds of civilized mankind are strangers. So it is clear that health may be enjoyed apart from my system. Only, it must be remembered that children and savages lead a perfectly natural life; plenty of open air and plenty of exercise, and no duties which involved unnatural postures of the body, late hours, or overwork . . . All good things suffer from exaggeration of their virtues.[87]

Sandow's critique of the baneful influence of civilization is echoed in all Mao's comments on physical culture. For Sandow was not an advocate of a 'return to nature' but of alternative forms of postural training that would correct and eliminate the impact of civilization on the national body.

Mao's demand in 1916 was for the ideology, if not the technique, of fencing, so that the Chinese body would become 'real Chinese' and not mere simulacra:

> At present, most people overemphasize knowledge . . . In the educational system of our country, required courses are as thick as the hairs on a cow. Even an adult with a tough, strong body could not stand it let alone those who have not reached adulthood, or those who are weak. Speculating on the intentions of the educators, one is led to wonder whether they did not design such an unwieldy curriculum in order to exhaust the students, to trample on their bodies and ruin their lives . . . How stupid![88]

Mao's view may well have been affected, if indirectly, by the role Zionist thought had in the development of nationalism in Asia. While there was only a marginal presence of Zionist views in China, as the historian of modern China Zhou Xun has argued, it is clear that Nordau's views were widely circulated after 1868 in the modernist reforms of Meiji Japan, where many Chinese thinkers had their first exposure to modernity and ideas of bodily reform. Many of the young revolutionaries had been educated or exiled in Japan, where German officers trained the army and a cult of bodily reform was already present. One of them, Sun Yat-Sen, the physician who led the revolt against the Dowager Empress, wrote in 1919: 'we live in an age of competition. The only way to survive is to defend . . . today we call for the promotion of people's strength. Because this is crucial to national salvation.'[89] The path to the new citizen was through postural reform, and this was understood in terms of training the new citizen as a soldier. The novelist Mao Dun remembered his schooling at the beginning of the twentieth century, in which 'the gymnastic lessons included spear drills, the horizontal bar, "pass the cross-over bridge" and marching. Actually, gymnastic lessons . . . were military training.'[90] This, of course, included only the young men. For young women, the transition to the new revolutionary body took quite another direction of postural reform, the reform of the female gait.

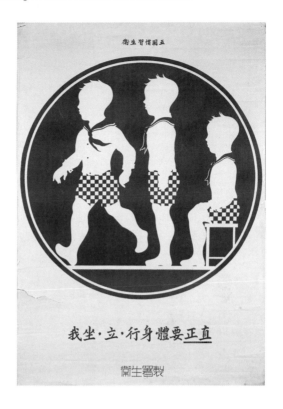

The Department of Health of the Republic of China, c. 1930. The caption states, 'I must keep my body *upright* while sitting, standing and walking.'

衛生習慣圖五

我坐·立·行身體要正直

衛生署製

Part of the struggle for the modern Chinese body had to do with the elimination of the foot-binding that had typified Imperial China, but which was now seen as an antiquated practice to control the bodies of women. In the United States, 'Chinese-American ladies' shoes' led to bad posture. Therefore, bad posture was not the result of foot-binding but of being Chinese: 'The foot is made too small and too high and is displaced forward. Its narrowness makes women unsteady in their gait like the Chinese.'[91] The bound foot causes women to walk 'like the Chinese'. Bad posture is a quality of the Chinese body.

Such views are not marginal in Chinese thought following the Xinhai Revolution that began with the Wuchang Uprising on 10 October 1911 and ended with the abdication of Emperor Puyi on 12 February 1912. By the 1920s the Nationalist government was demanding in its educational system, as had Mao, healthy posture and beautiful children.[92] One pamphlet published by the Republican government's Public Health Bureau teaches children how to stand up straight, how to sit and how to walk. It is headed: 'A good child must have correct posture.' No degenerate bodies; only healthy posture for the new citizens of the new China. Yet these 'beautiful' children, a demand of the eugenics of the time, are not simply Chinese but are the idealized future citizens of the new nation-state.

The Summer Olympic Games in Beijing in 2008 brought out the ongoing link between sports and nationalism in modern China. The People's Republic had bid for both the 1993 and the 2001 Games, but had not been successful. Chinese popular opinion, fuelled by the government's view of China as the perpetual victim of the West,

> felt that China was still treated by the u.s. as a third-rate country. They believed that the West was conspiring to keep China 'from taking its rightful place on the world stage'. When Beijing was awarded the 2008 Summer Olympic Games by the IOC in 2001, tens of thousands of people in China took to the streets to celebrate the success. 'Achieve the century-old dream of the Chinese nation' and 'the great rejuvenation of the Chinese nation' became popular mottos around China.[93]

There was a new fascination in China with sport and posture and with Chinese body culture, which included 'daily practices of health, hygiene, fitness, beauty, dress and decoration; postures, gestures, manners, ways of speaking and eating; ritual, dance, sports, and other kinds of bodily performance' and was heavily indebted to traditional models of Chinese medical culture.[94] The reality, however, is that from the 4 May 1919 movement that finalized the overthrow of the Qing monarchy through to the present, the nationalistic body had already been adapted into this model. Beginning with 4 May, 'anxiety about racial and national decline fueled a new craze among Chinese intellectuals for building the body, framed as collective responsibility. A healthy nation resided in a healthy population, and an advanced society expressed itself in the upright posture of its members.'[95] Pure biological definitions of the body come to be understood within the competing understandings of the Chinese body in the present world:

> Rejecting the vulgar anatomical model as too limited to resonate with the experience of the vast majority of people, it became popular during the 1980s to talk of a 'significant body', of the body inscribed, as an object imbued with cultural meaning. More recently, the body has been described as an

instrument by means of which personal and community identities are reinforced and through which new identities can emerge – through the *habitus* embodied; the regulation of personal regimen, in dress, adornment and, by extension, movement; through its balance, grace, power, precision, posture or gesture.[96]

The new national body in China shaped itself as the body with the best posture, in both biological and political terms. It was an embodiment of nineteenth-century national fantasies, on the left and the right, of the ideal new citizens, upright and forthright in their national identity.

TEN

Contemporary Posture and Disability Studies

OUR CONTEMPORARY IDEA of a 'normal' or normative posture was created during the Enlightenment, even though it evoked earlier Western ideas that had connected 'good' posture with health, beauty and morals – the values that made the good citizen. 'Bad' posture incorporated all the negative qualities: illness, ugliness, immorality and lack of patriotism. The twentieth-century French sociologist Georges Canguilhem noted that this complex shift from the idea of a bodily anomaly to pathology occurred at a very specific moment in the Enlightenment, when, 'between 1759, when the word "normal" appeared, and 1834 when the word "normalized" appeared, a normative class had won the power to identify – a beautiful example of ideological illusion – the function of social norms, whose content it determined, with the use that that class made of them.'[1] This is certainly in line with our sense that it is in the early Enlightenment, in the late seventeenth century, with the rise of a normative definition of posture defining a wide range of human activities, that posture begins to define the essence of what it means to be (or become) human. Canguilhem explores this 'within a sociological critique of normalizing social control'.[2] It is within this modern idea of social control of the body that the concept of disability arises. Social control of posture makes the idea of a 'normal' posture possible, but also postural disability comes to represent the very concept of the disabled.

By the twentieth century posture – which, as we have seen, includes uprightness, gait and mobility – had come to mark the image of disability. The classical Enlightenment categories that defined disability, the blind and the deaf, represented disability within the greater society; from the teacher of the blind, Louis Braille, to the symbol of mid-century American disability, the blind and deaf Helen Keller, disabled icons were the public image of disability.[3] Both these figures appeared on postage stamps across the world in the twentieth century. It was only in 1960, coincident with the opening of the 8th World Congress of the International Society for the Welfare of Cripples (now Rehabilitation International) in New York, that the United States issued a stamp showing a man in a wheelchair operating a drill press. The stamp, designed by Carl Bobertz, was intended to promote the employment of the physically handicapped and publicize the congress.

What disability is comes to be defined at this same juncture. The World Health Organization (WHO), in its *International Classification of Impairments, Disabilities, and Handicaps* (1980), made a seemingly clear distinction between impairment, disability and handicap. Impairment is an abnormality of structure or function at the organic level, while disability is the functional consequence of such impairment. A handicap is the social consequence of impairment and its resultant disability. Thus, cognitive or hearing impairments may lead to communication problems (disability), which in turn result in isolation or dependency (handicap). Such a functional approach (and this approach became the norm in American common and legal usage) seemed to be beyond any ideological bias. Yet it demanded a static notion of the world in which those with all functional impairments, visible or invisible, could never be completely accommodated within the same parameters as those without such functional impairment. Thus special schools for the blind and the deaf were created to provide accommodation outside the realm of the public school systems designed for children without such functional impairments. As with racial segregation in the United States before *Brown v. The Board of Education* (1953), 'separate' education was never truly 'equal'.

We can bracket for the moment the problems raised by the history of *mens sana in corpore sano*. For this tradition immediately visualized a healthy body, as defined by an erect, often male posture. When you imagine healthy minds linked to healthy bodies, what problems does this present for the visualization of disability as an abstraction? What icons represent the world of interiority, that of the developmentally or emotionally different? Many years ago I asked this question about the proliferation of 'ribbons' from the original red ribbon for HIV/AIDS and found no comfortable solution to this process of the visualization of the invisible.[4]

Such a visualization of the healthy body comes to be a reflex of the modern nation-state. A leading disability theorist, Lennard Davis, takes Benedict Anderson's thesis that 'language and normalcy come together under the rubric of nationalism' one step further: not only did language have to be standardized and normalized to create the modern nation-state, but bodies had to undergo the same treatment. Statistical reasoning, arising in the course of the nineteenth century and dominating both biological science and the new field of actuarial evaluation, then became the state's tool to enforce bodily norms: the concept of the bell curve encouraged people 'to strive to be normal, to huddle under the main part of the curve.'[5] The disabled body came to be defined as that of the individual who could never be included in the body politic: 'The crucial point taken from disability studies is that the inability to become a subject is not, in itself, a property of problem bodies. It is a property of exclusionary social and material organization.'[6] If the problem is the creation of the healthy citizen as an abstraction, then it is in the nation-state that some form of relief is to be found.

The most recent rethinking of disability draws this assumption into question and redefines disability on a scale of 'human variability' that understands the difficulties facing the disabled as resulting from the inflexibility of social institutions rather than from impairment. Such reconsideration formed the core of a new discipline: Disability Studies. Disability Studies had its roots in the idea of the pathological as defined within rehabilitation medicine and social work, but had come to be a part of the humanities by the twenty-first century. In 1986 the Section for the Study of Chronic Illness, Impairment, and Disability of the Social Science Association became the Society for Disability Studies. But as this field coalesced, the very definition of disability was being altered. Even with the passing of the Americans with Disabilities Act of 1990 and the United Nations Convention on the Rights of People with Disabilities of 2007, the WHO model of disability as 'impairment, restriction, dysfunctionality [and] abnormality' remained strongly in place.[7] Such views are radically rethought with the rise of Disability Studies in the academy. One of the creators of the field, Rosemarie Garland-Thomson, sees 'disability as a way of being in an environment' produced by the 'discrepancy between body and world, between that which is expected and that which is.'[8] Not only is disability the disjuncture between the world and the individual, but since all who age become disabled, 'disability is thus inherent in our being: What we call disability is perhaps the essential characteristic of being human.'[9] The 'ableist' view is centred in normality and understands disability as deviance or 'Other'. Garland-Thomson helpfully reversed this logic by defining the category of the 'normate' as merely labelling those defined as healthy and beautiful within specific historical bio-cultural norms.[10] Thus 'the disabled body' is truly a 'minority body', a 'merely different' body, rather than a pathological or defective body. 'Being disabled is primarily a social phenomenon – a way of being a minority, a way of facing social oppression, but not a way of being inherently or intrinsically worse off.'[11] Here the connection to other marginalized bodies discussed in this volume, from that of the civilian to that of the Jew, can be seen.

Thus the debate entered into by Erving Goffman in the 1960s about the stigmatization of all difference is joined through Disability Studies as a discipline to the societal obligation to include such differences by expanding its understanding of what makes a competent citizen. What Goffman had seen as the internalization of a 'spoiled' identity as defined by society's drive for 'normalcy', here on the part of the disabled, comes to be understood not as a 'special kind of relationship between attribute [condition] and stereotype', but as a clearly drawn antithesis between the experienced reality of each.[12] As Goffman noted, society 'expects the cripple to be crippled'.[13] He stressed that being seen as disabled defined one's 'spoiled' identity for oneself as well as for the world. Being 'crippled' is for Goffman one of the most salient categories of stigma, and he illustrates early on the effect of being perceived as belonging to such a category through a selection of extracts about disability defined as being 'crippled'. Thus he quotes a 'multiple sclerotic': 'Both healthy minds and healthy bodies may be crippled. The fact that "normal" people can get around, can see, can hear, doesn't mean that they are seeing or hearing. They can be very blind to the things that spoil their happiness, very deaf to the pleas of others for kindness; when I think of them I do not feel any more crippled or disabled than they.'[14] The argument now is that these very categories perpetuate the social isolation and stigma of those who are differently abled, but that such individuals also have an autonomous manner of dealing with the external world through their own disability perspective, defined more and more as postural disability.

Goffman offers the autobiographical account of a 'one-legged girl', whose wheelchair is seen to define her being:

> Whenever I fell, out swarmed the women in droves, clucking and fretting like a bunch of bereft mother hens . . . they assumed that no routine hazard to skating – no stick or stone – upset my flying wheels. It was a foregone conclusion that I fell because I was a poor, helpless cripple. Not one of them shouted with outrage, 'That dangerous wild bronco threw her!' – which, God forgive, he did technically. It was like a horrible ghostly visitation of my old roller-skating days. All the good people lamented in chorus, 'That poor, poor girl fell off!'[15]

The operative image in this anecdote is of being seen in the wheelchair as dependent and passive. The wheelchair defines the stigma attendant to the social stigma of disability. Goffman warns that the simple identification with the stigmatized does not suffice to undermine the power of such images; 'children stare', as he explains, at the physically different. Garland-Thomson will much later take this act of seeing difference as a form of empowerment of the disabled.[16] For Goffman it is the core moment of stigmatization.

The Wheelchair as the Icon of Postural Disability

Mapping postural concerns on to these shifting meanings, emphases and disciplines defining disability, we come to see the primacy of posture in much of the post-WHO evolution of public debates about disability, whether stated or not. While the traditional disabilities were crucial to the Enlightenment push for the creation of separate special educational institutions for the blind and the deaf, postural disabilities, exemplified by the icon of the wheelchair, have now become markers of 'access', 'integration' and 'flexibility'.[17] The wheelchair is a postural icon in the broadest sense: it represents an altered form of the upright body, an altered form of gait (or its compensation), as well as a radically visible, as opposed to an invisible, disability, such as deafness or blindness. It is also materially defined by the environment in a manner that the traditional disabilities are not.

Today it is the act of 'conceptualizing the environment' that comes to be 'crucial to the politics of disability research in delineating issues of access, a crucial dimension of a *socio-spatial model* of disability'.[18] Access, while seemingly a blanket term covering all disabilities, is a metaphor taken from the world of the wheelchair.[19] Paraplegia or other forms of disabled gait that require the use of a wheelchair are imagined rarely as postural disabilities, but instead as disabilities of mobility. It is true, as the quadriplegic anthropologist Robert Murphy notes, that a wheelchair 'cannot be hidden' because 'it is brutally visible.'[20] Yet its presence does not distinguish between those who use a wheelchair because of a transitory inability and those who have a previous, existing disability: 'And, indeed, using a wheelchair will eliminate one of the substantial difficulties (problems and pain when walking) of their original disability.'[21] Thus the wheelchair seems to become an icon of postural mobility limited only by the built environment, rather than answering the claim of the wheelchair as a harbinger of postural deficiency. The stigma we have seen associated with postural difference (as Goffman noted) is surpressed when the wheelchair is reduced to an icon representing all disabilities, visible or not, and no longer specifically references postural disabilities.

In what is both an early statement about the nature of disability and a comment on human difference, Tobin Siebers, then professor of English, Art and Design at the University of Michigan and a major disability theorist, reflected on how disability can be seen. Siebers observed in 1998 in a personal essay called 'My Withered Limb':

> To be crippled in America is not the American way. In a country where image is everything, it is hard to find an example for growing up crippled and hardly worth it when you do. The icon of the cripple is the paralytic, a double edge sword, but we desire role models all the same. They tried to make one of FDR last year, setting him in stone upon his wheelchair, condemning him to a double immobility. A wheelchair made of stone is an interesting object for any paralyzed person to contemplate.[22]

The 'cripple', then, is our modern image of the disabled according to Siebers, who was affected by his 'withered limb', caused by 'poliomyelitis [that] struck during my second year of life'. He wrote: 'I am the luckiest in my acquaintance – lungs intact, no arms affected, one leg not two – except for everyone in my acquaintance who was not struck down.'[23] Here, gait and its infirmities point to an impairment of posture.

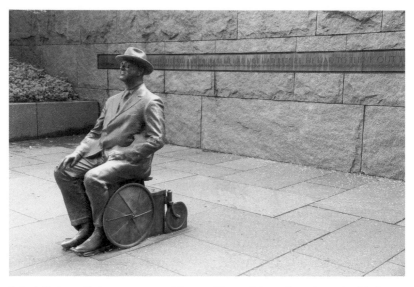

Robert Graham, *Prologue*, 2001, cast bronze. The sculpture of FDR in a wheelchair near the entrance of the Franklin Delano Roosevelt Memorial in Washington, DC, was added in January 2010. On a wall behind the figure is a 12-metre-long bronze bas-relief quotation by Eleanor Roosevelt: 'Franklin's illness gave him strength and courage he had not had before. He had to think out the fundamentals of living and learn the greatest of all lessons – infinite patience and never-ending persistence.'

How engrained this notion of exemplary disabilities is in the first half of the twentieth century can be judged by the National Assistance Act passed by the British Parliament in 1948. Clement Attlee's new Labour government, having swept the Conservatives and Winston Churchill from office in 1945, began a radical rethinking of the role of the state in the lives of those marginalized by society. The Act abolished the so-called Poor Laws first established by Elizabeth I to deal with the indigent and unemployed. The Victorian workhouse was exemplary of the moralizing attitudes towards the poor under this regime. The new social service network established by the National Assistance Act covered for the first time, among other classes, 'the handicapped'. Section 29 (1) of the Act mandated that the county and borough councils promote the welfare of the handicapped. Three categories define what the law understands under handicapped: 1) the blind and partially sighted; 2) the deaf or dumb, including the hard of hearing; and 3) the 'general classes of the handicapped', that is, everyone else. By the 1960s this image of the iconic disabled had begun to shift.

For Siebers and his generation, raised in the 1960s, it was the invisible wheelchair of Franklin Delano Roosevelt that was the mirror in which they saw themselves.[24] The American poet David Citino reflected on how the absence of any image of FDR's wheelchair in the public sphere forced him to deal with his own disability: 'America, thanks to a conspiracy of reporters and photog[rapher]s, saw him only from the waist up. My parents . . . weren't ready to march up a steep slope behind a lame leader.' This presence of an absence, the wheelchair never seen, is now read not as a sign of the strong military leader but as a reflection of Citino's own new state, the transfiguration of the poet into the use of the wheelchair:

> The polio that sat you down is gone. But here's another sneak attack. Doctors are saying MS to me, reading my lesions on the MRI. My legs move to strange music. I grip a cane to straighten my spine. How long before I sit in my own chair? The doctors don't know, but the state of Ohio labels me Disabled, issues me papers stamped H for Handicapped. I've been conscripted. I won't be alone, I know. We're mobilizing, an army ready to roll, to follow our leader out over shining fields of the republic to do what needs to be done.[25]

Being 'mobile' now reads as a new sign of action, of the mobilization into the new army of the disabled.

Germany's Icon of Disability

The newest 'sign' of disability comes to be the wheelchair, a material icon of mobility that is simultaneously a silent sign of postural disability. It is now called the International Symbol of Access (ISA), an international standard maintained by a committee of Rehabilitation International, which (in spite of the icon's ubiquity) owns its copyright. Not the 'three black dots' armband worn on the left upper arm so familiar in Germany from the Weimar Republic, nor indeed other potential icons of visible disability, defines the new discourse, but rather the wheelchair, an icon of posture.

The yellow armband with three black dots came to mark all those with disabilities in the German-speaking lands after the First World War. The symbol of three black dots on a yellow background had begun as a traffic sign during the war, forbidding entrance into an otherwise accessible space. In 1919 the reformer Konrad Plath attempted to appropriate the icon as an armband or pennant for the deaf and hard of hearing. It was quickly appropriated in a slightly different configuration by the blind. At first an inverted triangle was used to represent the deaf or hearing-impaired. As an upright triangle it came to signify a sightless or visually impaired person. The yellow armband made visible these classically invisible disabilities in a world more and more inhabited by the war wounded, with their mostly visible disabilities. They were ubiquitous, begging on the streets; by the end of 1918, as Evelyn Blücher noted in her diary, 'all the blind, the halt, the lame of Prussia seemed to have collected' in Berlin.[26] Over time the icon slowly took on the quality of identifying the disabled, whether war wounded or not. While present in the Weimar Republic, its status was heightened by state action in the Third Reich, a world in which disability came to have many contradictory meanings.

The situation of the icon for disability from the Weimar Republic to the Third Reich is a classic case of the complexity of mid-twentieth-century disability iconography.[27] The Germans on the home front were in no way prepared for the devastating loss of the First World War, believing to the last month that they were winning the war, and thus were forced to come to terms not only with a lost cause but with an overwhelming number of severely wounded ex-soldiers. They came, in work by such left-wing artists as George Grosz, Otto Dix and Max Beckmann during the Weimar Republic, to represent visually the futile nature of the war itself.[28] In 1919 Beckmann published a series of lithographs entitled *Hell*, in which the second, *The Street*, showed a blind man and an amputee in a wheelchair in a chaotic street scene echoing the result of the war's sudden end. Dix, in his *Men Playing the Card Game Skat* (1920), presents three badly disabled officers – so badly disabled that, as the disability historian Carole Poore notes, they could hardly have survived their wounds, but remain recognizable as

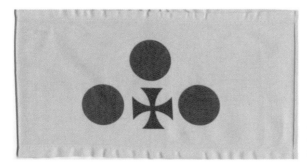

An armband for the blind war wounded with an 'Iron Cross', *c.* 1940.

German officers by their otherwise rigid posture and their chests full of medals. Dix's cynical representation of 'pompous military bearing' only highlighted the horrors that they had experienced.²⁹ But this stance is not merely one of pacifism, for the struggle against the war came to be defined by how one imagined the cause of the war: on the left, it was unbridled capitalism and the forces of imperial reaction; on the right, the betrayal of the nation by the left (who called forth various instantiations of the Republic on 9 November 1918) and the Jews. Thus disability becomes one with the struggle for political domination between left and right during the Weimar Republic. The politics of disability mirror the politics of the street. It is important that while visual and literary representations of disability haunted the arts after 1919, it was the damaged bodies of the soldiers that were seen as the image of this struggle.

Slowly, after 1919, the three black dots, more than wheelchairs or crutches or white canes, come to represent this struggle. In a little-known charcoal drawing from 1921, *Blind Man Crossing the Street*, the expressionist artist Albert Birkle presented 'a blind war veteran . . . pitted against a sea of roaring automobiles. Still clad in remnants of an army uniform, he wears the armband with three black circles that identified him as blind . . . The helpless soldier is articulated in fragile, white, attenuated forms against the massive black machines, the headlights of which oddly echo the dot pattern on the blind man's band.' Birkle's work is meant to evoke compassion: 'That the handicapped veteran has lost his eyesight for the cause of a country that now neglects his needs stresses the cruelty of his fate and indicts the society of which he is a discarded, powerless victim.'³⁰ (Birkle, as with some artists on the left who remained in Germany, found himself unable to work in the Nazi state. His work was officially removed from the Haus der Kunst in Munich on Hitler's orders.) The armband represents more than any other icon the abstraction of disability in the interwar period. By 1926 it featured in the public images of capitalist exploitation in leaflets by the Communist Party of Germany in its political attacks against the forces of the right. This abstraction surfaced in the world where being disabled had become a more and more clearly defined category of identity.

The reformer Otto Perl created the Selbsthilfebund der Körperbe-hinderten (League for the Advancement of Self-help for the Physically Handicapped; 1919–31) for these wounded veterans as well as for all

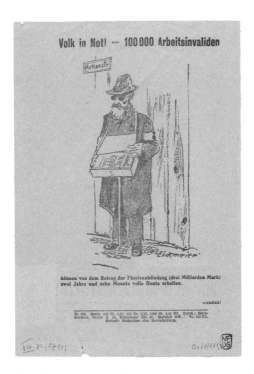

Peter Paul Eickmeier, *A People in Distress – 100,000 Invalids Unable to Work*, 20 June 1926. Poster from the Communist Party of Germany (KPD) in favour of the referendum to expropriate the property of the former ruling houses of the various German states, as well as the Imperial Hohenzollern family.

disabled. In 1926, after moving to an institute for special education in Nuremberg, Perl published *Krüppeltum und Gesellschaft im Wandel der Zeit* (Crippledom and Society Through the Ages), in which he fought against the institutionalization of the disabled and demanded the right to self-determination. He limited his demand for education and job training to the 'mentally normal' but physically handicapped person, in contrast to the disabled, who were 'mentally handicapped'. The year after the Nazis came to power in January 1933, he lobbied that the term *Krüppel* (cripple) should be replaced in official documents by the less stigmatizing *Körperbehinderte* (physically handicapped). How this specific category, that of the physically disabled, figured in the symbolic world of National Socialism is part of the tale of today's wheelchair icon.

By 1935 Perl, now closely following official state policy, had demanded the separation of the 'mentally sound' from the 'mentally degenerate', and unmistakably applauded the National Socialists for their measures to control hereditary biological problems. The key to his thinking seemed to be whether a disability, other than intellectual disability, was inherited or not. Thus when the teachers at the Berlin-Steglitz State School for the Blind petitioned as early as 1933 for the inclusion of the 'sightless' in the official state youth organizations, the question was raised as to the cause of the students' blindness. One of the teachers at Steglitz, Hellmuth Söllinger, an *SA-Mann* as early as 1928, was the singular force behind this movement to include those who were not *congenitally* blind in the Hitler Youth (Hitler-Jugend). This was the Nazi Party youth organization (begun in 1922) that was divided into the HJ (Hitler Youth) for boys and the BDM (Organization of German Girls) for teenage girls, with sections for pre-teen boys (*Jungvolk*) and girls (*Jungmädel*).

Immediately after the Nazis' seizure of power, in February 1933, a Hitler Youth group of 'genetically sound' (*erbgesund*) students had been created at Steglitz.[31] In 1934 Eduard Bechthold, director of the Institute for the Blind in Halle and a member of the Nazi Party, created a 'special section HJ-B' (*Sonderbann* HJ-B) for his 'genetically sound' blind students. The teacher Franz Bögge at Steglitz was its head and incorporated students of all ages, boys and girls. In December 1933 the periodical of the blind group, *Weckruf: Mitteilungsblatt für die Hitler-Jugend aller deutschen Blindenanstalten* (Awake! The Official Newsletter for the Hitler Youth in All German Schools for the Blind), was founded. Published in Braille, it had to be translated into print to pass party censorship. By 1934 it had become the official publication of the Reichs-jugendführung für die blinde Hitlerjugend (State Youth Organization for the Blind Hitler Youth). Thus all the accoutrements of the Hitler

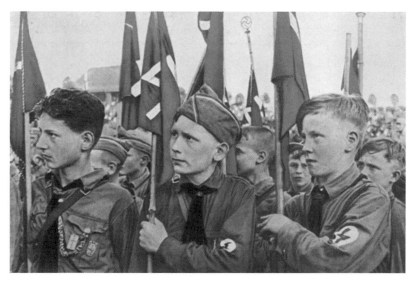

This is Germany's Future. The idealized Nazi Youth in a postcard from 1936.

Youth were present. All blind students admitted to this special group wore the standard HJ uniform, augmented by a yellow armband with three dots.[32] The HJ insignia signalled the inclusion of the students in the body politic; the armband signified their difference.

And different they were. For the Nazis had in July 1933 begun advocating and then officially sanctioning sterilization of the disabled with the 'Law for the Prevention of Hereditarily Diseased Offspring'. On 28 June 1933 the Nazi Minister of the Interior, Wilhelm Fricke, gave a speech lumping all 'defectives', from the mentally ill to the physically disabled, including those who were 'genetically sound', with those who had inherited their disability. The journal of the Reich League of the Physically Handicapped (Reichsbund der Körperbehinderten), *Der Körperbehinderte* (The Physically Handicapped), was full of discussions about the capacity of the healthy physically handicapped to function as valuable citizens of the new order.[33] By 1942 the only real question asked by the Nazi regime was how such individuals would be kept from reproducing, and the answer was clear: 'It is entirely irrelevant whether the elimination occurs by way of sterilization or celibacy, by death, or however it may be brought about.'[34] Such sterilization measures were even folded into the so-called Wannsee Protocol of January 1942, which outlined the elimination of European Jewry. Forced sterilization would be undertaken of any individual with Jewish ancestry; all others would be killed.

The so-called Hitler Youth Law, passed on 1 December 1936, amalgamated all youth groups in Germany under the single banner of the new unified state group, the Hitler Youth, which to that moment had been the official organization of the Nazi Party. It outlawed all other organizations, from the Boy Scouts to the various youth groups of the now forbidden political parties. Soon physically disabled children who were 'genetically sound' were allowed to join a special section called the 'Disabled and Infirm Hitler Youth', so long as they passed the eugenic and – of course – racial tests. Blind and deaf children were welcomed as well, provided their disability was not inherited and they did not have Jewish ancestry. Developmentally challenged children were not allowed to join the Hitler Youth, even if their parents were loyal party members and they were understood as 'genetically sound'.[35] Exempt from intensive sport competition and paramilitary training, the disabled Hitler Youth were trained in office skills and carpentry.[36] Thus the Hitler Youth groups 'G' (*Gehörlose und Taubstumme*, deaf and mute) and 'K' (*Körperbehinderte*, physically disabled) were created. In 1936 the hard of hearing were able to join the deaf and the mute, and this group was relabelled hearing-impaired (*Gehörgeschädigte*). But, and this is a vital moment in the state organization of the image of the disabled, the youth organization for the physically disabled was disbanded that same year, as its members' external appearance was held not to be helpful (*dienlich*) for the Hitler Youth.[37] Disabilities that were invisible but could be made visible through icons such as the three-dot armband were acceptable (within those limits noted); those marked by wheelchairs and crutches were permanently seen as different and thus excluded. The wheelchair became a sign of exclusion.

Young people, no matter what their status, had to have a healthy eugenic inheritance to be members of Nazi society, unless they were too visible as disabled. This was stressed in a letter to deaf congregants from the Reich Union of Pastors of the Protestant Deaf:

> The authorities have ordered that whoever is hereditarily diseased shall have no more children in the future, for our German fatherland needs healthy and sound persons . . . And you, dear friend, you are afflicted with deafness. How burdensome it is! . . . Now this is where the authorities want to help you. They want to protect you from transmitting your affliction . . . obey the authorities. Obey even when it is difficult for you. We know that all things turn out for the best for those who love God.[38]

How random the inclusion and exclusion in such programmes was cannot be stressed enough. 'Genetically sound' deaf and blind youth were involuntarily sterilized. When the so-called T4 action, mandated by Hitler in 1939 to murder the disabled, was undertaken, five blind children from the Frankfurt Institute of the Blind with no other disabilities were murdered at the psychiatric hospital at Hadamar, along with many other children with multiple disabilities. The old eugenic argument was augmented by an economic one: these people were drains on the German economy. The disabled were to be removed from society, since they could never truly contribute to it either genetically or economically.

The identical argument was used to remove Jews (as defined by the Nazis) from the body politic. Race clearly played a constant role among the disabled in the Third Reich. Laws limiting access to state structures of all types began with the Nazi seizure of power and continued in ever more detail throughout the 1930s. The 'Aryan paragraph' was introduced at a meeting of the Union of Blind Academics of Germany in July 1933. Its chairman, Carl Strehl, expressed his willingness to go along with the decision to exclude Jews from the union as follows: 'For the UBAG it was a matter of course that we would align ourselves with the fundamental principles of the new National Socialist government and carry them out as they related to the union's day-to-day activities.'[39] In the same year the organization of blind veterans excluded all Jewish members: 'Members of foreign races cannot hold any positions of authority or leadership in state government, and they must be kept out of the teaching profession.'[40] Jews were systematically excluded or marginalized in educational institutions for the blind and disabled along with the mentally disadvantaged and socially unacceptable, the official designation of individuals seen as misfits because of their criminal record or addictive behaviour.[41] The Jewish disabled were limited to special institutions and schools for Jews, such as the blind Oscar Weidt's Berlin Workshop for the Jewish Blind and the Hebrew Institute for Deaf-mutes, also known as the Israelite Institute for the Deaf in Berlin-Weissensee. Felix Reich, who had been the director of the school, was sent to the Sachsenhausen concentration camp in 1939. When he was released he fled with eleven of the children in his care on the *Kindertransport* to London. The 146 deaf Jewish students remaining were deported in 1942 and murdered.

The exemplary status of the 'acceptable' disabled demanded that they be 'healthy' members of society, even with their disability. In 1938 about 15 per cent of all the members of all Nazi youth organizations were evaluated as not being healthy enough to belong, so the criteria for the disabled were seen to be the same as for all other youth.[42] Being healthy became one of the mantras for the disabled. If the three-dot armband signified the minimal acceptance of the blind Hitler Youth as a member of civil society, it was no small result of the exemplary status of the blind in the Third Reich. The model disabled person in the Third Reich was, to no one's surprise, Adolf Hitler. Peter Plein, one of the leaders of the organization of blind veterans (Verband der Kriegsblinde), wrote:

> It is we, the blinded German veterans, who look to Reich Chancellor Adolf Hitler with particular trust; for, since he

was deprived of his eyesight for several weeks because of a gas-related injury during that critical November of 1918, he, like no one else, will know how to show his appreciation for the heavy sacrifice that we blinded veterans have made for the fatherland, a sacrifice which we must bear for the rest of our lives.[43]

Hitler, who had become the visual icon of the Nazi movement well before 1933 through the publication of highly selected photographs, also came to represent the disabled as now included in the 'healthy' Aryan body politic.[44] By 31 December 1933 the now 2,884-strong League of Blinded Veterans had thrown out seventeen of its members because of their non-Aryan origin. Thereafter, all the private organizations were either closed or merged into state groups, such as the Reich Union of the Deaf of Germany (Reichsverband der Gehörlosen Deutschlands), founded in 1927, which became the Nationalsozialistischen Reichsverbands der Gehörlosen Deutschlands. Its more than 3,900 members largely sympathized with the Nazis after 1933. In 1934 the organization, led by Fritz Albreghs, spontaneously excluded all deaf Jews. The Jewish disabled could in no way meet the expectations of the ideology of that exemplary disabled leader Adolf Hitler.

In 1937, with the war effort ramping up, the government seemed to advocate for the integration of the handicapped into the economy.[45] Indeed, the law of 1935 guaranteeing the special education of people with disabilities, in which the demand for 'race hygiene' was writ large, also stated that the purpose of the schools was to assure this productive economic integration. Beginning in 1937, *Der Körperbehinderte* evoked the slogan: 'Handicaps do not handicap!' and reported on disabled workers, 'including one who had learned to do all her housework from her wheelchair and another who used a wheelchair due to polio and was now an office worker. After the war began, the emphasis shifted to those described as "fighters on the home front", who were sent to work in the armaments industry.'[46] Yet the reality was very different.

The National Socialist People's Welfare organization, into which the Weimar organization founded by Perl had been forcibly integrated, continued to demand a reduction of economic support for the disabled, and insisted that they support themselves and their families. One must note the duplicitous narrative here concerning wheelchair users and the very idea of disability under the Nazis: the importance was to make the 'useless eaters' – the term used by Nazi eugenicists about the disabled – an integrated, 'productive' part of the economy. Become 'valuable' and you are a member of civic society. This is, of course, the lie that underpinned the ghastly gates at Dachau, Sachsenhausen and Auschwitz, emblazoned with the words 'Work will set you free!' (*Arbeit macht Frei!*). Nazi ideology argued that Jews, the Sinti and Roma, the disabled and the socially unacceptable were all shirkers. Such lies underpinned the exploitation of Jewish workers in the sweatshops in the ghettos such as Łódź, but their forced productivity in no way slowed their murder in the death camps. The claim was that the Jews, like the disabled, were 'parasites' on the body of the state. The high rate of death in the ghettos, the continued deportations from the ghettos to the death camps, and the eugenic frenzy of first sterilization and then the euthanasia of the disabled undertaken under the T4 plan vitiated any claim of achieving 'value' in such a society. The claims that such value was needed were linked to the ramping up of the war effort and then, after 1 September 1939, to the war itself. Hitler actually backdated his orders to euthanize the disabled to the first day of the war as a sign of their uselessness to his understanding of civil society. Indeed, the euthanasia continued during the war, even after public demonstrations against it organized by Bishop August von Galen in 1941 forced the Nazis to be more circumspect about their murders. Claiming to be valuable to the state did not outweigh the sense of vulnerability of the disabled.

Most striking in this complex ambivalence about disability in the Third Reich and its visualization is the question of the icon of disability. An effort was organized to forbid blind Jews to wear the yellow-and-black armband for the disabled, but this move was rejected on 13 July 1942, well after the compulsory icon of the Yellow Star had been introduced for Jews, in September 1941. In the concentration camp at Buchenwald, blind inmates were marked by an armband with a triangle in yellow with the ubiquitous three dots in a second triangle.[47] Deaf, blind and posturally disabled Jews were still required to wear the armbands for the disabled, because 'the protection of other road-users' was 'of primary importance': 'The truck-driver, bicyclist, etc., must acknowledge and take into account the sensory disturbance (deafness, blindness) or motor impairment of a person wearing this form of identification and must behave accordingly.'[48] The highly visible armband protected the observer against the disabled Jews' presence. By this point in the early 1940s there is no question that the yellow and black armbands signified all disabilities, including those of mobility and posture, even though the function representing the classic disabilities of blindness and deafness still dominated.

The three dots continue after the war as a sign of disability in both German states. In the novelist and activist Kay Boyle's fictive memoir of immediate post-war Germany, the protagonist sits on a train and sees 'the cane between the young man's legs, and the yellow brassard, marked with three dots, upon his sleeve'.[49] Boyle takes this almost as a fulfilment of her Cassandra-like prophecy in 1936, when she warned in her novel *Death of a Man* of the growing international danger of Nazi Germany. Her protagonist immediately thinks, 'with some emotion that he could not name (bitterness, irritation, it may have been) [,] that an entire division of men must have been blinded at the Russian front'. This was the ubiquitous sign of the war, the destruction of Germany by the Nazis,

> the blind were everywhere; they sat in every streetcar, in every train, in every university hall . . . even had they not carried canes and worn the yellow armbands, and even before the scarlet, empty button-holes of the eye sockets could be perceived, they were marked by their excessive cleanliness, their well-brushed clothing, their well-shined shoes, the hair so neatly trimmed and combed . . . [T]he absence of vision making them, forever children for women to dress, and comb, and need, and bathe in the warm fluid of their love.[50]

The yellow armband comes to be an icon for the dependent good Germans, clean, prosperous, but blinded to the reality of what had transpired, echoing the post-war German novelist Wolfgang Borchert, who supplied Boyle with the title for the novel.

The yellow armband with the three black dots seems ubiquitous among Borchert's contemporaries in immediately post-Second World War German literature. In the Austrian novelist Ingeborg Bachmann's controversial speech 'Ein Ort für Zufälle' (A Place for Coincidences), given in Berlin when she accepted the Georg Büchner prize in 1964, they appear to signal the world into which the inhabitants are now thrust, a world of many war wounded.[51] The narrator stands at the S-Bahn station Bellevue ('beautiful vista'), where the president of West

Germany has his mansion, and observes as the multitude of broken, crippled individuals spill out into the light with their white canes and their yellow armbands with black circles. It is a world, however, that – while overrun with such icons – seems not really to see the people attached to them. In the Swiss novelist Max Frisch's *Mein Name sei Gantenbein* (Let's Assume My Name is Gantenbein; translated as *A Wilderness of Mirrors*; 1964), perhaps they even include the narrator, who assumes new identities one after another beginning with that of Theo Gantenbein, a sighted person taking the role of a blind man wearing the yellow armband.[52] 'Even a blind man, he ought to have seen, is a member of society. Without the yellow armband he had no rights . . . Don't they trust his official armband?'[53] The irony is, of course, that as the wheelchair became more and more accepted as the icon of disability in the second half of the twentieth century, the yellow armband became less and less visible, being seen as stigmatizing and therefore less indicative of 'human rights'.

In the late 1940s the idea that blindness demanded an abstract signal beyond that written on the body was not universally accepted. In 1949 the Israeli physicist Moshé Feldenkrais – born an Eastern European Jew, educated in Paris and during the war part of the British scientific teams working against the Nazis – published his first book on his body awareness method, *Body and Mature Behavior: A Study of Anxiety, Sex, Gravitation and Learning*, in which posture is central.[54] Feldenkrais began to look at the disabled body as part of his examination of how thought, feeling, perception and movement were closely interrelated and influenced one another. His own disability, a long-standing knee injury, led to his examination of body maps as a source of bodily change. For Feldenkrais, posture is the product of a series of inputs, from both the vestibular system and the optic system, that monitor the body in the world. The subjective body, the body observing itself, is at the very centre of his work. This may mean that those with impaired systems of orientation have different postural responses to the world:

> If the conscious control or the optical righting reflexes are responsible for faulty posture, then their elimination should leave the lower centers in control, and a reduction of flexion should take place, and the carriage should become more erect. Under hypnotism and spontaneous somnambulic states, the

head is, in fact, lifted and the pelvis straightened, so that the person stands taller than in his normal waking state. Blind people, too, carry their head higher than the average.[55]

What appears to be 'good' posture is easily read by the sighted observer as a sign of blindness. This is late 1940s London, where the blind and disabled were a permanent part of the public sphere. Blindness could be read in bodily posture, Feldenkrais claimed; it did not need to be 'signalled' with any external sign such as a yellow armband. The blind, for Feldenkrais and his contemporaries, remained the touchstone for understanding the idea of disability.

The blind disability theorist Rod Michalko notes that standard rehabilitation models understand

> sight as embodied in an 'ideal actor'. This ideal actor is some-one who is like every other sighted person insofar as he or she can see, and potentially do, what everyone else can see and do. This ideal actor is an actor who 'fits in' and, ideally, cannot be distinguished from any other actor on the basis of 'looking like' he or she can see. Rehabilitation's ideal actor moves through the world looking like everyone else who can see.[56]

The standard model reproduces not a blind person but, as Feldenkrais writes, 'a sighted person whose sight is missing'.[57] How is this to be undertaken?

> [An] astonishing amount of 'training' and 'rehabilitation' of the blind deals with . . . the visible manifestations of blindness. Eliminate 'blindness', the experts say, the physical traits to which the blind are allegedly prone – the wobbly neck, uneven posture, shuffling gait, unblinking gaze. Discoloured or bulging eyes should be covered with patches or dark glasses, empty sockets filled with prosthetics.[58]

Correct posture to the normative manner by which the sighted move and you have made the blind vanish. This is precisely what Feldenkrais began to argue against in the 1940s. Not prescriptive posture, but rather the idea that each individual's posture is appropriate for him or her. While Feldenkrais argues that posture can be made more efficient in terms of mobility (he worked with individuals with cerebral palsy), he never assumed that posture needed to be corrected – only maximized.

The Origin of the Wheelchair Icon

The passage of time in Germany and the ageing of the youngest generation born at the very end of the war or in its immediate aftermath – those who had no conscious awareness of the Nazi period and were shaped largely by the Cold War and the gradual Americanization, for good or ill, of West Germany – led to a sudden and rather startling confrontation with the past, producing what historians have called the generation of 1968. But the question had first been formulated in 1967, when two German psychoanalysts, Margarete and Alexander Mitscherlich, published their study *The Inability to Mourn*.[59] An immediate best-seller in Germany, the text seemed to focus all the anxiety about the past felt by the youngest generation on the to-that-point-unspoken question: 'What did you do in the war, Daddy?' (And it really was 'Daddy' who was asked.) It is only with the rise of this generation of 1968 that the symbolic language of disability shifts and the wheelchair comes to be the visual sign of modern disability.

The history of posture becomes a structuring moment of difference within this post-war discourse of biopower.[60] The normal, Canguilhem noted in biology, is defined by the nature of the organism itself: 'To say that "no doctor proposes to produce a new kind of man, with a new arrangement of eyes or limbs", is to recognize that an organism's norm of life is furnished by the organism itself, contained in its existence.'[61] It is striking that Canguilhem, writing (like Feldenkrais) in the 1940s, sees the 'new man' never imagined by biomedicine as consisting of eyes and limbs. While, he notes, medical dictionaries define the normal as 'that which conforms to the rule, regular', he expands the notion: '(1) normal is that which is such that it ought to be; (2) normal, in the most usual sense of the word, is that which is met in the majority of cases of a determined kind, or that which constitutes either the average or standard of a measurable characteristic.'[62] His metaphor is the transitional moment between the older model of iconic images of disability and the emerging one. The presence of the 'limbs' as a marker of difference equivalent to that of the 'eyes' in our 'new man' is a sign of the shift from the older markers, such as blindness, to the newer or perhaps ever-present markers, those of posture.

Julien Hébert's disability icon for the International and Universal Exposition or Expo '67, Montreal, Canada, 1967.

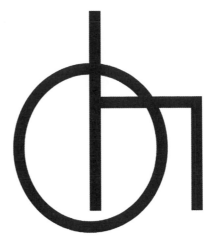

Post-war society rejected symbols that were contaminated by the euthanasia and genocide of the mid-twentieth century, and a proliferation of icons began to appear, mostly variants of the wheelchair, such as the sign developed for the Montréal Expo in 1967 with a highly stylized icon of a wheelchair.[63] The International Symbol of Access, a white stylized wheelchair on a blue background, first appeared in 1968. That year the international charity Rehabilitation International (RI) held its Pan-Pacific Rehabilitation Conference, 'Promotion of Non-handicapped Physical Environments for Disabled People', and its director-general, Norman Acton, felt that there was a need for a new logo. Acton, also the Director of UNICEF's U.S. committee, recalled some years later that 'a number of different symbols were beginning to appear and several of us could see a messy situation developing with multiple symbols – so there was some urgency'.[64] One might add that national and pan-European symbols, such as the German three-dot armband, had their own complex and unacceptable history. The new logo was designed by the Danish design student Susanne Koefoed at a conference held by the Scandinavian Design Students' Organization, influenced by the work of the Austrian-American designer Victor Papanek, who had fled Austria as a sixteen-year-old after the Anschluss in 1938.

Papanek stressed in his work in the 1960s, and in his *Design for the Real World* (1971), the need to address the physically and developmentally disabled as well as the 'normative' body as the object of design. His work was clearly an answer to the technological models that had dominated German design in the 1930s and 1940s. He evokes Friedrich

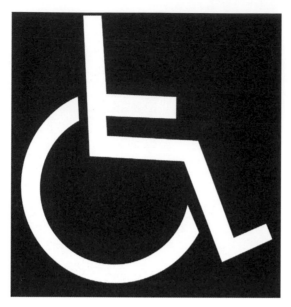

Susanne Koefoed's design was one of six submitted to a nine-person jury of representatives from various international organizations in the fields of architecture, design and disability advocacy in 1968. In 1969 a clear majority of the ICTA-convened jury voted for the Scandinavian design.

Porsche and the Nazi design of the Volkswagen, as well as Bruno Bettelheim and his image of the concentration camps.[65] Papanek is aware that the drive for a technology that dominated the human being had led to the mass factories of death of the concentration and death camps. Yet underlying much of his argument is the notion of the adaptability of technology as a key to providing the greatest access to the disabled. His example is the development of a wide range of wheelchairs, such as 'racing wheelchairs that permit some of the handicapped to participate in marathons . . . [and] exercising vehicles specifically designed for children'.[66] The wheelchair is that adaptive technology that defines modern mobility in the light of its use to destroy life in the Third Reich.

While Koefoed's initial design showed only a stylized wheelchair with a stick figure, the International Commission of Technology and Accessibility adapted the symbol with an added semicircle signifying a seated figure. Karl Montan, first director of the Swedish Handicap Institute and chair of the RI International Commission for Technical Aids (ICTA), modified the image, since the original symbol, with its lines of equal thickness, could have been indecipherable as a meaningless monogram of letters. All the Scandinavian countries had adopted the German symbols for disability well before Denmark and Norway were occupied in 1940. Although 'modern', the new design was also a clear repudiation of the German iconic tradition and an enhancement of

During committee discussion, however, an important modification was suggested by the chair of the committee, Karl Montan, and approved. A stylized head was added to the symbol for aesthetic purposes. Montan noted: 'A slight inconvenience with the symbol is the equally thick lines, which may give an impression of a monogram of letters. With a "head" on the symbol this inconvenience would disappear.'

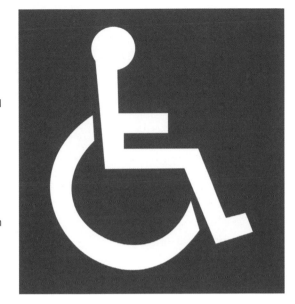

the wheelchair as an abstraction in the place of the three dots. Taking the original copy of the submitted design, Montan 'humanized' it further by adding a circle to the top of the seated figure, giving it a 'head'. Thus anthropomorphized, the symbol was no longer illegible. With the addition of the head, the ICTA panel gave its enthusiastic endorsement to the new symbol.

One of the major reasons for this alteration was the complaint that the initial design was indecipherable. As the architect Selwyn Goldsmith, who was central to the adoption of the wheelchair icon in another arena (we will come to that below), commented in 1969, the figure was 'ambiguous – it is not apparent whether the upper component of the device implies a person (in which even the symbol ought to be categorized as image-related) or whether, as seems more probable on account of the lack of a "head", it represents the frame of a wheelchair.'[67] Goldsmith surveyed a range of possible abstract symbols in his study in 1969, from which this quotation is taken, rejecting an assortment of images that were simply too abstract. For him, this image was virtually unreadable, especially to someone who was trying to move the iconic reference to the actual wheelchair from the abstraction of the three dots that had been used to signify disability in the recent past. In an article in *The Times* in 1967, he was already quoted as advocating 'replacing abstract symbols to identify special facilities (which are meaningless to the uninitiated) by pictorial signs. If special

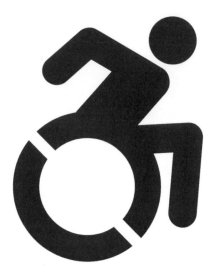

Sara Hendren and Brian
Glenney, 'The "Accessible
Icon" Project', www.
accessibleicon.org.

facilities and these signs were used regularly in public buildings they would finally be regarded as normal facilities for ordinary people with special needs.'[68] The rejection of abstraction may well also lie in the yellow armband with its abstract three dots, now associated irreparably with a defeated Germany. The new wheelchair should not be abstract; it should be a concrete representation of the postural and mobility disabilities of 'normal people'.

At first, as we have seen, the wheelchair icon was unreadable to those for whom older icons of disability, such as the three dots, had become natural. They expected an icon that was redolent of the blind/deaf nexus in representing the nature of disability. One can note in this context that the new international icon for blindness is a blue sign with a white male figure holding a cane, a variation on the wheelchair icon (except in Austria, where this traffic sign is black on a yellow background, clearly evocative of the older three-dot armband).

Indeed, the classic wheelchair icon of disability, the International Symbol of Access, universally adapted and advocated by governments across the world, was challenged with the rise of disability activism as too 'rigid' and too evocative of the passivity implicated in the very concept of the 'handicapped'. There has been an ongoing critique of the modified wheelchair symbol. Does the image imply a notion that mobility is the sole sign of disability and that the wheelchair user is otherwise a 'normate'. Jenny Morris has stated that the symbol seems to imply that 'the typical disabled person is a young man in a wheelchair who is fit, never ill, and whose only need is a physically accessible

environment.'[69] Or is it the wheelchair as icon itself that is the problem?
Liat Ben-Moshe and Justin Powell have noted that

> the symbol produces ambiguity over the centrality of 'disability'
> or 'person'. Although the figure in the symbol refers to a human
> being, the contour represents mostly the wheelchair, which
> reinforces a common cultural misconception that people with
> mobility impairments are 'confined' or 'bound' to their wheel-
> chairs. In line with what happens on a daily basis in social
> interactions, disability becomes an all-encompassing feature
> stigmatizing and dehumanizing the person bearing it.[70]

This, as we will see, can historically be claimed of any iconic abstraction that becomes *the* symbol of disability. One self-identified disabled
commentator noted, 'Disabled people are not confined to wheelchairs;
they are liberated by them . . . Yet none of these things are possible
without the presence of visible symbols of disability, symbols that evoke
strong feelings from everyone around the symbol carrier. It was only
through a willingness to be identified as disabled that I gained access
to the tools of my self-care.'[71] One must add to all these comments that
icons are never naturalized equivalents to the meanings attached to
them. We only learn and internalize their meanings over time. When
we do, they may seem incomplete or contradictory to some.

In 1994 Brendan Murphy, an Irish graduate student at the University of Cincinnati, suggested a more activist revision by pushing the
figure's posture forward and putting the arm behind the body, as if he
or she had just pushed off on the wheel. For Murphy, the chair was no
longer a sign of the imprisonment of individuals but of their liberation
through access. This was seen as 'disrupting [the] ableist conception
of humanity' by the conceptual artist Sara Hendren, who discovered
his work that year at the Museum of Modern Art in New York City.[72]
She and the philosopher Brian Glenney subsequently replaced Murphy's version with 'a revised symbol that included a wheelchair in
motion':

> Hendren and Glenney thought the symbol made the chair look
> more important and visible than the person sitting on it. So
> they came up with their own version, in which the figure was
> leaning forward, elbows out, as if about to push off in some

direction. The pair went around pasting a transparent sticker featuring their redesign over the old symbol in public places, so that people could see both old and new.[73]

This act of guerrilla street art superimposed the new icon on the traditional signage in Boston in 2010.

The new version was a more socially acceptable icon that is yet 'faster' and thus a more integrative image of an activist notion of disability. Hendren observed, following the rhetoric of disability activism,

> I think disability is partly a medical identity, and partly a political identity. What our culture needs to hear, though, is how disability is a political identity, because we live in a time where disability exclusively exists on the body. Your legs don't work, so therefore you are disabled. Actually, you are not disabled by your legs not walking, you are disabled by infrastructure and cities and towns that are built with stairs and without ramps.[74]

In the twenty-first century the 'Accessible Icon' project thus put forward a yet more 'engaged' image, which placed greater emphasis on the figure in movement as a symbol of this new politics of access, rather than the mechanism of transportation. This further revision had immediate cultural (if not political) acceptance. The Museum of Modern Art also added it to its design archive. Speed and access were signs of liberation; being seated, the postural content of this sign went without comment. It is clear that the way that 'speed' and 'access' are signposted is through alteration in *posture* and posture alone. Wheelchair icons in the end are comments on our understanding of posture.

The Posture of the Normate Body in Space

The wheelchair icon created in 1969 has its parallel in the development of a visual vocabulary of 'universal design'. Ever since the Renaissance, the icon of a body within a square and a circle proposed by Vitruvius, whose work had been 'rediscovered' by Poggio Bracciolini in 1414 (even though it was well known in the Middle Ages), became the basis of the iconography of proportional, ideal and healthy bodies in both architecture and medicine. Such bodies were a fantasy of implausibility. They presented an image of upright posture reaching towards the gods as much as any other of the wide range of postural icons we have examined so far.

We retain such images in the ubiquitous reworkings of Leonardo da Vinci's *Vitruvian Man* (1490), which haunted architecture as a model for the ideal user of space even when not concerned with proportionality.[75] Indeed, Leonardo's image becomes the way the Western imagination conceives of upright posture across the widest range of sources. Toby Lester notes in the conclusion of his book on this image:

> The picture is reproduced so often today, and in so many different contexts, that it's hard not to think of it as ubiquitous, timeless, and inevitable . . . It all made me reflect on the utter contingency of the image, which could so easily not have

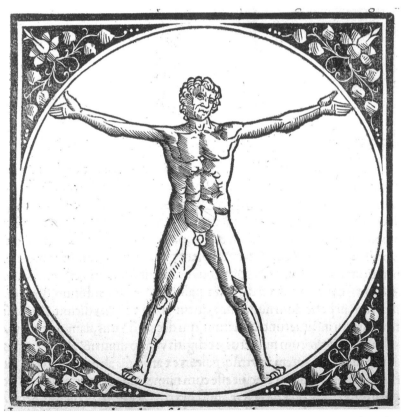

'Vitruvian Man'. From the illustrated edition of *De architectura M. Vitrvvivs per Iocvndvm solito castigatior factvs cvm figvris et tabvla vt iam legi et intelligi possit* (Venice, 1511).

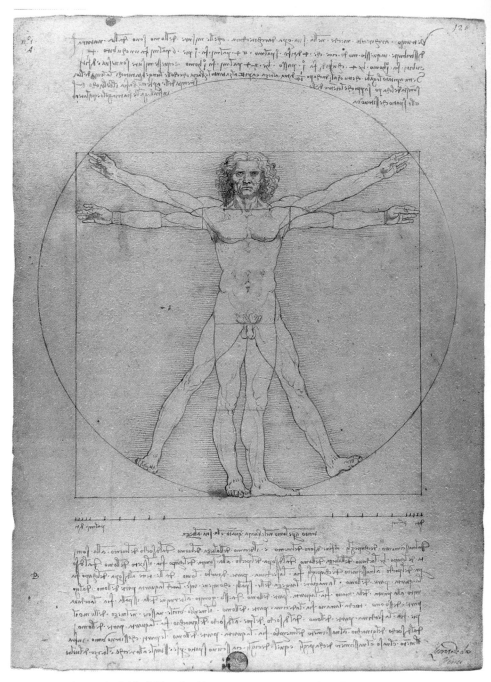

Leonardo da Vinci, *Vitruvian Man*, *c.* 1490, pen on ink with wash over metalpoint.

existed. What if the Greeks had defined beauty and the nature of the cosmos differently? What if Vitruvius had never written the *Ten Books*, or if medieval scribes, flummoxed by the difficulty of the text, had quit copying it? What if Christian theologians and mystics hadn't incorporated elements of Vitruvian Man into their worldview? What if Leonardo hadn't ...turned to the study of architecture and anatomy in Milan?[76]

And we can add: what if we had not learned to see upright posture in the world of built space to no little degree through the power of this icon? It is Vitruvius made real for our world.

For Vitruvius' world defined posture in its own way. In the *Ten Books on Architecture* (*De architectura*), written in the first century BC, Vitruvius, following in the classical tradition, outlines *how* the human being came to be *Homo faber*, the builder of buildings:

Therefore, because of the discovery of fire, there arose at the beginning, concourse among men, deliberation and a life in common. Many came together into one place, having from nature this boon beyond other animals, that they should walk, not with head down, but upright, and should look upon the magnificence of the world and of the stars. They also easily handled with their hands and fingers whatever they wished. Hence after thus meeting together, they began, some to make shelters of leaves, some to dig caves under the hills, some to make of mud and wattles places for shelter, imitating the nests of swallows and their methods of building.[77]

Fire allows the creation of society, which then encourages humans to stand upright and look towards the heavens. Only then are human beings capable of using tools with their suddenly freed hands. For the upright body as the creation of the gods was the ideal for the Graeco-Roman world as well as, with a different inflection, for Christianity. That built space came to be understood in terms of the posture of the upright human is also not surprising. But that it implied a rigid, erect posture is. Vitruvius is known in the ancient world as much as a mathematician as an architect. The measurement of time, as he illustrates in his work, is a fundamental obligation of the architect. One recent critic has observed that

The *gnomon*, sundial pointer, is essentially the same tool as the architect's *norma*, set square. Both pointer and set square are referred to by the Greek word *gnomon* (generically, any upright), from which the Latin *norma* derives. Both, interchangeably, are agents of the 'squaring' that establishes the 90-degree relation between verticals and horizontals without which there can be neither sundials nor cities nor buildings, nor yet the exclusively human upright posture that makes a man in his prime architecture's fundamental human referent.[78]

The notion of the upright human as the rigid, Vitruvian figure defined by the plumb line comes then from the very origin of the notion of the normative. But because it is an artificial construct of the body, as are all the Greeks' images of the body in art, it is an artificial measure of the human being in the world of space as well as of time. It is the measure placed on nature, not arising from nature.

Thus bodies and buildings come to be linked in the Renaissance as the Vitruvian ideal is rediscovered as the new, normative body. In his anatomy of 1543, Vesalius employs architectural metaphors for the body, since he assumes that the upright body is analogous to the built space that has been seen as an idealization and extension of the normative body.[79] His reference seems often to be the built environment, as when he sees the excretory process of the body as equivalent to a well-constructed building with good sewers that remove waste as far as possible away from the senses of its occupants.[80] Thus the ideal posture of the upright human as imagined within built space mirrored the very nature of his divinely created body, but it also reflected that space.

Again, it is only after the horrors of the Second World War, the death camps, the bombing of European cities and the displacement of their inhabitants, that people began to think about the ideal space for bodies in other ways. We should remember that the iconic high modernist building at this moment was Philip Johnson's Glass House (1949), which had its roots in Johnson's flirtation with Fascism and his exposure to burnt-out homes with only their chimneys standing during the German invasion of Poland, as much as in his debt to Ludwig Mies van der Rohe's earlier Barcelona Pavilion and his post-war Farnsworth House.[81] High Modernism makes the buildings transparent, but for all the wrong reasons. They are housing for the bodies of the elites, revealing in their openness and their absences the power now invested in them.

After the Second World War the members of the Royal Institute of British Architects (RIBA) in the United Kingdom were heavily involved in both post-war reconstruction and the radical rethinking of the city that led to Le Corbusier-like Brutalist public housing. The iconic structures of the time were Denys Lasdun's Keeling House (1958) and Ernő Goldfinger's Balfron Tower (1965) housing estates, both in the East End of London. They bore absolutely no relationship to the transparent architectural machines of Mies and Johnson. They were not merely 'cities in the sky', but self-contained social environments, intended to create both social cohesion and access for all members of a society displaced from its original environment either by bombing or by urban renewal. They were also bunkers that sought to defend the bodies of their inhabitants and provide a modicum of safety, or at least the illusion of safety, through built space – more medieval tower than hidden garden.

It is often overlooked that part of this rethinking of public spaces in the late 1960s was the establishment of a new national standard for the definition of the human bodies that were to inhabit these spaces. In 1963 Goldsmith's book *Designing for the Disabled* provided new icons seemingly quite independent of the concern about public icons for disability, based on existing anthropometric data employed by architects drawing blueprints and catalogued in the *Architectural Graphic Standards.*[82] Goldsmith's own experience was central to his rethinking of the icon of disability. He was hemiplegic from having acquired polio on holiday in 1958, immediately after his training as an architect at Trinity Hall, Cambridge, and then the Bartlett School of University College London. Unable to draw with his right hand, he quickly learned to use his left, and after recuperating he moved to London to practise architecture. The resulting pronounced weakness in his legs left him unstable for the rest of his life, and so mobility defined his understanding of disability.

In 1961, while working for the South East Metropolitan Regional Hospital Board, Goldsmith was appointed by RIBA and the Polio Research Fund to produce *Designing for the Disabled*, the first architectural guidance manual in the United Kingdom concerning access. It was published by RIBA in 1963. As had been the case with virtually all work done in this field, the manual contained suggestions for the incorporation of the disabled, not guidelines for their incorporation, even though the National Assistance Act mandated the building of homes for the elderly and the adaptation of existing dwellings for the handicapped. Goldsmith later noted that 'wheelchair access was not then an item which anyone would have thought to put on the agenda.'[83] It was he whose engagement meant that the wheelchair became the icon of access in architecture. The blind and the deaf, with their own specific demands, were to be written out of such codes, since postural access seemed most relevant to Goldsmith's world view.

In his work, Goldsmith rethinks what the very idea of disability in the British public sphere could be:

> No commonly accepted definition of the term disability exists which would enable individuals to be categorized as either disabled or non-disabled. The dictionary definition is loose: 'inability, incapacity, impotence'. Now that severely disabled people, including many obliged to use wheelchairs, are regularly rehabilitated to comparative or complete independence such definitions are obsolete . . . Many disabled people who are socially and economically independent would be unwilling to regard themselves as handicapped.[84]

What Goldsmith accomplishes here is to redefine disability primarily in terms of posture and mobility. His primary distinction is between 'ambulant' and 'non-ambulant, i.e., wheelchair users'.[85] (Although he does qualify this as he works out the spaces that the disabled inhabit, and thus adds the 'semi-ambulant' to his categories, that is, people with crutches and walking frames.[86]) The wheelchair is the key to his understanding of access, even though he acknowledges peripherally the need for special accommodation for the blind in his understanding of the built environment.

While building on work done in Denmark and Sweden, much of Goldsmith's work was indebted to Timothy J. Nugent's American Standard of 1961, a design standard for making buildings accessible to disabled people – not those falling into specific categories of disability, but for all disabled people. Nugent's view was that facilities could be adapted by expanding on accepted architectural features that were 'hitherto accepted in Britain . . . that disabled people should be treated virtually as normal people, and that provision for them – ramps, wider doors, etc., – should deviate as little as possible from normal facilities.'[87] Goldsmith disagreed vehemently: 'It is impossible to design facilities which are useable by everyone; in practice it means that people who are not normal are excluded.'[88] His approach was much more limited; it began with specific questions of access for wheelchair users and moved on to other categories of disability, such as the blind and the deaf. No 'macro-solution' was conceived under this model. *Designing for the Disabled* stressed disabilities of mobility, beginning with wheel-chair users and users of crutches and other aids to mobility.

Goldsmith subsequently became the assistant buildings editor – a research architect, as he called it – at RIBA's *Architects' Journal*, a position he held from 1968 to 1972. In 1972 he joined the Department of the Environment, where he produced the reports 'Wheelchair Hous-ing' and 'Mobility Housing', which became widely accepted as standards for public sector housing. His impact thereafter was marked, not only in the UK but globally. The wheelchair came to be the icon of disability for Goldsmith and, through him, for the accessible built environment.

Forced by the adoption in the UK of the metric system, the very nature of the 'normal' inhabitants of these buildings was also being rethought under Goldsmith's influence. In 1968 the *Architects' Journal*, the quasi-official journal of British architecture, devoted three issues to creating a standardized metric model of 'normal' humans and their relationship to the built environment to resolve 'many areas of confu-sion and doubt among those responsible for the change to metric.'[89] The anthropometric data in this project was written and compiled by Goldsmith, who defined 'normal' as being at the 95th percentile of the population. He supplied a new 'Vitruvian Man' (and woman) in 1968, representing the 'normal' British citizen. This figure mirrored in every way the ideal upright posture associated with built space.

It is striking that by 1968 the Vitruvian figures were accompanied by male and female figures in wheelchairs, even though Goldsmith noted, in his very pragmatic style, that 'it may not be possible to obtain a solution to a specific design problem which is equally efficient for a typical ambulant person and a person in a wheelchair.'[90] Goldsmith simply converted images that had been in feet and inches in his earlier work *Designed for the Disabled* into the 'basic metric data' he produced for the handbook. But what was vital was that in the anthropometric data the bodies in a wheelchair were considered as parallel to and different from those of the ambulant person. While this had been

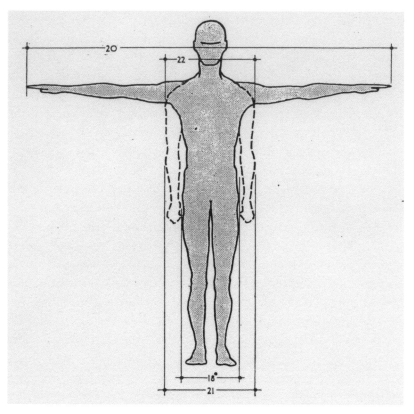

The metric Vitruvian man. From the *Architects' Journal*, CXLVII/3 (13 March 1968).

common in handbooks for the design of hospital rooms (and indeed was also the case in this handbook), the image of the Vitruvian man came to be paired with that of wheelchair man (and woman).

Goldsmith's work had highlighted the fact that, like the insurance data of the time, mid-century architectural icons rested on '[anthropometric] data . . . based on the average, young, white, and able-bodied male.'[91] Goldsmith generated an anthropometric figure of a wheelchair user, showing the proportions of the body and such measurements as reach, seated height and the width of the chair. By the 1980s, well after the wheelchair had come to be the iconic representation of disability, firms such as Henry Dreyfuss Associates, who provided the anthropometric data for the later *Architectural Graphic Standards* figures, had changed its edition of *Humanscale 1/2/3* of 1981 to include adult and child wheelchair users.[92] It was only in 1997 that the 'Principles of Universal Design' were developed under the leadership of Ron Mace, FAIA, which advocated for 'environments usable by all people, without the need for adaptation or specialized design'. The final of their seven points stressed uses 'regardless of user's body size, posture, or mobility'.[93] Posture, that hidden quality inscribed in the new icons of disability, finally surfaces in the demands for a universal definition of the human.

But is the wheelchair truly an icon of posture, or is it an icon of gait or mobility? As we have seen, these have been overlapping categories throughout our history of posture. How we walk is a version of how we stand. Very few, if any at all, commentators or even members of the general public – now so acculturated to the sign of the wheelchair – see it as an icon of posture. The wheelchair, speedy or not, is a sign of disability since it is, for the moment, the icon that defines 'disability' broadly, not solely as a 'person who cannot stand and move without aid'.

The twenty-first-century discourse on posture and disability, or indeed on disability defined through direct or hidden models of posture, has its origins in even older models of the meaning of posture than the mid-twentieth-century French sociology, where it is typically rooted by contemporary disability scholars. In this discourse, self-awareness of the body is not a sign of the pathological, but, to use Michel

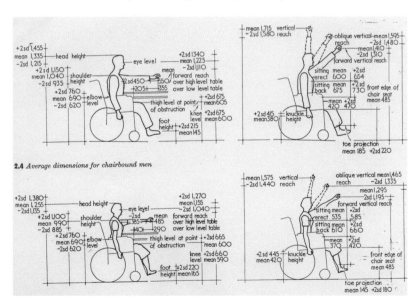

2.4 *Average dimensions for chairbound men*

Selwyn Goldsmith's incorporation of the wheelchair user into his first biometric rethinking of architectural space, 1968. This and other images first appeared in feet and inches in his *Designing for the Disabled* (1963). The second edition also employs these figures, but their direct source in Goldsmith's initial work is removed, giving an even greater sense that these are simply analogous bodies, not specific to any rethinking of questions of access. From the *Architects' Journal*, CXLVII/3 (13 March 1968).

Foucault's term, an anomaly. This is a trope from the world of Sigmund Freud as well as that of Friedrich Nietzsche, whom Freud had read as a young medical student in Vienna.

For, as Nietzsche noted, one is aware of one's own body only when it is ill, or perhaps here when it is discordant with the world in which it must function. He writes in *Human, All Too Human* about the 'Usefulness of sickliness':

> He who is often sick does not only have a much greater enjoy-
> ment of health on account of the frequency with which he gets
> well: he also has a greatly enhanced sense of what is healthy
> and what sick in works and actions, his own and those of
> others: so that it is precisely the sickliest writers, for example
> – and almost all the great writers are, unfortunately, among
> them – who usually evidence in their writings a much steadier
> and more certain tone of health, because they understand the
> philosophy of physical health and recovery better and are
> better acquainted with its teachers – morning, sunshine, forests
> and springs – than the physically robust.[94]

Health is what one has when one is no longer ill. As the philosopher Hans-Georg Gadamer noted, 'we need only reflect that it is quite mean-ingful to ask someone "Do you feel ill?" but it would be quite absurd to ask someone "Do you feel healthy?" Health is not a condition that one introspectively feels in oneself. Rather, it is a condition of being involved, of being in the world, of being together with one's fellow human beings, of active and rewarding engagement with one's every-day tasks.'[95] Thus, if such an argument is followed one must be or have been physically ill in order to feel 'healthy'. Nietzsche had commented long before Gadamer that 'One must comfort the patient's fantasy as he suffers more from the idea of his illness, than from the illness itself.'[96] We sense our posture only when we imagine ourselves ill and we subscribe meaning to our altered sense of our bodies.

Postural disability comes to define posture, and good posture is the result when one is no longer posturally disabled. Yet the icons of the wheelchair visually define disability without any overt reference to the complex history of the idea of posture; indeed, these images seem to bracket any sense of postural difference. As Lennard Davis noted, 'the fact is that no one is or can be normal, as no one is or can be equal. Everyone has to work hard to make it seem they conform, so the person with disabilities is singled out as a dramatic case of not belonging. This identification makes it easier for the rest to think they fit the paradigm.'[97] Thus disability is a social category of stigmatization, as Goffman made clear in his own work. But it is an unrecognized stigma defined within postmodern theory that refuses to take physical disability, here the disability of the wheelchair, into account. For postmodern theory, Davis argued:

> the body is seen as a site of *jouissance,* a native ground of pleasure, the scene of an excess that defies reason, that takes dominant culture and its rigid, power-laden vision of the body to task . . . The nightmare of that body is the one that is deformed, maimed, mutilated, broken, diseased . . . Rather than face this ragged image, the critic turns to the fluids of sexuality, the gloss of lubrication, the glossary of the body as text, the heteroglossia of the intertext, the glossolalia of the schizophrenic. But almost never the body of the differently abled.[98]

At the core of Davis's vision of the disabled is the physicality of wheelchair as icon, not the classical figures of the deaf and blind, and certainly not, as Foucault had done, building on half a century of cultural fascination with difference, the 'mad'.[99] Davis argues that the corporeal body, represented by the wheelchair, becomes invisible when it is transformed into an icon that is the abstraction of 'disability'.

Thus the therapeutic force that propelled disability into the public sphere was called 'universal design', the functional symbol of which came to be the wheelchair. Initially it was the discussion in the 1980s about barrier-free design that reflected the 1990 Americans with Disabilities Act's focus on technical accessibility standards for specific disabilities (exemplified by wheelchair access). The broader appeal of universal design was that it ideally included all bodies, those of the disabled as well as the normate. The architect Ronald Mace coined the term to describe accessibility that goes beyond the scope of barrier-free design.[100] Mace, reflecting his own experience of disability as a wheelchair user, defined universal design as 'a way of designing a building or facility, at little or no extra cost, so it is both attractive and functional for all people, disabled or not. The idea is to remove that expensive, "special" label from products and designs for people with mobility problems, and at the same time, eliminate the institutional appearance of many current accessible designs."[101] The idea was to eliminate any specific response to specific disabilities and have a space that could be accessed by all people without the special pleading for 'special needs'. This is the antithesis of Goldsmith's view in 1963, which had led to the wheelchair and its implications becoming the ideal icon for postural and mobility disabilities. But by then this image could no longer be questioned.

The Sitpoint Theory of Disability

For 'special needs people', the wheelchair, with its unspoken evocation of postural disability, stood as the icon of difference, encapsulated in the feminist disability concept of 'sitpoint theory', which stresses the postural impact on 'knowing' from the position of sitting in a wheelchair, as opposed to standing, as productive of a different epistemology. Indeed, it was the late Emory University theologian Nancy Mairs, who had multiple sclerosis and used a wheelchair, who evolved the notion that human beings are defined by their literal view of the world as they acquire upright posture. She noted that human grandiosity had its roots in the ability of the child to move from crawling to walking, 'and at this momentous point in the practicing stage, upright locomotion permits such vista, such possibilities, such triumphs, that a child can grow drunk on omnipotence and grandeur'.[102] This is the claim of the 'normal' seeing the world from a new perspective, that of upright posture, as we develop as adults a sense of pathological posture parallel to a generalized sense of our own body as normate. The normate was defined by the difference between those who were able to stand and those 'for whom the very thought of ever being like me so horrifies them that they can't permit themselves to put themselves on my wheels even for an instant'.[103] To be 'on my wheels' defines the new perspective of Disability Studies. For the key to seeing anew – and this brings us back to our discussion about posture as a Christian theological concept – is to contest the moral claims of uprightness, as Mair notes:

> the fact that the soundness of the body so often serves as a metaphor for its moral health, its deterioration thus implying

moral degeneracy, puts me and my kind in a quandary. How can I possibly be 'good'? Let's face it, wicked witches are not just ugly (as sin); they're also bent and misshapen (crooked). I am bent and misshapen, therefore ugly, therefore wicked. And I have no way to atone.[104]

And, she stresses, no reason to do so, for she, like Kant's notion of the 'crooked wood' from which we are all made, is aware of her own moral posture. It is the power of metaphor and yet seems to transcend this:

Nancy Mairs . . . comments on the way that one 'healthy', 'normal' and 'proportional' body shapes even our idea of moral-ity. She grounds her examination of metaphor in a study of the 'dead' metaphors that align morality with physicality. Her examples, such as the way that 'keeping your chin up' signifies courage, show that in everyday language, good traits are equated with 'upstanding', negative traits are 'looked down on'. It then so happens that a woman in a wheelchair, waist-high, is offered little access to the metaphors that might construct her morality in a positive light. The body that shapes the lan-guage is not hers – in fact, the language negates her body.[105]

And yet we evoke the moral power of concepts such as being 'mor-ally upright', unaware of their attachment to normative bodies.

Siebers, in his highly acclaimed work on the nature of disability, carried the image of the 'withered limb' into the academic discussion of the appropriateness of the Foucauldian model for the study of disabilities:[106]

Disability exposes with great force the constraints imposed on bodies by social codes and norms. In a society of wheel-chair users, stairs would be nonexistent, and the fact that they are everywhere in our society seems an indication only that most of our architects are able-bodied people who think un-seriously about access. Obviously, in this sense, disability looks socially constructed . . . But disability may also trouble the theory of social construction. Disability scholars have begun to insist that strong constructionism either fails to account for the difficult physical realities faced by people with disabilities or presents their body in ways that are conventional, conformist, and unrecognizable to them . . . The disabled body seems difficult for the theory of social construction to absorb: disability is at once its best example and a significant counter-example.[107]

Thus disabled bodies, exemplified by the wheelchair user, are neither simply extensions of our collective imaginations nor the simple by-product of the built environment. In Siebers's rejection of Foucault's romanticization of docile bodies, of disability and marginality as the true centre of human organization and existence, the disabled are no longer ideal alternatives but problems for body theory. They are to be taken seriously, but here posture becomes the symbolic representation of disability within Siebers's theory. He argues: 'If the docile body is disabled, however, it means that recent body theory has reproduced the most abhorrent prejudices of ableist society.'[108] His goal is the politics of representation as a politics of change:

> The central issue for the politics of representation is not whether bodies are infinitely interpretable but whether certain bodies should be marked as defective and how the people who have these bodies may properly represent their interests in the public sphere. More and more people now believe that disabled bodies should not be labeled as defective, although we have a long way to go, but we have not even begun to think about how these bodies might represent their interests in the public sphere for the simple reason that our theories of representation do not take account of them.[109]

For Siebers, the wheelchair comes to have clearly political significance as a symbolic representation of disability that has transcendental power. The difficulty is that this kind of metaphoric use of disability, especially postural difference, often serves, David Mitchell and Sharon Snyder argue, as 'an opportunistic metaphorical device' that creates the illusion of intersectionality among categories of difference.[110] The irony is that Mitchell, who is a wheelchair user, sees such metaphors as a 'crutch upon which literary narratives lean for their representational power, disruptive potentiality, and analytical insight'.[111] Postural differences both are the force of metaphor and represent the force of metaphor, whether with a positive or a negative tone. It is in the end a metaphor lodged in the rhetoric of posture as well as disability. For the imagined individual sitting in the abstract representation of disability that is simultaneously a real wheelchair has a double burden. That person becomes the disabled body incarnate: the wheelchair a sign of both new mobility and postural difference.

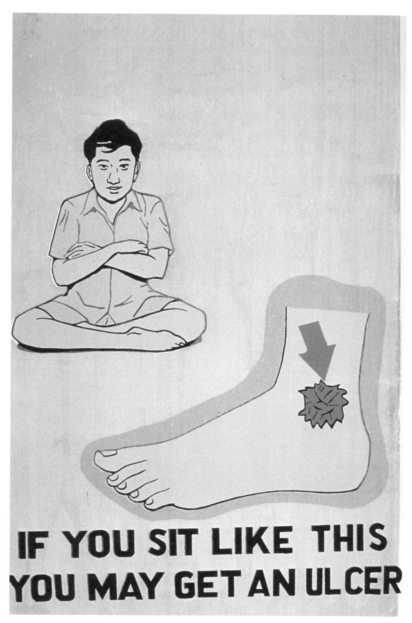

IF YOU SIT LIKE THIS YOU MAY GET AN ULCER

Global ideas of posture vary, but all are part of a metaphysics of the body as conceived in various postural systems. When systems collide (such as in India, where traditional posture is seen as leading to a pathology of posture), such models of the body become self-conscious: 'If you sit like this you may get an ulcer.' Christian Medical College (Vellore, India), 20th century.

Conclusion:
Maps of Moral Posture

HOW EXOTIC IS IT to think about posture as a means of defining what society understands as human? While we have focused in this book on Western notions of posture (and their importation into China through Western models of nineteenth-century nationalism), we could have spread our net more widely – from worshipping practices in Islam to the iconography of Buddha to postural codes in the Pacific islands. The anthropologist Clifford Geertz comments about Bali that 'speech style, posture, dress, eating, marriage, even house-construction, place of burial, and mode of cremation are patterned in terms of a precise code of manners which grows less out of a passion for social grace as such as out of some rather far-reaching meta-physical considerations.'[1] Indeed, our book has at its core the idea that posture is a concept in action representing various such 'metaphysical considerations' in all societies.

Pierre Bourdieu, the sociologist of habitus (the way we are shaped by the worlds in which we are situated), observed in his classic study of taste in 1984 that status in his world of late twentieth-century Paris is determined in society by a range of things, including 'bearing, posture, presence, diction and pronunciation, manners and usage', which define one's status in the middle class.[2] Even though Bourdieu analyses other forms of what he labels our habitus in his study of male domination through codes of posture in the indigenous north African Kabyle people, such codes are not strange to his own world.[3] Posture is thus for him one of the 'mutually reinforcing and infinitely redundant signs of which each body is the bearer'.[4] But it is specific to a 'typically bourgeois deportment [that it] can be recognized by a certain breadth of gesture, posture and gait, which manifests by the amount of physical space that is . . . occupied in social space'.[5] Paris is thus not really much different from Bali or Algeria in that there are 'metaphysical considerations' that shape posture. Actually, as we have seen, systems of posture permeate all disciplines of the body in every possible corner of social interaction: it is the metaphysical or at least the transcendental implications of posture, often contradictory and even more often unstated, that we have tracked in this book.

Posture shapes and shaped our sense of culture just as our culture shapes our sense of the body. Oswald Spengler, a fervent believer in the truths of physiognomy, observed in *The Decline of the West* (1922–3) that 'the visible foreground of all history has the same significance as the external appearance of the human being, such as physique, facial expression, posture, gait; not what is spoken, but the speaking; not what is written, but the handwriting.'[6] Here we try to use our readings of posture as clues to 'an understanding of those large scale human organisms that I call cultures'.[7] Without agreeing with Spengler's pessimism, it is possible still to imagine understanding cultures from their postures (in all senses of that word).

Mental Maps

Since posture, broadly defined, is a universal category of organization that society uses to define the human, we should examine whether there are mechanisms underlying its wide and contradictory practices. With the rise of modern brain science in the nineteenth century, posture came to be understood as our unconscious psychological map of our bodies – omnipresent, yet always elusive. We have, as the British neurologist Sir Henry Head first noted in 1911, a 'postural model of the body', ever unconsciously shifting in response to our environment and our self-awareness, yet providing a consistent reference for our sense of self at each and every moment. He noted that a feather in a lady's hat could become part of her body map as much as the hammer in the hand of the worker, even though they represent very different aspects of human activity.[8] Habituation is at the core of posture, but habituation also contains some level of social meaning.

Head's model of a 'body schema' located that map strictly in 'the sensory cortex [that] is also the storehouse of past impressions'. There are bodily maps that may rise into consciousness as images, but more often, as in the case of spacial impressions, remain outside central consciousness. Here they form organised models of ourselves which may be termed 'schemata'. Such schemata modify the impressions produced by incoming sensory impulses in such a way that the final sensations of position, or of locality, rise into consciousness charged with a relation to something that has happened before.[9]

We can see how this works in patients who have suffered 'a lesion of the cortex [that] renders impossible all recognition of posture or of the locality of a stimulated spot in the affected part of the body'.[10] Experience generates a memory (at least the memory of an affect) associated with posture to create an internal map of our bodies, and such maps can be lost if the brain is damaged.

Head's work built on that of Carl Wernicke, the German neurologist working in the latter half of the nineteenth century on brain localization and aphasia, who realized that the brain cortex generated a 'somatopsychic' map of the body in time and space.[11] Wernicke contrasted this realm with the 'allopsychic' (our cortical map of the external world) and 'autopsychic' (our representation of ourselves) realms. Yet neither Head nor Wernicke saw the symbolic function of posture rooted in a metaphysics of cultural meaning as a core constituent of our mental maps. In other words, that the lady's feather or the worker's tool could become part of the mental map was clear, but what abstract symbolic and affective function the feather or the hammer had in the mental lives of their possessors was not a feature on these mental maps.

Even with such insights into human neurology, as the Viennese psychoanalyst Paul Schilder observed in 1935, 'Our own body is in no way better known to us than the bodies of others. We should not use the mirror so eagerly if it were otherwise'.[12] Schilder, who trained as a psychiatrist in Vienna during the First World War (working with Sigmund Freud, who had exposed him to the idea that the ego is primarily a body ego) and also as a philosopher, was then working at Bellevue Hospital in New York City.[13] He turned his hand to examining the nature of our complex relationship with our own bodies or, perhaps better, to our own *sense* of our bodies. Our bodies are physiological, psychological and phenomenological. They are not out of our control, but inhabit the space between the external world and our own self-awareness. Schilder argued that our posture plays the fundamental role of the body image in man's relation to himself, to his fellow human beings and to the world around him.[14] Posture was, for Schilder, the primary criterion for understanding the interrelationship among these internal as well as external categories in the creation of our body image.

Schilder's phenomenological understanding of posture as simultaneously psychological, physiological and social came to dominate debates about postural mapping. As Erwin Straus observed, 'Upright posture pre-establishes a definite attitude toward the world; it is a specific mode of being-in-the-world'.[15] Consciousness and posture seem to be inherently intertwined: 'There is no moment in our conscious life when we are completely unaware of our bodily posture, of the fact that we are walking, standing, sitting, lying down'.[16] The phenomenologist Maurice Merleau-Ponty notes that we map our own body according to our 'global awareness of . . . posture in the inter-sensory world, a form in Gestalt psychology's sense of the word'.[17] We sense ourselves as form. Yet, as we have seen, the unconscious too seems to have its own sense of our posture.

Schilder also undermined the notion that posture is more than simply a fixed position at rest. Indeed, he argues that it is only in the act of moving the body that posture becomes actualized. For him, the ideal body map is both fixed and dynamic:

> As soon as we leave the state of rest and start movement, it is much more difficult to remain in the attitude of what Kant has called, 'Interesseloses Wohlgefallen'. We are immediately stirred up to a more energetic action. It is true that when we build up our own body-image and the body-image of others, we always tend to build up something static and then to dissolve it again. We always return to the primary positions of the body. When we think about a person running, we see him changing from one primary position into another primary position. Primary positions are positions of relative rest.[18]

This image of the static body at rest is, as we have seen in our discussion of philosophers, theologians and posture, the core definition of aesthetic man. Schilder's formulation presents this as a given of our subjective

Our body maps reflect ourselves, but we are a mix of our biology and our socialization. Public health authorities, such as here in the Republic of Ireland (Eire) in the late 20th century, came to see poor posture as a quality defining 'bad mental health', since it limits the male's ability to attract a mate.

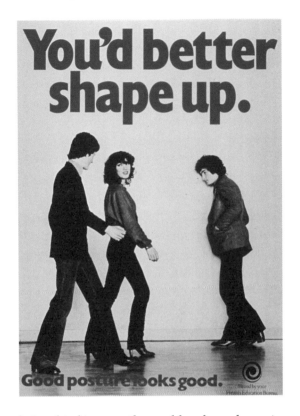

understanding of the relationship between the world and our dynamic selves. Here we begin to sense the structure of a 'normal' body that can also be extended to *all* bodies. The notion that there is an objective, 'normal' posture is dismissed since all bodies map themselves on the world as they experience movement.

Schilder insisted that our inner postural map is also configured in terms of the metaphysics of the world in which we live. Posture is part of our relationship to the structures of power in our world, as the Nobel Prize-winning author Elias Canetti remarked:

> Rank and power are traditionally connected with certain postures and from the way in which men group themselves we can deduce the amount of authority which each enjoys. We know what it means when one man sits raised up while everyone round him stands; when one man stands and everyone else sits; when everyone in a room gets up as someone comes in; when one man falls on his knees before another; when a new arrival is not asked to sit down.[19]

The 'individual significance' of these meanings associated with our posture creates the maps through which our psyche comprehends our bodies. These meanings are superimposed upon us, Canetti argues, because of the social relationships in which we stand. As with Michel Foucault writing in a very different tone, posture is shaped by power working across time and space. While it may have its origin in some aspects of human development, its key is how humans interact in collectives.[20] For Canetti, such maps of human interaction are responses to past practices of posture, for 'every new posture a man adopts is related to the one which precedes it and can be properly understood only if this is known.'[21] It is this history of posture reflecting power that we have also examined in the present book. These histories also shape our mental maps.

Certainly even the remembered whisper of 'stand up straight' brings us to attention. Whether uttered by parent, teacher or sergeant, it is a call to be self-aware, or at least aware of how we are seen. Posture, that code for the way we stand, is used over and over again as a marker for a way to be. It is, as John Schumacher observes, a code for our 'incarnation' – 'to-be-in-flesh' – how we become human in our physical bodies.[22] We are the way we stand – ideally. Indeed, 'standing up straight' evokes the image of the plumb line, an imaginary rigid line dropped through our bodies from the top of the head through the ear hole, the shoulder and the knees, down to the ankle. This image of a rigid posture also has a history: 'Physiologists, anatomists, and orthopedists, to say nothing of specialists in physical education, have dealt exhaustively with a few "ideal" postures – principally the fairly rigid attention stance beloved of the drillmaster, and student's or stenographer's habits of sitting at desks.'[23] The latter, as we have seen, has recently returned to our cultural obsession with posture. Our interest in this present study has been to expand that history and show how complex the interrelationship between the various histories of posture can be.

How We Stand Defines Who We Are

Whatever meaning we give to our bodies, our bodies (and our character) are malleable. They change with age and with the demands we place on them. Our bodies may well be inherently different at birth from our bodies at the end of life. The stories they tell may be radically different, and how we map our sense of self on such shifts of posture is the result of our relationship with the dynamic world that we inhabit. Indeed, our bodies may show radically different forms, from the 'normative' to the 'disabled', at every stage of our lives. How we stand – our posture – defines us to the world. It defines us as human or not human. How do these shifting ideas of posture provide insights into the claims society makes on who we are and what we are able to do?

For posture is not a fixed concept any more than the meaning of the very word 'posture' is fixed: sometimes it has been understood as either part of fixed physiognomy, the inherent structures of the body, determined by inheritance, or that of mobile physiognomy, determined by either pathology or by culture. We stand the way we do because of the inherent inability to distinguish between our sense of innate posture and the postural meanings of the worlds in which we exist. It is neither 'nature' nor 'nurture' but both simultaneously that is our postural self. We are, as Karen Barad notes, 'responsible for the world of which we are a part, not because it is an arbitrary construction of our choosing but because reality is sedimented out of particular practices that we have a role in shaping and through which we are shaped'.[24] Posture is a set of such 'particular practices', but these are never clearly demarcated one from the other. Dancing seems to have very different trajectories from the various forms of yoga; the military's idea of posture seems very different from those evoked in the competing forms of medical gymnastics; and nineteenth-century race science and its evocation of posture seems very different from contemporary anthropology's attempt to trace the evolution of upright posture. Yet the reality is that these are all 'entangled genealogies',[25] and we internalize the confused, overlapping and contradictory uses and meanings associated with the very term 'posture' based on who we are, where we are and what is expected from us in such circumstances. In the 1920s, during the official college 'Posture Week', Vassar College appointed a 'Posture Police' who wore a badge with SUS (Stand Up Straight) emblazoned on it.[26] (Vassar was one of the colleges where William Herbert Sheldon compiled his archive of nude posture photographs of incoming freshman in the 1950s.) They were the posture police and they knew what good posture had to be.

The entangled genealogies of posture are reflected in virtually every discussion of the nature and form of the human – from race to gender, from pathology to beauty. It is, to use Donna Haraway's term, a 'corporeal fetish' that mistakes 'heterogeneous relationality for a fixed, seemingly objective thing'. Of equal importance in confusing our cultural presuppositions with objective or functional definitions in studying the history of posture is the assumption that posture 'denies the ongoing action and work that it takes to sustain technoscientific material-semiotic bodies in the world'.[27] Posture is a slippery concept, as Judith Butler observed of corporeality in *Bodies that Matter*:

> Not only did bodies tend to indicate a world beyond them-selves, but this movement beyond their own boundaries, a movement or boundary itself, appeared to be quite central to what bodies 'are.' I kept losing track of the subject. I proved resistant to discipline. Inevitably, I began to consider that per-haps this resistance to fixing the subject was essential to the matter at hand.[28]

Looking at attempts to discipline posture tells us about broader attempts to discipline bodies, as well as about the resistance coming from the people disciplined. Thus the postural tension of gendered bodies becomes part of any understanding of the very categories of gender themselves. The study of bodily discipline draws bright lines between male and female bodies seen as sites defined by posture, and reflects the very debates about race and gender inherent in the posture discussions of earlier ages.[29] When these bright lines are exam-ined, as in Gayle Salamon's investigation of posture and transgen-dered bodies, we see how necessary and yet how fragile these posture maps really are.[30] In a discussion of the debates about bodily materi-ality and disability, Simon Williams noted in the 1990s that 'bodily processes are not simply static (i.e. homeostasis) or "fixed" (i.e. genes), they are also developmental, pliable and contingent. Seen in these terms, human biology is not constant, rather it is in a state of considerable indeterminacy, flux and transformation.'[31] The entangled genealogies of posture provide a means of teasing out these relationships in new and surprising ways.

I might add here that the present project examining the interlock-ing Venn diagram of the various meanings and disciplines of posture is contingent on my own sense of my posture, which may be why I undertook it in the first place. My father's voice still echoes – after seven decades – in my memory, urging me to 'stand up straight!' Perhaps this book is my own answer to his order admonishing me to stand up and not slump, about being upright in all senses of the word. About being a man, not a child in braces. This is not my memory alone.

For being 'upright' still has complex and contradictory meanings in our world. In 1984 the disability theorist Robert S. Williams, Jr, asked:

> Yet, what happens with those who are deprived of their 'upright-ness' in either the literal or moral sense (as in 'not to stoop to anything'), through becoming Dis-abled? Getting up, rising in opposition to the 'other' implies a moral dimension in the case of human Dis-ability, which is tied to the leitmotiv established by the upright posture of *anthropos*. The suggestion that there is a moral dimension to Disability is a radical notion in a culture whose health professionals have become very sensitive to any idea that suggests we are blaming those who through no fault of their own have become in some way disadvantaged as compared to the mainstream of society.[32]

The idea of the *anthropos* (ανθρωπος), which is at the core of this volume, has been brought now full circle. The Japanese post-colonial theorist Nishitani Osamu critiques the global idea of the *anthropos* much as disability theorists interrogate the notion of the normate, as that object to be studied and examined through a Western epistemology. Here we can see the constitution of the Other as the subject of study, a theme that has run through this volume. In contrast for Osamu is *humanitas*, the self-knowing subject. This self-knowing is both meta-physical and physical, mapped by society, but also mapped within each of us as brain functions.

The old dichotomy of nature/nurture is clearly disproven by our sense of posture: it is experienced internally and shaped externally without any true boundary between these aspects of lived experience. This, as Osamu points out, creates a moral distance between two defin-itions of the human: one defined by the observed uprightness of the *anthropos* as categorized by society; the other by our self-consciousness as an 'object of knowledge, in this case the object of knowledge [that] is not natural or physical human being, but the knowing subject itself' – a subject that is beyond 'posturing'.[33] This moral dimension is an omnipresent thread through all of our discussion of posture.

We think of being upstanding as the preferable moral position. To the Victorians, there was no problem inherent in seeing an erect person as 'a tall, upstanding man of spare figure',[34] or indeed seeing 'a white-headed clergyman . . . called upon to say prayers, which he did upstanding'.[35] This was hardly differentiated from the moral upright-ness of 'a lot of game upstanding chaps, that acted like men'.[36] Upright men are at the core of such images, with their moral presence writ large on their posture. But the Romantic reversal is also true. In spite of a misshapen posture, moral action is also possible, indeed may prove the radical falsity of uprightness being the equivalent of morality.

Posture covers all bases: it is the world of the human but also the world of the interpretation of that which is human. In this study we have traced the multiple overlapping images of posture, images that shape the way we see our bodies and are shaped by the moral over-tones given to that selfsame body. We are, in the end, an accretion of all notions of posture, whether we accept or reject them, that we map on our own sense of self.[37] We posture in the world, but are never sure whether our posturing is real or self-consciously feigned. We are sus-pended between Charles Darwin and Uriah Heep, between Plato and Isadora Duncan. Thus we hear in our dreams that call to 'stand up straight!', and know not what to make of it as we rearrange our limbs and straighten our backs.

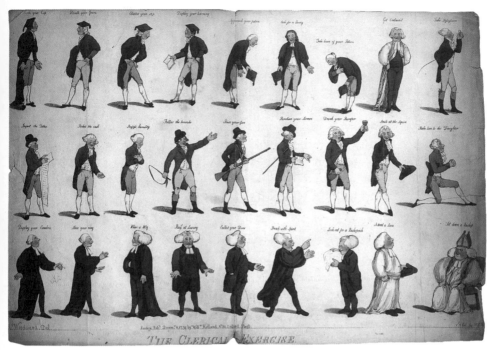

Posture can be a system of dissemblance that can be both seen and learned over a lifetime, as in this caricature of a preacher's postural education, from his initial role as a student 'observing his step' (3) to a stance of 'professed humility, standing, fashionably dressed, his hands crossed on his breast' (12), to his final stage seated as a 'gross, corpulent, ugly bishop, his hands placed arrogantly on his knees' (27). F. G. Broyn, after George Murgatroyd Woodward, 'The Clerical Exercise', 1791, etching with watercolour.

REFERENCES

PREFACE

1 Michael Lynch, 'Discipline and the Material Form of Images: An Analysis of Scientific Visibility', *Social Studies of Science*, XV (1985), p. 43.

INTRODUCTION: POSTURE BEYOND THE WORKPLACE

1 Jane Brody, 'Good Posture May Better your Position', *New York Times* (28 December 2015), p. D5.
2 Quoted by Anson Rabinbach, *The Human Motor: Energy, Fatigue, and the Origins of Modernity* (Berkeley, CA, 1992), p. 6.
3 Kelly Starrett and Glen Cordoza, *Deskbound: Sitting Is the New Smoking* (Las Vegas, NV, 2016).
4 James A. Levine, *Get Up!: Why Your Chair is Killing You and What You Can Do about It* (New York, 2014), p. 1.
5 Matt Lubshansky, 'Let Me Tell You About My Standing Desk', www.the-toast.net, 10 November 2015.
6 S.A.D. Tissot, *Sermo inauguralis de valetudine litteratorum* (Lausanne, 1766); *De la Santé des gens de lettres* (Lausanne, 1768).
7 S. A. Tissot, *An Essay on Disease Incident to Literary and Sedentary Persons*, ed. J. Kirkpatrick (London, 1769), p. 65.
8 Thomas Beddoes, *Hygëia, or, Essays, Moral and Medical, On the Causes Affecting the Personal State of our Middling and Affluent Classes* (Bristol, 1802–3), vol. II, p. 94.
9 Bede, *Expositio in Evangelium S. Lucae, Patrologiae cursus completus. Series latina*, ed. Jacques-Paul Migne (Paris, 1862), vol. XCII, col. 633–936, here 734c.
10 John Armstrong, *The Art of Preserving Health: A Poem* (London, 1744), p. 72.
11 William Buchan, *Domestic Medicine, or the Family Physician* (Philadelphia, PA, 1772), p. 82.
12 Ibid., p. 83.
13 Xenophon of Athens, *Oeconomicus*, trans. E. C. Marchant and O. J. Todd (Cambridge, MA, 1923), vol. IV, p. 415.
14 Ibid., p. 419.

15 Michel Foucault, *The History of Sexuality*, vol. II: *The Use of Pleasure*, trans. Robert Hurley (New York, 1985), 'Ischomachus' Household', pp. 152–66; Leo Strauss, *Xenophon's Socratic Discourse: An Interpretation of the Oeconomicus* (Ithaca, NY, 1970).

16 Jerome Perzigian, 'Lift your Head Up!', *New York Times* (27 February 2017), p. A18.

17 See www.uprightpose.com, accessed 25 March 2017.

ONE: POSTURE IN THE WORLD OF MOVEMENT

1 Matthew B. Roller, *Dining Posture in Ancient Rome: Bodies, Values and Status* (Princeton, NJ, 2006), p. 10.

2 Bernd Jürgen Warneken and Anka Blashofer-Hrusa, eds, *Der aufrechte Gang: Zur Symbolik einer Körperhaltung* (Tübingen, 1990).

3 Mark L. Latash and Vladamir M. Zatsiorski, eds, *Classics in Movement Science* (Champaign, IL, 2001), p. 384.

4 Z. J. Koles and R. D. Castelain, 'The Relationship between Body Sway and Foot Pressure in Normal Man', *Journal of Medical Engineering Technology*, XVIII (1980), pp. 279–85.

5 Oliver Sacks, *A Leg to Stand On* (New York, 1984), p. 107. See also his case study 'On the Level', in *The Man who Mistook His Wife for a Hat and other Clinical Tales* (New York, 1970), pp. 71–6. He uses J. Purdon Martin's *The Basal Ganglia and Posture* (London, 1967), with its account of the pathologies of proprioception to ground his accounts in human physiology, noting constantly how such postural changes amplify his and his patients' sense of psychological disorientation.

6 Sacks, *A Leg to Stand On*, p. ix.

7 Fernando Poyatos, *New Perspectives in Nonverbal Communication: Studies in Cultural Anthropology, Social Psychology, Linguistics, Literature, and Semiotics* (Oxford, 1983), p. 191.

8 Gordon W. Hewes, 'World Distribution of Certain Postural Habits', *American Anthropologist*, LVII (1955), p. 242.

9 A.W.S. Watson and C. MacDonncha, 'A Reliable Technique for the Assessment of Posture: Assessment Criteria for Aspects of Posture', *Journal of Sports Medicine and Physical Fitness*, XL/3 (2000), p. 270.

10 Arthur Frank, *The Wounded Storyteller: Body, Illness, and Ethics* (Chicago, IL, 1995), p. 27.

11 On disability in Shakespeare's England, see Allison P. Hobgood, ed., *Recovering Disability in Early Modern England* (Columbus, OH, 2013).

12 Phyllis Rackin, 'Shakespeare's Boy Cleopatra, the Decorum of Nature, and the Golden World of Poetry', *PMLA*, LXXXVIII (1972), pp. 201–12.

13 Terry Eagleton, *The Function of Criticism* (New York, 1984), p. 15.

14 Ibid., p. 35.

15 The complexity of gender and the cultural ambiguity of the hunchback are central motifs in David T. Mitchell and Sharon L. Snyder, *Narrative Prosthesis: Disability and the Dependencies of Discourse* (Ann Arbor, MI, 2000).

16 That this becomes problematic in the twenty-first century can be seen in the new Reform Jewish High Holidays text, entitled *Mishkan HaNefesh*

in Hebrew, or 'Sanctuary of the Soul'. 'Among the additions is a prayer acknowledging those with disabilities. Alongside a prayer that calls God "the straightener of bent backs", the new one asks, "But what of those who cannot stand up?" and then answers, "Those whose bodies cannot rise possess the same divine essence, the same potential."' Michelle Boorstein, 'Revised Jewish Prayer Book Speaks to Gay Equality, Women and Doubt', *Washington Post* (9 March 2015), available at www.washingtonpost.com.

17 See Allison P. Hobgood, 'Teeth before Eyes: Impairment and Invisibility in Shakespeare's *Richard III*', in *Disability, Health, and Happiness in the Shakespearean Body*, ed. Sujata Iyengar (New York, 2015), pp. 23–40.

18 John Wright, *Child from Home: Memories of a North Country Evacuee* (Stroud, 2009), p. 104.

19 Søren Kierkegaard, *Papers and Journals: A Selection*, trans. Alastair Hannay (Harmondsworth, 1996), p. 347.

20 Roger Poole, *Kierkegaard: The Indirect Communication* (Charlottesville, VA, 1993), pp. 178–80.

21 Barbara Korte, *Body Language in Literature* (Toronto, ON, 1997), p. 165.

22 George Mosse, *The Image of Man: The Creation of Modern Masculinity* (New York, 1996), p. 27.

23 Victor Hugo, *Notre-Dame de Paris*, trans. Isabel F. Hapgood (New York, 1888), p. 309.

24 Jenny Morris, *Pride against Prejudice: Transforming Attitudes to Disability* (Philadelphia, PA, 1991), p. 100.

25 Charles Dickens, *The Posthumous Papers of the Pickwick Club* (London, 1837), p. 153.

26 Philip Larkin, *Selected Letters of Philip Larkin, 1940–1985*, ed. Anthony Thwaite (London, 1992), p. 242.

27 Kingsley Amis, *I Like It Here* (London, 1958), p. 200.

TWO: POSTURES OF THE MIND: THEOLOGY AND PHILOSOPHY EXPLAIN HUMAN POSTURE

1 Edmund Hill, ed. and trans., *The Works of Saint Augustine* (Brooklyn, NY, 1996), vol. III, pt. 4, p. 272.

2 Marjorie O'Rourke Boyle, *Senses of Touch: Human Dignity and Deformity from Michelangelo to Calvin* (Boston, MA, 1998), pp. 31–3.

3 All references are to Pavel Gregorić, 'Plato's and Aristotle's Explanation of Human Posture', *RHIZAI*, II/2 (2005), pp. 183–96.

4 Aristotle, *History of Animals*, trans. A. L. Peck (Cambridge, MA, 1965), vol. I, p. 55.

5 Aristotle, *Parts of Animals*, trans. A. L. Peck and E. S. Forster (Cambridge, MA, 1937), p. 217.

6 Ibid., p. 371.

7 Plato, *Timaeus*, trans. R. G. Bury (Cambridge, MA, 1929), p. 101.

8 Ibid., p. 253.

9 Plato, *Laws II*, trans. R. G. Bury (Cambridge, MA, 1926), p. 553.

10 Gabriela Roxana Carone, *Plato's Cosmology and its Ethical Dimensions* (Cambridge, 2005), p. 155.

11 Werner Jaeger, *Paideia: The Ideals of Greek Culture*, trans. Gilbert Highet (New York, 1945), p. 13.

12 Xenophon of Athens, *Apology*, trans. E. C. Marchant and O. J. Todd (Cambridge, MA, 1923), vol. IV, p. 685.

13 Juvenal, *Satires*, ed. and trans. George Gilbert Ramsey (Cambridge, MA, 1965), pp. 396–7.

14 William Heinemann, *Xenophon*, trans. E. C. Marchant (Cambridge, MA, 1968), pp. 57–8.

15 It seems to be a late anecdote, as can be seen when Sextus Empiricus notes mockingly that 'Plato declares that "Man is a featherless two-footed animal with broad nails, receptive of political science." Sextus Empiricus, *Outlines of Pyrrhonism*, trans. R. G. Bury (Cambridge, MA, 1933), p. 169. Its origins may well be in the so-called Pseudo-Platonic *Definitions*; see Alice Swift Riginos, *Platonica: The Anecdotes Concerning the Life and Writings of Plato* (Leiden, 1976), p. 149.

16 'We ought at that time to have divided walking animals immediately into biped and quadruped, then seeing that the human race falls into the same division with the feathered creatures and no others, we must again divide the biped class into featherless and feathered, and when that division is made and the art of herding human beings is made plain, we ought to take the statesmanlike and kingly man and place him as a sort of charioteer therein, handing over to him the reins of the state, because that is his own proper science.' Plato, *The Statesman*, trans. Harold North Fowler and W.R.M. Lamb (Cambridge, MA, 1925), p. 41.

17 Quoted in Diogenes Laertius, *Lives of Eminent Philosophers*, trans. R. D. Hicks (Cambridge, MA, 1925), vol. II, p. 43.

18 Boyle, *Senses of Touch*, p. 32.

19 Richard Boyd, 'Introduction', in *The Philosophy of Science*, ed. Richard Boyd, Philip Gasper and J. D. Trout (Cambridge, MA, 1991), p. 16.

20 Bertrand Russell, 'Early Drafts on the Theory of Types' [1906–8], in *The Collected Papers*, ed. Gregory H. Moore (New York, 2014), vol. V, pp. 554ff.

21 Anatole France, *Penguin Island*, trans. A. W. Evans (London, 1921), p. 21.

22 Ibid., p. 312.

23 Ovid, *Metamorphoses*, trans. Frank Justus Miller, revd G. P. Goold (Cambridge, MA, 1916), vol. I, p. 9. See Erwin Straus, 'Born to See, Bound to Behold: Reflections on the Function of Upright Posture in the Esthetic Attitude', *Tijdschrift voor Philosophie*, XXVII (1965), p. 659 n.1.

24 Theodore Silverstein, 'The Fabulous Cosmogony of Bernard Silvestris', *Modern Philology*, XLVI (1948–9), pp. 92–116, esp. p. 97 n.28.

25 Even though Philo is clearly attuned to the meaning of posture in the cultures in which he lived, as in his discussion of Melchisedek's posture of prayer after the victory of Abraham over the kings who kidnapped Lot. Jutta Leonhardt, *Jewish Worship in Philo of Alexandria* (Tübingen, 2001), p. 136.

26 *BeReshit Rabbah* 8:11, in H. Freedman, trans., *Midrash Rabba* (London, 1939), vol. I, p. 61.

27 Isidore, *Etymologiae sive Origines*, ed. W. M. Lindsay (Oxford, 1911), vol. II, 1.5. See also *Disability in the Middle Ages: Reconsiderations and Reverberations*, ed. Joshua Eyler (Burlington, VT, 2010).

28 Gregory of Nyssa, 'On the Making of Man', in *Dogmatic Treatises, etc.*, ed. William Moore (Grand Rapids, MI, 1976), pp. 398–9. See also A. H. Armstrong, 'Platonic Elements in St Gregory of Nyssa's Doctrine of Man', *Dominican Studies*, I (1948), pp. 112–26.

29 David Appleby and Teresa Olsen Pierre, 'Upright Posture and Human Dignity According to Bernard of Clairvaux', in *On the Shoulders of Giants: A Festschrift in Honor of Glenn W. Olsen*, ed. David Appleby and Teresa Olsen Pierre (Toronto, ON, 2016), p. 177.

30 Walter Pater, *The Works of Walter Pater* (Cambridge, 1900), vol. I, p. 76.

31 MacDonald Critchley, *Silent Language* (London, 1975), p. 112.

32 Boyle, *Senses of Touch*, p. 81.

33 Quoted in Roy J. Deferrari, trans., *Fathers of the Church* (Washington, DC, 1977), vol. XXXVI, p. 181.

34 Paul Oskar Kristeller, 'The Dignity of Man', in *Renaissance Thought and its Sources*, ed. Michael Mooney (New York, 1979), p. 170.

35 Esther Dotson, 'An Augustinian Interpretation of Michelangelo's Sistine Ceiling', *Art Bulletin*, LXI (1979), pp. 223–56, 405–29.

36 Julien Klaczko, *Rome and the Renaissance: The Pontificate of Julius II*, trans. J. Dennie (New York and London, 1903), p. 292.

37 Leo Steinberg, 'Who's Who in Michelangelo's Creation of Adam: A Chronology of the Picture's Reluctant Self-revelation', *Art Bulletin*, LXXIV (1992), p. 554.

38 Johann Gottfried Herder, *Outlines of a Philosophy of the History of Man*, trans. T. Churchill (London, 1800, repr. New York, n.d.), pp. 67–8.

39 Ibid., p. 67.

40 Sander L. Gilman, *On Blackness without Blacks: Essays on the Image of the Black in Germany* (Boston, MA, 1982), pp. 30–36.

41 Ibid., p. 49.

42 Quoted by Marjorie Grene and David Depew, *The Philosophy of Biology: An Episodic History* (Cambridge, 2004), p. 325.

43 Ibid., p. 70.

44 For an odd, almost mechanical reading of this notion of posture, see Frank Ardolino, 'Satan's "Ups and Downs": Posture and Posturing in Books I and II of *Paradise Lost*', *Journal of Evolutionary Psychology*, XIV (1993), pp. 53–9.

45 Susannah B. Mintz, *Threshold Poetics: Milton and Intersubjectivity* (Newark, DE, 2003), p. 237.

46 Georgia Christopher, 'Milton and the Reforming Spirit', in *The Cambridge Companion to Milton*, ed. Dennis Danielson (Cambridge, 1989), pp. 200–201.

47 Maharal, *Tiferet Israel*, ed. Avigdor Shiloh (Merkaz Shapira, 5770 [2010]), chapter 16, p. 3; trans. Hannah Tzuberi with my thanks.

48 See Cathy S. Gelbin, *The Golem Returns: From German Romantic Literature to Global Jewish Culture, 1808–2008* (Ann Arbor, MI, 2010).

49 Astrid Gesche, *Johann Gottfried Herder: Sprache und die Natur des Menschen* (Würzburg, 1993), p. 87.

50 Kant used this phrase from Horace's *Epistles* 1.2.40 to define the Enlightenment in his 'An Answer to the Question: "What Is Enlightenment"', first published in the *Berlinische Monatsschrift*,

December 1784. See James Schmidt, ed., *What Is Enlightenment? Eighteenth-century Answers and Twentieth-century Questions* (Berkeley, CA, 1996), p. 58.

51 Immanuel Kant, 'Idea for a Universal History with a Cosmopolitan Aim', in *The Cambridge Edition of the Works of Immanuel Kant: Anthropology, History and Education*, ed. Günter Zöller and Robert B. Louden, trans. Allen Wood (Cambridge, 2007), p. 113.

52 Immanuel Kant, 'Idee zu einer allgemeinen Geschichte in weltbürgerlicher Absicht', in *Kant: Gesammelte Schriften: Akademie Ausgabe* (Berlin, 1912), vol. VIII, p. 23.

53 Kant, 'Idea for a Universal History', p. 113. Woods translates *künstlich* as 'artificial'. While certainly true, it is clear that what Kant is stressing is the potential for human malleability.

54 Ibid.

55 Isaiah Berlin, *The Crooked Timber of Humanity* (New York, 1991), p. 50. Oddly, these questions are not discussed in Angelica Nuzzo, *Ideal Embodiment: Kant's Theory of Sensibility* (Bloomington, IN, 2008).

56 Mark Poster, 'Kant's Crooked Stick', *Psychoanalytic Review*, LXI (1974), p. 477.

57 David Blackbourn, *The Conquest of Nature: Water, Landscape and the Making of Modern Germany* (New York, 2006), p. 40.

58 Ibid., p. 44.

59 Stephen Jeffries, 'The Conflict Surrounding Ferdinand von Mueller's Scientific Botanic Garden as a Site of Spiritual Elevation', in *Die Lektüre der Welt: Zur Theorie, Geschichte und Soziologie kultureller Praxis/Worlds of Reading: On the Theory, History and Sociology of Cultural Practice*, ed. Helmut Heinze and Christiane Weller (Frankfurt am Main, 2004), pp. 55–62.

60 Rafael Ziegler, 'Crooked Wood, Straight Timber – Kant, Development and Nature', *Public Reason*, II (2010), p. 67.

61 *Goethes Werke – Im Auftrag der Großherzogin Sophie von Sachsen* (Weimar, 1887–1919), section 1, vol. XXVII, pp. 175–90.

62 Michael Mack, 'The Other', in *The Oxford Handbook of German Philosophy in the Nineteenth Century*, ed. Michael N. Forster and Kristin Gjesdal (Oxford, 2015), p. 744.

63 Hans S. Reiss, ed., *Kant: Political Writings*, trans. H. B. Nisbet (Cambridge, 1991), p. 203.

64 Kant cites Rousseau's *Émile* (1762) as his model for human moral development, a text that begins in that same metaphoric garden.

65 Immanuel Kant, *Conjectural Beginning of Human History*, in *Toward Perpetual Peace and Other Writings on Politics, Peace, and History*, ed. Pauline Kleingeld (New Haven, CT, 2006), p. 25.

66 Ibid., p. 29.

67 Herder, *Outlines of a Philosophy of the History of Man*, p. 200.

68 'Of the Corporeal Essential Differences between the Structure of Humans and Animals', trans. Gunter Zoller, *Kant: Anthropology, History and Education*, pp. 79–81.

69 John H. Zammito, *Kant, Herder, and the Birth of Anthropology* (Chicago, IL, 2002), p. 302.

70 Immanuel Kant, *Lectures on Anthropology*, ed. Allen W. Wood and Robert B. Louden, trans. Robert R. Clewis and G. Felicitas Munzel (Cambridge, 2013), pp. 533–4.

71 Poster, 'Kant's Crooked Stick', p. 478.

72 See Leah Hochman, *The Ugliness of Moses Mendelssohn: Aesthetics, Religion and Morality in the Eighteenth Century* (New York, 2014), pp. 19–20.

73 Michael Mack, *German Idealism and the Jew: The Inner Antisemitism of Philosophy and German Jewish Responses* (Chicago, IL, 2003).

74 Johann Gottlieb Fichte, *Foundations of Natural Right in Accordance with the Principles of Wissenschaftslehre*, ed. Frederick Neuhouser, trans. Michael Baur (Cambridge, 2000), pp. 78–9.

75 Ibid.

76 Ibid.

77 Karl Rosenkranz, *Aesthetik des Hässlichen* (Königsberg, 1853), p. 51. See Werner Jung, *Schöner Schein der Häßlichkeit oder Häßlichkeit des schönen Scheines* (Frankfurt am Main, 1987), pp. 187–244 (translation by author).

78 Rosenkranz, *Aesthetik des Hässlichen*, p. 52.

79 R.W.B. Lewis, *The American Adam: Innocence, Tragedy and Tradition in the Nineteenth Century* (Chicago, IL, 1955), p. 35.

80 All references are to Oliver Wendell Holmes, *Elsie Venner: A Romance of Destiny*, in *The Poetical Works of Oliver Wendell Holmes* (Boston, MA, 1895), vol. V, pp. 248–9. See also Justine Murison, *The Politics of Anxiety in Nineteenth Century American Literature* (Cambridge, 2013), pp. 5–6; and Jane Thrailkill, *Affecting Fiction: Mind, Body, and Emotion in American Literary Realism* (Cambridge, MA, 2007), pp. 10–14.

81 Robert Ernest Spiller, ed., *The Early Lectures of Ralph Waldo Emerson* (Cambridge, MA, 1969), vol. III, p. 189. In this context, see David van Leer, *Emerson's Epistemology: The Argument of the Essays* (Cambridge, 1986) on Emerson as a Kantian.

82 G.W.F. Hegel, *Hegel's Aesthetics: Lectures on Fine Art*, ed. and trans. T. M. Knox (Oxford, 1988), vol. II, p. 739.

83 Susan Buck-Morss, *Hegel, Haiti and Universal History* (Pittsburgh, PA, 2009), pp. 21–78.

84 Alexandre Kojève, *Introduction to the Reading of Hegel, Lectures on the Phenomenology of Spirit*, ed. Allan Bloom, trans. James H. Nichols, Jr (Ithaca, NY, and London, 1980), p. 47.

85 Oscar Wilde, 'The Decay of Lying', in *The Complete Writings of Oscar Wilde* (New York, 1909), vol. VII, pp. 48–9.

86 Anon., 'Correct Posture', *The Lancet*, CCV/5291 (1925), p. 193.

87 Joel E. Goldthwait, 'An Anatomic and Mechanistic Conception of Disease', *Boston Medical and Surgical Journal*, CLXXII (1915), p. 891.

88 Nigel Spivey, *Greek Sculpture* (Cambridge, 2013), p. 37. See also Robin Osborne, *The History Written on the Classical Greek Body* (Cambridge, 2011).

89 Suzanne L. Marchand, *Down from Olympus: Archeology and Pan-Hellenism in Germany, 1750–1970* (Princeton, NJ, 1996), p. 15.

90 George Mosse, *The Image of Man: The Creation of Modern Masculinity* (New York, 1996), p. 35.

91 G.W.F. Hegel, *Hegel's Philosophy of Mind*, ed. and trans. Michael J. Inwood (Oxford, 2012), p. 143.
92 Ibid., p. 149.
93 Frantz Fanon, *Black Skin, White Masks*, trans. Richard Philcox (New York, 1967), p. 220.

THREE: CHEST OUT! POSTURE'S MILITARY MEANINGS

1 John Taylor, *An apology for private preaching in which those formes are warranted or rather justified, which the maligannt sect contemne and daily by prophane pamphlets make ridiculous: viz. preaching in a tub: teaching against the backe of a chaire: instructing at a tables end: revealing in a basket: exhorting over a buttery hatch: reforming on a bad side or, indeed, any place according to inspiration, since it is knowne, the spirit moves in sundry places: whereunto is annexed, or rather conjoyned or furthermore united, or moreover knit the spirituall postures, alluding to that of musket and pike / by T. J.* (London, 1642), p. [6].
2 All these references are from 'Posture' in the *Oxford English Dictionary Online*. See www.oed.com, accessed 7 November 2013.
3 E. M. Curley, ed., *The Collected Works of Spinoza* (Princeton, NJ, 1985), vol. I, p. 373.
4 Flavius Vegetius Renatus, *The Military Institutions of the Romans*, trans. John Clarke (1767). See www.digitalattic.org, accessed 10 September 2016.
5 Sara Elise Phang, *Roman Military Service: Ideologies of Discipline in the Late Republic and Early Principate* (Cambridge, 2008), p. 103.
6 Pierre Bourdieu, *Masculine Domination*, trans. Richard Nice (Cambridge, 2001), pp. 171–4.
7 George Mosse, *The Image of Man: The Creation of Modern Masculinity* (New York, 1996), p. 192.
8 Phang, *Roman Military Service*, p. 100.
9 Pierre Bourdieu, *The Logic of Practice*, trans. Richard Nice (Palo Alto, CA, 1990), p. 71.
10 Anthony Corbeill, *Nature Embodied: Gesture in Ancient Rome* (Princeton, NJ, 2004), pp. 70–72.
11 MacGregor Knox and Murray Williamson, eds, *The Dynamics of Military Revolution, 1300–2050* (Cambridge, 2001), p. 49.
12 Elias Canetti, *Crowds and Power*, trans. Carol Stewart (New York, 1962), p. 312.
13 Klaus Theweleit, *Male Fantasies*, trans. Erica Carter and Chris Turner (Minneapolis, MN, 1989), vol. II, p. 160.
14 Michel Foucault, *Discipline and Punish: The Birth of the Prison*, trans. Alan Sheridan (New York, 1995), pp. 135–6.
15 Tobin Siebers, *Disability Theory* (Ann Arbor, MI, 2008), p. 58.
16 Susan Griffin, *A Chorus of Stones: The Private Life of War* (New York, 1993), p. 238.
17 Mary Mosher Flesher, 'Repetitive Order and the Human Walking Apparatus: Prussian Military Science versus the Webers' Locomotion Research', *Annals of Science*, LIV (1997), p. 466.

18 Geoffrey Parker, *The Military Revolution: Military Innovation and the Rise of the West, 1500–1800* (Cambridge, 1988), pp. 18–19.

19 Susanne J. Walker, 'Arms and the Man: Constructing the Soldier in Jacques de Gheyn's "Wapenhandelinghe"', *Nederlands Kunsthistorisch Jaarboek*, LVIII (2007/8), p. 142.

20 Johann Friedrich von Flemming, *Der vollkommene Teutsche Soldat welcher die gantze Kriegs-Wissenschafft, insonderheit was bey der Infanterie vorkommt, vorträgt, von Hannss Friedrich von Fleming* (Leipzig, 1726; repr. Graz, 1967).

21 Walker, 'Arms and the Man', pp. 138–61.

22 Ibid., p. 144.

23 See Herman Roodenburg, ed., *A Cultural History of Gesture from Antiquity to the Present Day* (Ithaca, NY, 1992), pp. 88–9.

24 Herman Roodenburg, *The Eloquence of the Body: Perspectives on Gesture in the Dutch Republic* (Zwolle, 2004).

25 Walker, 'Arms and the Man', p. 161: 'compared to the task of the fencing masters, who dealt in an activity that encompassed a wider variety of possible situations, with a relatively undeveloped descriptive language. Chapter four of [Domenico] Angelo's book, "Sword Fighting: Vocabulary and Taxonomy" [1763] (119–147) is a fascinating case study of the use of words, pictures, and abstract concepts to communicate the activity of fighting.'

26 Ben Jonson, *The Workes of Benjamin Jonson* (London, 1640), p. 38.

27 All cited in the *Oxford English Dictionary Online*, www.oed.com, accessed 24 January 2013.

28 Immanuel Kant, 'Idea for a Universal History with a Cosmopolitan Aim', in *The Cambridge Edition of the Works of Immanuel Kant: Anthropology, History and Education*, ed. Günter Zöller and Robert B. Louden, trans. Allen Wood (Cambridge, 2007).

29 Robert D. Eagleson and C. T. Onions, *A Shakespeare Glossary* (Oxford, 1986), p. 324.

30 Karl Gaulhofer, *Die Fusshaltung. Ein Beitrag zur Stilgeschichte der menschlichen Bewegung* (Kassel, 1930), p. 62.

31 'Art militaire, exercice', in *Encyclopédie méthodique ou Dictionnaire raisonné des sciences, des arts, et des métiers*, ed. Denis Diderot and Jean d'Alembert (Paris, 1762), vol. XVIII, plate 10, 1.

32 Christian von Mechel, *Soldaten- und Plotons-Schule für die Infanterie, aus dem französischen Reglement vom 1. August 1791, übersetzt. Herausgegeben mit 13 meist neu gezeichneten Kupfer-Tafeln* (Basle, 1799), p. 5 (translation by author).

33 Carney Lake, *Reflected Glory* (London, 1990), p. 14.

34 Vegetius, *The Military Institutions of the Romans*.

35 Larry H. Addington, *The Patterns of War through the Eighteenth-century* (Bloomington, IN, 1990), p. 122.

36 [Friedrich Christoph von Saldern,] *Elements of Tacticks, and Introduction to Military Evolutions for the Infantry by a Celebrated Prussian General*, trans. Isaac Landmann (London, 1787), p. 2.

37 Ibid., pp. 3–4.

38 Ibid.

39 Azar Gat, *A History of Military Thought: From the Enlightenment to the Cold War* (Oxford, 2001), pp. 38–9.

40 William O. Shanahan, *Prussian Military Reforms: 1786–1813* (New York, 1945), p. 35.

41 Reginald Thoumine, *Scientific Soldier: A Life of General Le Marchant, 1766–1812* (Oxford, 1968).

42 Colonel David Dundas, *Principles of Military Movements, Chiefly Applied to Infantry. Illustrated by Manoeuvres of the Prussian Troops* (London, 1788), p. 41.

43 Roodenberg, ed., *A Cultural History of Gesture*, p. 47.

44 James Fenimore Cooper, *The Spy* (New York, 1821), vol. I, p. 3.

45 The implications of this revelation are explored in Melissa Fegan, *Wuthering Heights: Character Studies* (New York, 2008), pp. 79–81.

46 Arthur Conan Doyle, *The Complete Sherlock Holmes* (Garden City, NY [1959]), p. 14.

47 Thomas Wilkinson Speight, 'By Devious Ways', *Gentleman's Magazine Christmas Annual*, CCLXV (1888), p. 2.

48 Victor L. Whitechurch, 'The Mystery of the German Dispatch-box', in *Vintage Mystery and Detective Stories*, ed. David Stuart Davis (London, 2006), p. 345.

49 Gaulhofer, *Die Fusshaltung*, pp. 62ff.

50 Flesher, 'Repetitive Order and the Human Walking Apparatus', pp. 463–87.

51 E. H. Weber, 'Anatomisch/physiologische Untersuchung über einige Einrichtungen im Mechanismus der menschlichen Wirbelsäule', *Archiv für Anatomie und Physiologie* (1827), pp. 240–71 (with plates).

52 Christopher Duffy, *The Military Experience in the Age of Reason* (New York, 1987), p. 112.

53 Wilhelm and Eduard Weber, *Mechanik der menschlichen Gehwerkzeuge: Eine anatomisch–physiologische Untersuchung* (Göttingen, 1836), p. 99 (translation by the author).

54 Ibid., p. 401.

55 Ibid., p. 9.

56 Franz Carl Naegele, *Das weibliche Becken: Betrachtet in Beziehung auf seine Stellung und die Richtung seiner Höhle: Nebst Beyträgen zur Geschichte der Lehre von den Beckenaxen* (Karlsruhe, 1825).

57 Carl von Clausewitz, *On War* (Ware, UK, 1997), p. 83.

58 'Progress in anatomy is most likely to occur when its problems include the study of growth and function, as well as of structure.' Reinhard Hildebrand, 'Über den Anatomen und Physiologen Ernst Heinrich Weber (1795–1878) und über Wilhelm His (1831–1904), seinen Nachfolger auf dem Lehrstuhl für Anatomie an der Universität Leipzig', *Annals of Anatomy*, CLXXXVII (2005), pp. 439–59.

59 Christian Wilhelm Braune and Otto Fischer, *Über den Schwerpunkt des menschlichen Körpers mit Rücksicht auf die Ausrüstung des deutschen Infanteristen* (Leipzig, 1889), pp. 3–4. The English translation is *On the Centre of Gravity of the Human Body as Related to the Equipment of the German Infantry Soldier* (Berlin and New York, 1985).

60 Christian Wilhelm Braune and Otto Fischer, *Der Gang des Menschen* (Leipzig, 1899). The English translation is *Human Mechanics* (Springfield, VA, 1963).

61 Nathan Zuntz and Wilhelm Schumberg, *Studien zu einer Physiologie des Marsches* (Berlin, 1901). On the single step in marching, see pp. 290–91. On the context of the history of physiology, see Anson Rabinbach, *The Human Motor: Energy, Fatigue, and the Origins of Modernity* (Berkeley, CA, 1991), p. 189.

62 William Hardy McNeill, *Keeping Together in Time: Dance and Drill in Human History* (Cambridge, MA, 1995), p. 1.

63 Braune and Fischer, *Über den Schwerpunkt des menschlichen Körpers*, pp. 6–7.

64 Oliver Wendell Holmes, 'The Stereoscope and the Stereograph', *Atlantic Monthly*, III/20 (1859), p. 740.

65 Joseph Grigely, 'Postcards to Sophie Calle', in *The Body Aesthetic: From Fine Art to Body Modification*, ed. Tobin Siebers (Ann Arbor, MI, 2000), p. 32.

66 Eadweard Muybridge, *Animal Locomotion: An Electro-photographic Investigation of Consecutive Phases of Animal Movements. Prospectus and Catalogue of Plates* (Philadelphia, PA, 1887).

67 Sarah Gordon, *Indecent Exposures: Eadweard Muybridge's Animal Locomotion Nudes* (New Haven, CT, 2015), p. 117.

68 Quoted in George Mather, *The Psychology of Visual Art: Eye, Brain, and Art* (Cambridge, 2014), p. 93.

69 Quoted ibid.

70 Quoted in Tom Gunning, 'New Thresholds of Vision: Instantaneous Photography and the Early Cinema of Lumiere', in *Impossible Presence: Surface and Screen in the Photogenic Era*, ed. Terry Smith (Chicago, IL, 2001), p. 89.

71 Quoted in Katherine Kuh, ed., *The Artist's Voice: Talks with Seventeen Modern Artists* (New York, 1962), p. 83.

72 Lawrence Rainey, Christine Poggi and Laura Wittman, eds, *Futurism: An Anthology* (New Haven, CT, 2009), p. 314.

73 Bernd Martin, *Japan and Germany in the Modern World* (Providence, RI, 1995), pp. 40ff.

74 'Medicine: Posture Lady', www.time.com, 5 April 1937.

75 Robin Veder, 'Seeing your Way to Health: The Visual Pedagogy of Bess Mensendieck's Physical Culture System', *International Journal of the History of Sport*, XXVIII (2011), pp. 1336–52.

76 Karl Toepfer, *Empire of Ecstasy: Nudity and Movement in German Body Culture, 1910–1935* (Berkeley, CA, 1997), pp. 38ff.

77 'Medicine: Posture Lady'.

78 Mike Huggins and Mike O'Mahony, *The Visual in Sport* (New York, 2012), pp. 252ff.

79 Liaquat Ahamed, *Lords of Finance: The Bankers Who Broke the World* (New York, 2009), p. 130.

80 Bess M. Mensendieck, *It's Up to You* (New York, 1931), pp. 193–4.

81 Ana Carden-Coyne, *Reconstructing the Body: Classicism, Modernism and the First World War* (Oxford, 2009), p. 307.

82 Katharina von Ankum, *Women in the Metropolis: Gender and Modernity in Weimar Culture* (Berkeley, CA, 1997), p. 40.

FOUR: MEDICINE AS THERAPY FOR AN UNHEALTHY POSTURE

1 Hippocrates of Kos, *Prognostic*, trans. W.H.S. Jones (Cambridge, MA, 1924), vol. II, p. 13.
2 Carolyn Smith-Morris, *Diagnostic Controversy: Cultural Perspectives on Competing Knowledge in Healthcare* (New York, 2015), pp. 1–2, 19.
3 E. S. Vasiliadis, T. B. Grivas and A. Kaspiris, 'Historical Overview of Spinal Deformities in Ancient Greece', *Scoliosis*, IV/6 (2009), pp. 1–13.
4 Hippocrates, *Prognostic*, vol. II, p. 283.
5 Galen, *De affectorum locorum notita* (Cambridge, MA, 1990), iv.6.
6 Martha L. Rose, *The Staff of Oedipus: Transforming Disability in Ancient Greece* (Ann Arbor, MI, 2003), pp. 43–4.
7 Jean-Paul Vernant and Pierre Vidal-Naquet, *Myth and Tragedy in Ancient Greece*, trans. Janet Lloyd (New York, 1988), p. 136.
8 Ibid., p. 211.
9 René Girard, *Oedipus Unbound: Selected Writing on Rivalry and Desire*, ed. Mark R. Ansbach (Stanford, CA, 2004), p. 110.
10 Harold Bloom, ed., *Sophocles' Oedipus Rex* (New York, 2007), p. 58.
11 Louis Fu, 'Hippocratic Medicine in China: Comparison with a 9th Century Chinese Manual on Bone Setting', *Journal of Orthopaedics, Trauma and Rehabilitation*, XVIII (2014), pp. 128–35.
12 The ancients also knew the triple curvature of the spine, as we can see in the Hippocratic corpus in *De articulis*. See Hippocrates, *The Genuine Works of Hippocrates*, ed. Charles Darwin Adams (New York, 1868), 45.24ff.
13 Vesalius cites *De ossibus* in the margin. 'The tenth . . . is the only vertebra to have not only its upward apophyses but also its downward terminating in condyloid ends.' (§760 of Galen, *De ossibus ad tirones*. See Charles Singer, trans., 'Galen's Elementary Course on Bones', *Proceedings of the Royal Society of Medicine*, XLV [1952], pp. 25–34.) See also Galen, *On the Usefulness of the Parts of the Body. De usu partium*, trans. Margaret Tallmadge May (Ithaca, NY, 1968), 4.79.1ff. In this work, Galen describes the unique articulation that he ascribes to the tenth thoracic vertebra: 'Just as this vertebra has a special position and a special posterior outgrowth not shared with the others, so its articulations are special too; for in order that the whole spine might bend uniformly it was of course necessary for the middle vertebra to remain in place while all the others withdrew gradually from one another and from it, the upper ones retiring upward and the lower ones down' (p. 588). This is what Vesalius means when he quotes Galen as saying this vertebra 'is supported above and below', *supra infraque suscipi*. But we are unable to find a passage in either of the Galenic works where it is stated that transverse processes in thoracic vertebrae 10–12 would have interfered with lateral motion of the spine. In the edition of 1555 Vesalius rewrote the parenthesis as follows: 'Which Galen said is received from the adjacent vertebrae by its ascending and descending processes, as we shall say more explicitly a little later.'

14 Maude Gleason, 'Shock and Awe: The Performance Dimension of Galen's Anatomy Demonstrations', in *Galen and the World of Knowledge*, ed. Christopher Gill, Tim Whitmarsh and John Wilkins (Cambridge, 2009), p. 112.

15 Reinhard Hildebrand, 'Attic Perfection in Anatomy: Bernhard Siegfried Albinus (1697–1770) and Samuel Thomas Soemmerring (1755–1830)', *Anatomischer Anzeiger*, CLXXXVII (2005), pp. 555–73.

16 Ibid., p. 558.

17 Ibid., p. 561.

18 Robert Herrlinger and Edith Feiner, 'Why Did Vesalius not Discover the Fallopian Tubes?', *Medical History*, VIII (1964), pp. 335–41.

19 Hildebrand, 'Attic Perfection in Anatomy', p. 561.

20 Beth Linker, 'A Dangerous Curve: The Role of History in America's Scoliosis Screening Programs', *American Journal of Public Health*, CII/4 (2012), pp. 606–16.

21 George T. Stafford, 'First Problem in Education to Prevent or Correct Physical Defects', *School Life*, X (1925), pp. 114–15.

22 Joel E. Goldthwait, *Body Mechanics in the Study and Treatment of Disease* (Philadelphia, PA, 1934), p. 31.

23 Joel E. Goldthwait, 'An Anatomic and Mechanistic Conception of Disease', *Boston Medical and Surgical Journal*, CLXXII (1915), pp. 881–98.

24 Ibid.

25 Ibid., p. 897.

26 Irving Fisher and Eugene Lyman Fisk, *How to Live: Rules for Healthful Living, Based on Modern Science* (New York, 1915), p. 57. See also Laura D. Hirschbein, 'Masculinity, Work and the Foundation of Youth: Irving Fisher and the Life Extension Institute, 1914–1931', *Canadian Bulletin of Medicine*, XVI (1999), pp. 89–124.

27 Fisher and Fisk, *How to Live*, p. 57.

28 Ibid., p. 147.

29 Office of the Surgeon General, *Defects Found in Drafted Men* (Washington, DC, 1920). See also Beth Linker, *War's Waste: Rehabilitation in World War I America* (Chicago, IL, 2011).

30 Constance Malpas, 'Jules Guerin Makes his Market: The Social Economy of Orthopaedic Medicine in Paris, 1825–45', in *Cultural Approaches to the History of Medicine: Mediating Medicine in Early Modern and Modern Europe*, ed. Willem de Blécourt and Cornelie Usborne (New York, 2004), pp. 187–213.

31 Valerie Steele, *The Corset: A Cultural History* (New Haven, CT, 2001), p. 56.

32 Lynne Sorge-English, *Stays and Body Image in London: The Staymaking Trade, 1680–1810* (London, 2011), p. 124.

33 Frank Drake Dickson, *Posture: Its Relationship to Health* (Philadelphia, PA, and London, 1931), p. 112.

34 John Spargo, *The Bitter Cry of the Children* (London, 1916), p. 5.

35 Charles Elgood, 'A Note on the Etiology of Rickets', *The Lancet*, CLIV/3964 (1899), p. 488.

36 Alfred Adler, 'The Development of the Child: Preventing the Inferiority Complex', in *The Collected Clinical Works of Alfred Adler*, ed. Henry T. Stein (Bellingham, WA, 2006), vol. XI, p. 141.

37 William G. Niederland, 'Clinical Observations on the "Little Man" Phenomenon', *Psychoanalytic Study of the Child*, XI (1956), pp. 381–95.

38 William James, *The Principles of Psychology* (New York, 1899), vol. II, p. 468.

39 Heikki Lempa, *Beyond the Gymnasium: Educating Middle-class Bodies in Germany* (Lanham, MD, 2007), p. 67.

40 Daniel Gottlieb Moritz Schreber, *Das ärtzliche Zimmergymnastik*, 30th edn (Leipzig, 1905), pp. 27–8.

41 See the discussion in the anonymous essay 'Das Turnen in der Volksschule', *Volksschulblatt*, V/43 (1858), p. 676.

42 Moritz Schreber, *Illustrated Medical In-door Gymnastics*, trans. Henry Skelton (London and Edinburgh, 1856), p. 5.

43 Daniel Gottlieb Moritz Schreber, *Die schädlichen Körperhaltung und Gewohnheiten der Kinder: Nebst Angabe der Mittel dagegen* (Leipzig, 1853).

44 Such as *Kallipädie oder Erziehung zur Schönheit: Durch naturgetreue und gleichmässige Förderung normaler Körperbildung, lebenstüchtiger Gesundheit und geistiger Veredelung und insbesondere durch mögliche Benutzung specieller Ersiehungsmittel; Für Aeltern, Erzieher und Lehrer* (Leipzig, 1858).

45 Ibid., p. 51.

46 Thomas Szasz, 'The Psychology of Bodily Feelings in Schizophrenia', *Psychosomatic Medicine*, XIX (1957), p. 14.

47 Morton Schatzman, *Soul Murder: Persecution in the Family* (New York, 1973); this was rebutted in Zvi Lothane, *In Defense of Schreber: Soul Murder and Psychiatry* (Hillsdale, NJ, and London, 1992). On the implications of gender and race here, see also Jonathan Dollimore, *Sexual Dissidence: Augustine to Wilde, Freud to Foucault* (Oxford, 1991), pp. 169–90. For my detailed reading of this text, see my *Freud, Race, and Gender* (Princeton, NJ, 1993), pp. 140–61.

48 Daniel Paul Schreber, *Denkwürdigkeiten eines Nervenkranken nebst Nachträgen und einem Anhang über die Frage: 'Unter welchen Voraussetzungen darf eine für geisteskrank erachtete Person gegen ihren Willen in einer festgehalten werden?'* (Leipzig, 1903). All references are to Daniel Paul Schreber, *Memoir of My Nervous Illness*, trans. Ida Macalpine and Richard A. Hunter (New York, 2000), here pp. 113, 106.

49 Ibid., p. 280.

50 Ibid., p. 133.

51 Letter from Sigmund Freud to Carl Gustav Jung, 31 October 1910, in *The Freud/Jung Letters: The Correspondence Between Sigmund Freud and C. G. Jung*, ed. William McGuire, trans. Ralph Manheim and R.F.C. Hull (Princeton, NJ, 1979), p. 368.

52 Friedrich Eduard Bilz, *Das neue Naturheilverfahren mit Einschluß der Biologie und aller verwandten Heilmethoden* (Leipzig, 1888), p. 454.

53 Eike Reichardt, 'Health, "Race" and Empire: Popular-scientific Spectacles and National Identity in Imperial Germany, 1871–1914', PhD thesis, Stony Brook University, 2006, p. 111, www.lulu.com, accessed 15 January 2014; and Paul Weindling, *Health, Race and German Politics between National Unification and Nazism, 1870–1945* (Cambridge, 1989), p. 22.

54 Nils Hansson and Anders Ottosson, 'Nobel Prize for Physical Therapy? Rise, Fall, and Revival of Medico-Mechanical Institutes', *Physical Therapy*, XCV (2015), pp. 1184–94.

55 J. H. Kellogg, *The Art of Massage* (Battle Creek, MI, 1909), p. v.

56 See Carol Thomas Neely, *Distracted Subjects: Madness and Gender in Shakespeare and Early Modern Culture* (Ithaca, NY, 2004), esp. pp. 167–212.

57 Sander L. Gilman, *Seeing the Insane: A Cultural History of Psychiatric Illustration* (New York, 1982; repr. Brattleboro, VT, 2013), pp. 12–22, 214–22.

58 Sander L. Gilman, *Health and Illness: Images of Difference* (London, 1995), p. 156.

59 Hippolyte Bruyères, *La Phrenologie, la Geste, et la Physiognomie, démontrés par 120 Portraits* (Paris, 1847).

60 Joseph Simms, *Physiognomy Illustrated: Or, Nature's Revelations of Character. A Description of the Mental, Moral, and Volitive Dispositions of Mankind, as Manifested in the Human Form and Countenance* (New York, 1887), p. 267.

61 Ibid., p. 397.

62 George Combe, *Elements of Phrenology* (Philadelphia, PA, 1826), p. 48.

63 Christopher Lukasik, *Discerning Characters: The Culture of Appearance in Early America* (Philadelphia, PA, 2010), p. 12.

64 Archibald Church and Frederick Peterson, eds, *Nervous and Mental Diseases* (Philadelphia, PA, and London, 1919), p. 19.

65 Frederick Peterson, 'Idiocy', ibid., p. 887.

66 Anon., 'The Stereotyped Attitudes and Postures of the Insane in Regard to Diagnosis and Prognosis', *The Lancet*, CLIX/4094 (1902), pp. 465–6.

67 A. Ross Diefendorf, *Clinical Psychiatry*, adapted from Emil Kraepelin, *Lehrbuch der Psychiatrie*, 7th edn (New York, 1915), p. 241.

68 H. C. Rümke, 'The Nuclear Symptom of Schizophrenia and the Praecox Feeling' [1941], trans. Jan Neeleman, *History of Psychiatry*, I (1990), pp. 331–41.

69 L. J. King, 'A Sensory Integrative Approach to Schizophrenia', *American Journal of Occupational Therapy*, XXVIII (1974), pp. 529–36.

70 Kristin S. Cadenhead, Yulya Serper and David L. Braff, 'Transient versus Sustained Visual Channels in the Visual Backward Masking Deficits of Schizophrenia Patients', *Biological Psychiatry*, XLIII (1998), pp. 132–8.

71 Aulikki Ahlgrén-Rimpiläinen, et al., 'Effect of Visual Information on Postural Control in Patients with Schizophrenia', *Journal of Nervous and Mental Disorders*, CXCVIII (2010), pp. 601–3.

72 American Psychiatric Association, ed., *Diagnostic and Statistical Manual of Mental Disorders*, 5th edn (Washington, DC, 2013), p. 157.

73 'Minutes', *Bulletin of the International Psycho-Analytic Association*, III (1922), p. 133.

74 See, for example, George Frederick Drinka, *The Birth of Neurosis: Myth, Malady and the Victorians* (New York, 1984), pp. 108–22. See also Esther Fischer-Homburger, *Die traumatische Neurose: Vom somatischen zum sozialen Leiden* (Bern, 1975).

75 John Eric Erichsen, *On Concussion of the Spine, Nervous Shock, and Other Obscure Injuries to the Nervous System in their Clinical and Medico-legal Aspects* (New York, 1886), p. 94.

76 C.-É. Brown-Séquard, 'On the Hereditary Transmission of Effects of Certain Injuries to the Nervous System', *The Lancet*, CV/2679 (1875), pp. 7–8.

77 Hans Schmaus, 'Zur Casuistik und pathologischen Anatomie der Rückenmarkserschütterung', *Archiv für klinische Chirurgie*, XLII (1891), pp. 112–22, with plates.

78 Daniel Hack Tuke, *Chapters on the History of the Insane in the British Isles* (London, 1882), p. 183.

79 Charles M. Tipton, ed., *History of Exercise Physiology* (Windsor, ON, 2014).

80 Francis Galton, 'Eugenics: Its Definition, Scope, and Aims', *American Journal of Sociology*, X/1 (1904), www.mugu.com.

81 Quoted ibid.

82 Christine Rosen, *Preaching Eugenics: Religious Leaders and the American Eugenics Movement* (New York, 2004), p. 113.

83 Francis Galton, 'Eugenics and the Jew', *Jewish Chronicle* (29 July 1910), p. 16.

84 University of Minnesota Libraries Archives, 'The Relation of Posture to Health', *The Minnesota Children's Home Finder* (1922), box 40, folder 40-8, homefinder 8.

85 Henry G. Beyer, 'The International Hygiene Exhibition at Dresden', *Popular Science Monthly*, LXXX (1912), p. 122.

86 Ibid., p. 120.

87 Martin Vogel, 'Das Deutsche Hygiene-Museum Dresden', in *Grosse Ausstellung Düsseldorf 1926 für Gesundheitspflege, Soziale Fürsorge und Leibesübungen* (Düsseldorf, 1926), p. 66 (translation by the author).

88 Klaus Vogel, 'The Transparent Man: Some Comments on the History of a Symbol', in *Manifesting Medicine: Bodies and Machines*, ed. Robert Bud, Bernard Finn and Helmuth Trischler (Amsterdam, 1999), p. 45.

89 Charles Loring and Edward Robinson, *Greek and Roman Sculpture* (New York, 1891), p. 225.

90 Simon Richter, *Laocoon's Body and the Aesthetics of Pain: Winckelmann, Lessing, Herder, Moritz, and Goethe* (Detroit, MI, 1992).

91 Nigel Spivey, *Enduring Creation: Art, Pain and Fortitude* (Berkeley, CA, 2002), p. 251.

92 Elena Canadelli, 'The Diffusion of a Museum Exhibit: The Case of the Transparent Man', in *Understanding Cultural Traits: Multidisciplinary Perspective on Cultural Diversity*, ed. Fabrizio Panebianco and Emanuelle Serrelli (New York, 2016), pp. 61–80.

93 Paul Schultze-Naumburg, *Nördische Schönheit: Ihr Wunschbild im Leben und in der Kunst* (Munich, 1937), pp. 34–6 (translation by the author).

FIVE: DANCE AND THE SOCIAL TAMING OF POSTURE

1 William Hardy McNeill, *Keeping Together in Time: Dance and Drill in Human History* (Cambridge, MA, 1995), p. 2.

2 Norbert Elias, *The Civilizing Process*, trans. Edmund Jephcott (Oxford, 1978), p. 92.

3 Cas Wouters, 'The Integration of Classes and Sexes in the Twentieth Century: Etiquette Books and Emotion Management', in *Norbert Elias and Human Interdependencies*, ed. Thomas Saluments (Montreal, 2001), pp. 71ff.

4 Kellom Tomlinson, *The Art of Dancing Explained by Reading and Figures* (London, 1735), p. 64.

5 M. Franko, 'Archaeological Choreographic Practices: Foucault and Forsythe', *History of the Human Sciences*, xxiv (2011), pp. 97–112.

6 Michel Foucault, *Discipline and Punish: The Birth of the Prison*, trans. Alan Sheridan (New York, 1995), p. 168.

7 Richard Watson, *Descartes's Ballet: His Doctrine of the Will and his Political Philosophy (with a Transcript and English Translation of La Naissance de la Paix)* (South Bend, IN, 2007).

8 Kate van Orden, *Music, Discipline and Arms in Early Modern France* (Chicago, IN, 2004), pp. 187–8.

9 Ibid., p. 188.

10 Karl Gaulhofer, *Die Fusshaltung: Ein Beitrag zur Stilgeschichte der menschlichen Bewegung* (Kassel, 1930), pp. 113–14.

11 G. Yvonne Kendall, 'Le Gratie d'Amore 1602 by Cesare Negri: Translation and Commentary', PhD thesis, Stanford University, 1985.

12 Claire Paolacci, 'Serge Lifar and the Paris Opera during World War II', *Journal of the Oxford University History Society*, II (2004), pp. 1–9.

13 Jennifer Nevile, *The Eloquent Body: Dance and Humanist Culture in Fifteenth-century Italy* (Bloomington, IN, 2004), p. 77.

14 Quoted ibid., p. 84.

15 Laura S. Youenes, 'Dance Music', in *The Routledge Encyclopedia of Tudor England*, ed. Arthur F. Kinney and David Swain (New York, 2001), pp. 175–7.

16 Quoted in Kendall, 'Le Gratie d'Amore', p. 88.

17 Ibid.

18 Ibid., p. 92.

19 Nevile, *The Eloquent Body*, p. 2.

20 Ibid., p. 45.

21 Richard Leppert, *Music and Image: Domesticity, Ideology and Socio-cultural Formation in Eighteenth-century England* (Cambridge, 1988), p. 76.

22 Ibid., p. 82.

23 Matthew McCormack, *Embodying the Militia in Georgian England* (Oxford, 2015), p. 59.

24 Ibid., p. 101.

25 Ibid., p. 99.

26 William Hogarth, *Analysis of Beauty, Written with the Idea of Fixing the Fluctuating Ideas of Taste* (London, 1753), p. viii. See also Ronald Paulson's interpretations of this work, *Hogarth: His Life, Art, and Times* (New Haven, CT, and London, 1971), pp. 2, 153–87, 439–42, as well as his *Hogarth* (Cambridge, 1993), vol. III, pp. 56–151.

27 Hogarth, *Analysis of Beauty*, p. vi.

28 Sarah Waters, '"The Most Famous Fairy in History": Antinous and Homosexual Fantasy', *Journal of the History of Sexuality*, VI (1995), p. 198.

29 Hogarth, *Analysis of Beauty*, p. 58. See also Anne Bloomfield and Ruth Watts, 'Pedagogue of the Dance: The Dancing Master as Educator in the Long Eighteenth Century', *History of Education*, XXXVII (2008), pp. 605–18.

30 Hogarth, *Analysis of Beauty*, p. 144.

31 See the discussion of 'Devices to correct posture and upright stance and "straightness"' in Alun Withey, *Technology, Self-fashioning and Politeness in Eighteenth-century Britain: Refined Bodies* (London, 2016), pp. 18–40.

32 Hogarth, *Analysis of Beauty*, p. 145.

33 Ibid., p. 49.

34 Lynne Sorge-English, *Stays and Body Image in London: The Staymaking Trade, 1680–1810* (London, 2011), p. 38.

35 Tobin Siebers, *Disability Aesthetics* (Ann Arbor, MI, 2010), pp. 4–5.

36 Ato Quayson, *Aesthetic Nervousness: Disability and the Crisis of Representation* (New York, 2007).

37 Tonya Howe, '"All Deformed Shapes": Figuring the Posture-master as Popular Performer in Early Eighteenth-century England', *Journal for Early Modern Cultural Studies*, XII (2012), pp. 26–47.

38 Samuel Johnson, *A Dictionary of the English Language: In which the Words are Deduced from their Originals, and Illustrated in their Different Significations by Examples from the Best Writers*, 8th edn (London, 1799), vol. II, p. 331. See also Henry Hitchings, *Defining the World: The Extraordinary Story of Dr Johnson's Dictionary* (New York, 2005), p. 166.

39 Joseph Addison and Sir Richard Steele, *The Spectator: A New Edition*, ed. Henry Morley (London, 1891), vol. II, p. 375.

40 *Daily Post*, 3081 (5 August 1729).

41 Anonymous, 'Of the Posture-master', *Philosophical Transactions of the Royal Society*, XX (1753), p. 262.

42 Henry Wilson, *The Book of Wonderful Characters: Memoirs and Anecdotes of Remarkable and Eccentric Persons in All Ages and Countries* (London, 1869), p. 145.

43 Henry Fielding and William Guthrie, *The Life and Adventures of a Cat* (London, 1760), p. 106.

44 Walter Scott, *The Waverley Novels* (London, 1893), vol. XII, p. 359.

45 H. Montgomery Hyde, *A History of Pornography* (New York, 1965), p. 100. One of the greatest ironies is that the *Oxford English Dictionary* provides a secondary entry for 'posture girl' following the model of 'posture master' in the 'posture' entry. This seems in an embarrassed way to want to repress the core meaning, defining it only as 'a female acrobat or contortionist'. Two of the three citations clearly mean a sexual exhibitionist and the third is a masked reference to this meaning. See www.oed.com, accessed 24 January 2013.

46 Such as those at the Beggar's Benison, the club to which David Stevenson in *The Beggar's Benison: Sex Clubs of Enlightenment Scotland and their Rituals* (East Linton, 2001) devotes his attention, which was dedicated to 'the convivial celebration of male sexuality'. This is parallel to clubs such as the Hellfire Club, the first of which by this name was founded in London in 1718, where such spectacles also took place.

47 Stevenson, *The Beggar's Benison*, p. 37.

48 Iwan Bloch, *The Sexual Extremities of the World* (New York, 1964), pp. 200, 239. See also Bloch's *Der Einfluss äusserer Faktoren auf das Geschlechtsleben in England* (Berlin, 1903), p. 100.

49 Quoted in the entry for 'Posture Girls', Gordon Williams, *A Dictionary of Sexual Language and Imagery in Shakespearean and Stuart Literature* (Atlantic Highlands, NJ, 1994), vol. II, p. 1077.

50 Anon., *The History of the Human Heart, or, The Adventures of a young Gentleman* (London, 1749), p. 128. See also Tassie Gwilliam, 'Female

Fraud: Counterfeit Maidenheads in the Eighteenth Century', *Journal of the History of Sexuality*, VI (1996), pp. 518–48.

51 Georg Christoph Lichtenberg, *Schriften und Briefe*, ed. Wolfgang Promies (Munich, 1972), vol. III, p. 556. See also Friederike Felicitas Günther, 'Explanations on the Edge of Reason: Lichtenberg's Difficulties Describing Hogarth's View of Bedlam', *Comparative Critical Studies*, V (2008), pp. 235–47; and Franz H. Mautner, 'Lichtenberg as an Interpreter of Hogarth', *Modern Language Quarterly*, XIII (1952), pp. 64–80.

52 Quoted in Williams, *A Dictionary of Sexual Language and Imagery*, vol. II, p. 662.

53 There is a longer tradition of calling her 'Posture Nan', as in David Kunzle, 'Plagiaries-by-memory of the *Rake's Progress* and the Genesis of Hogarth's Second Picture Story', *Journal of the Warburg and Courtauld Institutes*, XXIX (1966), p. 327.

54 Ann Louise Wagner, *Adversaries of Dance: From the Puritans to the Present* (Urbana, IL, 1997), p. 58.

55 Hunter Dickson Farish, ed., *Journal and Letters of Philip Vickers Fithian: A Plantation Tutor of the Old Dominion, 1773–1774* (Charlottesville, VA, 1983), p. 177.

56 Ibid., p. 33.

57 John Locke, *Some Thoughts Concerning Education*, ed. John W. Yolton (Oxford, 1989), p. 124.

58 Ibid., p. 252.

59 Ibid., p. 82.

60 Ibid., p. 102.

61 Ibid., p. 256.

62 Quoted in Roy Mullen, *Degas: His Life, Times, and Work* (London, 1985), p. 377.

63 All quotations are from Jean Sutherland Boggs, ed., *Degas* (New York, 1989), pp. 210–11.

64 Douglas Druick, 'La Petite Danseuse et les criminels: Degas moraliste?' in *Degas inédit: Actes du colloque Degas, Musée d'Orsay 18–21 avril 1988* (Paris, 1989), pp. 224–50.

65 Paul Mantz, 'Exposition des œuvres des artistes independants', *Le Temps* (23 April 1881), p. 3 (translation by the author).

66 Sophie von La Roche, *The History of Lady Sophia Sternheim*, trans. Christa Baguss Britt (Albany, NY, 1991), p. 160.

67 John F. Kasson, *Rudeness and Civility: Manners in Nineteenth-century Urban America* (New York, 1990), esp. chap. 4; Eliza Leslie, *Miss Leslie's Behavior Book* (Philadelphia, PA [*c.* 1859]), p. 69; Bernard Wishy, *The Child and the Republic: The Dawn of Modern American Child Nurture* (Philadelphia, PA, 1968), p. 38; Mrs H. O. Ward, *Sensible Etiquette of the Best Society* (Philadelphia, PA, 1878), pp. 138–9; Marion Harland, *Eve's Daughters; or, Common Sense for Maid, Wife, and Mother* (New York, 1882); *The School of Good Manners* (Providence, RI, 1828), pp. 9–10; Emma Parker, *Important Trifles: Chiefly Appropriate for Females on their Entrance into Society* (London, 1817); *Blunders in Behaviour Corrected . . . (by an Observer of Men and Things)* (London, 1855), p. 22.

68 Adrienne L. McLean, *Dying Swans and Madmen: Ballet, the Body, and Narrative Cinema* (New Brunswick, NJ, 2008), p. 39.

69 Cited in Michael Cowan, *Cult of the Will: Nervousness and German Modernity* (University Park, PA, 2008), p. 150.

70 F. Matthias Alexander, *Man's Supreme Inheritance: Conscious Guidance and Control in Relation to Human Evolution in Civilization* (New York, 1918), p. vii.

71 Ibid., pp. xv–xvi.

72 Ibid., pp. 148–9.

73 Ibid., p. 335.

74 Ibid., pp. 126–7.

75 Patricia Vertinsky, 'Transatlantic Traffic in Expressive Movement: From Delsarte and Dalcroze to Margaret H'Doubler and Rudolf Laban', *International Journal of the History of Sport*, XXVI (2009), pp. 2031–51.

76 Nancy Lee Chalfa Ruyter, 'The Delsarte Heritage', *Dance Research: The Journal of the Society for Dance Research*, XIV (1996), pp. 62–74.

77 Robin Veder, 'Seeing your Way to Health: The Visual Pedagogy of Bess Mensendieck's Physical Culture System', *International Journal of the History of Sport*, XXVIII (2011), pp. 1336–52.

78 See Sander L. Gilman, ed., *'Zettelwirtschaft': Briefe Friedrich Gundolfs und Hermann Brochs an Gertrude von Eckardt-Lederer. Mit Briefen von Elisabeth Gundolf, Bertold Vallentin und Joachim Ringelnatz* (Berlin, 1992).

79 Mark Knowles, *The Wicked Waltz and Other Scandalous Dancing: Outrage at Couple Dancing in the 19th and early 20th Centuries* (Jefferson, NC, 2009), p. 38.

80 Marguerite Agniel, *The Art of the Body: Rhythmic Exercise for Health and Beauty* (London, 1931), p. 93.

81 Ana Carden-Coyne, *Reconstructing the Body: Classicism, Modernism and the First World War* (Oxford, 2009), p. 307.

82 Ibid.

83 Ibid., p. 61.

84 Kimerer L. LaMothe, *Nietzsche's Dancers: Isadora Duncan, Martha Graham, and the Revaluation of Christian Values* (New York, 2006), p. 187.

85 Abraham Walkowitz, *Isadora Duncan in her Dance* (Girard, KS, 1945), p. 9.

86 Cowan, *Cult of the Will*, p. 153.

87 Quoted in LaMothe, *Nietzsche's Dancers*, p. 186.

88 Ibid., p. 56.

89 Lawrence Rainey, Christine Poggi and Laura Wittman, eds, *Futurism: An Anthology* (New Haven, CT, 2009), p. 237.

90 Rosalind Krauss, 'Corpus Delecti', *October*, XXXIII (1985), p. 40.

91 I am grateful for the work of Adrien Sina, ed., *Feminine Futures – Valentine de Saint-Point – Performance, Dance, War, Politics and Eroticism* (Paris, 2011).

92 Nils Jockel, 'Aus dem Moment des Empfindens: Die Hamburger Tänzerinnen Gertrud und Ursula Falke', *Tanzdrama*, VII (1989), pp. 19, 83; Rebecca Loukes, 'Body Awareness in Performer Training: The Hidden Legacy of Gertrud Falke-Heller (1891–1984)', *Dance Research Journal*, XXXIX (2007), pp. 75–90.

93 Cowan, *Cult of the Will*, p. 151.

94 Karl Toepfer, *Empire of Ecstasy: Nudity and Movement in German Body Culture, 1910–1935* (Berkeley, CA, 1997), p. 217.

95 Susan Manning, *Ecstasy and the Demon: Feminism and Nationalism in the Dances of Mary Wigman* (Berkeley, CA, 1993). Posture is at the centre of Wigman's conceptualization of modern dance. The dancer has 'to place [the] feet, to displace [the] hips, to regulate the posture of the torso in order to achieve the abstract form of rotation and to be able to bring these turns back to the sphere of their ecstatic experience' (p. 94). Her choreography stressed her 'wave-like body posture' (p. 53).

96 Karen Bell-Kanner, *The Life and Times of Ellen von Frankenberg* (New York, 1991), p. 57.

97 É. Jaques-Dalcroze, *Rhythm, Music, and Education* (New York, 1972), p. 252.

98 Alfred Berchtold, *Émile Jaques-Dalcroze et son temps* (Lausanne, 2005), p. 99.

99 Ernst Bloch, *The Principle of Hope*, trans. Neville Plaice, Stephen Plaice and Paul Knight (Cambridge, MA, 1986), vol. I, p. 394.

100 Ibid. See also Vincent Geoghegan, *Ernst Bloch* (London, 1996), pp. 60–61.

101 Adorno writes evoking the posture of Franz Kafka's giant insect that 'The jitterbug looks as if he would grimace at himself, at his own enthusiasm and at his own enjoyment which he denounces even while pretending to enjoy himself . . . it is quite unlikely that the ceaseless repetition of the same effects would allow for genuine merriment . . . In order to become a jitterbug or simply to "like" popular music, it does not by any means suffice to give oneself up and to fall in line passively. To become transformed into an insect, man needs that energy which might possibly achieve his transformation into a man.' Theodor Adorno, 'On Popular Music', in *Essays on Music*, ed. Richard Leppert, trans. Susan Gillespie (Los Angeles, CA, 2002), pp. 467–8. See also the section of Rebecca Comay's essay 'The Siren Song' on the 'Antimonies of the Upright Posture' in Renée Heberle, *Feminist Interpretations of Theodor Adorno* (University Park, PA, 2006), pp. 43–7.

102 Hans Blüher, *Secessio Judaica: Philosophische Grundlegung der historischen Situation des Judenthums und der antisemitischen Bewegung* (Berlin, 1922), p. 19 (translation by the author).

103 Ernst von Sydow, *Die deutsche expressionistische Kultur und Malerie* (Berlin, 1920), p. 13 (translation by the author).

104 Julie M. Johnson, *The Memory Factory: The Forgotten Women Artists of Vienna 1900* (West Lafayette, IN, 2012), p. 102.

105 Kurt Peters, '"Du musst einfach eine Stil finden": Das Tanz – Duo Gertrud und Ursula Falke', *Ballet Journal/Das Tanzarchiv*, XXXI (1983), p. 52.

106 Manning, *Ecstasy and the Demon*, p. 57.

107 James Lei, 'Dalcroze: Eurythmics in Early Modern Theatre and Dance', PhD thesis, Texas Tech University, 2003.

108 Hedwig Müller, *Mary Wigman: Leben und Werk der grossen Tänzerin* (Berlin, 1992), p. 74.

109 Peters, '"Du musst einfach eine Stil finden"', p. 54 (translation by the author).

110 Max Tepp, *Gertrud und Ursula Falke: Tänze* (Hamburg, 1920, and Lauenberg, 1924).

111 Hans Brandenburg, *Der moderne Tanz* (Munich, 1921), pp. 36–8.
112 Quoted in Toepfer, *Empire of Ecstasy*, p. 218.
113 Ibid., p. 8.

SIX: EDUCATION SHAPES A HEALTHY AND BEAUTIFUL POSTURE

1 Nicolas Andry de Bois-Regard, *Orthopedia or the Art of Correcting and Preventing Deformities in Children* (London, 1743), vol. I, p. 211. This was a translation of Nicolas Andry, *L'orthopédie, ou l'art de prévenir et de corriger dans les enfants les difformités du corps* (Paris, 1741). See also Remi Kohler, 'Nicolas Andry de Bois-Regard (Lyon 1658–Paris 1842): The Inventor of the Word "Orthopedics" and the Father of Parasitology', *Journal of Childhood Orthopedics*, IV/4 (2010), pp. 349–55; Leonard F. Peltier, *Orthopedics: A History and Iconography* (San Francisco, CA, 1993), pp. 35–7; L. P. Fischer, C. Fischer-Athiel and B. S. Fischer, 'One Hundred Years of Bone Surgery in the Lyons Teaching Hospitals (1897–1997)', *Annales de chirurgie*, LII (1998), pp. 264–78; Ignacio V. Ponseti, 'History of Orthopaedic Surgery', *Iowa Orthopaedic Journal*, XI (1991), pp. 59–64; J. Ruhrah, 'Nicolas Andry 1658–1742', *American Journal of Diseases of Children*, XLIV (1932), pp. 1322–6. I am especially grateful to the essay by one of my students in our special issue on *Posture, Literature, and Culture*. See Rachel Weitzenkorn, 'Orthos and its Underlying Curves: A Close Reading of Nicolas Andry's 1741 *L'Orthopedie*', *Jahrbuch Literatur und Medizin*, VI (2014), pp. 93–106.
2 Andry, *Orthopaedia*, vol. I, pp. 72–3.
3 Ibid., p. 122. See also Lynne Sorge-English, *Stays and Body Image in London: The Staymaking Trade, 1680–1810* (London, 2011), p. 126.
4 'The Greek women were wholly unacquainted with those frames of whalebone in which our women distort rather than display their figures. It seems to me that this abuse, which is carried to an incredible degree of folly in England, must sooner or later lead to the production of a degenerate race. Moreover, I maintain that the charm which these corsets are supposed to produce is in the worst possible taste; it is not a pleasant thing to see a woman cut in two like a wasp – it offends both the eye and the imagination.' Jean-Jacques Rousseau, *Émile, or On Education*, trans. Barbara Foxley (London, Toronto, ON, and New York, 1921), p. 278. See Valerie Steele, *The Corset: A Cultural History* (New Haven, CT, 2001), p. 29.
5 Paolo Palladino, 'Life . . . On Biology, Biography, and Bio-power in the Age of Genetic Engineering', *Configurations*, XI (2003), p. 84.
6 Quoted in Georges Vigarello, 'The Upward Training of the Body from the Age of Chivalry to Courtly Civility', in *Fragments for a History of the Human Body*, ed. Michel Feher (New York, 1990), vol. II, p. 173.
7 'Quin etiam, si quis est paulo ad voluptates propensior, modo ne sit ex pecudum genere (sunt enim quidam homines non re, sed nomine), sed si quis est paulo erectior, quamvis voluptate capiatur, occultat et dissimulat appetitum voluptatis propter verecundiam.' (Nay, even if a man is more than ordinarily inclined to sensual pleasures, provided, of course, that he be not quite on a level with the beasts of the field [for some people are men only in name, not in fact] – if, I say, he is a little

too susceptible to the attractions of pleasure, he hides the fact, however much he may be caught in its toils, and for very shame conceals his appetite.) Cicero, *De officiis*, trans. Walter Miller (Cambridge, MA, 1913), pp. 106–9.

8 Andrew R. Dyck, *A Commentary on Cicero's* De Officiis (Ann Arbor, MI, 1996), p. 268.

9 All quotations are from Erasmus, 'On Good Manners for Boys', in *Collected Works of Erasmus*, ed. J. K. Sowards, trans. Brian McGregor (Toronto, ON, 1985), vol. XXV, p. 277.

10 Max Horkheimer and Theodor Adorno, *Dialectic of the Enlightenment*, ed. Gunzelin Schmid Noerr, trans. Edmund Jephcott (Stanford, CA, 2002), p. 194.

11 Peter Burke, *The Fortunes of the Courtier: The European Reception of Castiglione's 'Cortegiano'* (State College, PA, 2013), p. 123.

12 Baldassare Castiglione, *The Book of the Courtier*, trans. Leonard Eckstein Opdycke (New York, 1903), p. 37.

13 Ibid., p. 28.

14 Ibid., pp. 74–5.

15 Ibid., pp. 84–5.

16 Vigarello, 'The Upward Training of the Body', p. 183.

17 Lester G. Crocker, 'Order and Disorder in Rousseau's Social Thought', *PMLA*, XCIV (1979), pp. 247–60; and Mark S. Cladis, 'Lessons from the Garden: Rousseau's Solitaires and the Limits of Liberalism', *Interpretation*, XXIV (1997), pp. 183–200.

18 Eva M. Neumeyer, 'The Landscape Garden as a Symbol in Rousseau, Goethe and Flaubert', *Journal of the History of Ideas*, VIII (1947), p. 187.

19 Ibid., p. 191.

20 Ibid., p. 189.

21 Rousseau, *Émile*, p. 5. See Fernand de Girardin, *Iconographie des oeuvres de Jean-Jacques Rousseau* (repr. Geneva, 1971), p. 113.

22 Ibid., p. 104.

23 Ibid., p. 112.

24 See the essays in Klas Roth and Chris W. Surprenant, eds, *Kant and Education: Interpretations and Commentary* (New York, 2012), especially Joseph R. Reister, 'Kant and Rousseau on Moral Education', pp. 12–25.

25 Paul Guyer, 'The Crooked Timber of Mankind', in *Kant's Idea for a Universal History with a Cosmopolitan Aim: A Critical Guide*, ed. Amélie Oksenberg Rorty and James Schmidt (Cambridge, 2009), pp. 129–49.

26 Robert B. Louden, trans., 'Lectures on Pedagogy (1803)', in *The Cambridge Edition of the Works of Immanuel Kant: Anthropology, History and Education*, ed. Günter Zöller and Robert B. Louden (Cambridge, 2007), p. 443.

27 Johann Bernhard Basedow, *Das Basedowische Elementarwerk* (Leipzig, 1785), vol. I, p. 166 (translation by the author).

28 Johann Bernhard Basedow, *Das in Dessau errichtete Philanthropinum* (Leipzig, 1774), p. viii (translation by the author).

29 Daniel Chodowiecki and Johann Bernhard Basedow, *Des Elementarwerks: Ein geordneter Vorrath aller nöthigen Erkenntniß* (Dessau, 1774), plate 19a.

30 Immanuel Kant, *Gesammelte Schriften: Akademie-Ausgabe*, ed. Erich Adickes (Berlin, 1913), vol. XV, p. 974.

31 Immanuel Kant, *Gesammelte Schriften: Akademie-Ausgabe,* ed. Friedrich Berger (Berlin, 1934), vol. XIX, p. 92.

32 Karl Rosenkranz, *Pedagogics as a System*, trans. Anna C. Brackett (St Louis, MO, 1872), p. 12.

33 Ibid., p. 36.

34 Henry Barnard, 'Rosenkranz and his Pedagogy', *American Journal of Education*, XXVIII (1878), pp. 25–32.

35 Rosenkranz, *Pedagogics as a System*, p. 32.

36 Paul Miner, 'Contemplations on Iconography: Blake's Frontispieces and Tailpiece to *Songs of Innocence and Experience*', *Notes and Queries*, LXII (2015), pp. 378–9.

37 William Blake, *The Complete Poetry and Prose*, ed. David V. Erdman (New York, 1988), p. 9.

38 Kathleen Raine, 'Blake and the Education of Childhood', *Southern Review*, VIII (1972), pp. 253–72.

39 Blake, *The Complete Poetry and Prose*, p. 28.

40 Friedrich Nietzsche, *Anti-education; or, the Future of Our Educational Institutions*, trans. Damion Searls (New York, 2016), p. 7. Nietzsche's philosophy has haunted both ends of the political spectrum of our contemporary views of education, from Allan Bloom, *The Closing of the American Mind* (New York, 1987), who curses the aristocratic, anti-university, anti-system Nietzsche, whom Bloom sees as arguing for a complete dismantling of the German educational system, to Martin Simons, 'Montessori, Superman, and Catwoman', *Educational Theory*, XXXVII (1988), pp. 341–9, who claims that Nietzsche remains sympathetic to education, advocating as he does an aristocracy of the self.

41 Dena Goodman, *Becoming a Woman in the Age of Letters* (Ithaca, NY, 2009), pp. 112–13.

42 Ibid., p. 108.

43 Maria Edgeworth, 'The Good French Governess', in *Works* (Boston, MA, 1825), vol. IX, p. 342.

44 Mona Narain, 'Not an Angel in the House: Intersections of the Public and Private in Maria Edgeworth's *Moral Tales* and *Practical Education*', in *New Essays on Maria Edgeworth*, ed. Julie Ash (Aldershot, 2006), p. 64.

45 Erasmus Darwin, *A Plan for the Conduct of Female Education, in Boarding Schools, Private Families, and Public Seminars* (Philadelphia, PA, 1798), p. 113.

46 Jane Austen, *The Works of Jane Austen*, ed. R. W. Chapman (Oxford, 1954), vol. VI, p. 421.

47 William Cowper, 'On Conversation', *Connoisseur*, 138 (16 September 1756). Reprinted in Robert Southey, ed., *The Works of William Cowper in Eight Volumes* (London, 1854), vol. IV, pp. 385–6.

48 William H. Gilman, ed., *The Journals and Miscellaneous Notebooks of Ralph Waldo Emerson* (Cambridge, MA, 1982), vol. XV, p. 34.

49 Quoted in Heikki Lempa, *Beyond the Gymnasium: Educating Middle-class Bodies in Germany* (Plymouth, 2007), p. 4.

50 Adolf Freiherr von Knigge, *Social Life; or, The Art of Conversing with Men*, trans. Peter Will (Troy, MI, 1805), p. 31.

51 Quoted in Edmund Wilson, ed., *Hufeland's Art of Prolonging Life* (Philadelphia, PA, 1870), pp. 222–3.

52 Friedrich Froebel, *The Education of Man*, trans. Josephine Jarvis (New York, 1885), p. 27.

53 Philip Stanhope, 4th Earl of Chesterfield, *Letters of Advice to his Son* (New York, 1775), p. 177; also cited in C. Dallett Hemphill, 'Middle-class Rising in Revolutionary America: The Evidence from Manners', *Journal of Social History*, XXX (1996), pp. 317–44.

54 Francis Galton, 'Measurement of Character', *Fortnight Review*, XXXVI (1884), p. 184.

55 Ellen D. Kelly, *Teaching Posture and Body Mechanics* (New York, 1949), p. 188.

56 Robin Veder, 'The Expressive Efficiencies of American Delsarte and Mensendieck Body Culture', *Modernism/modernity*, XVII/4 (2010), pp. 819–38. See also Robin Veder, 'Seeing the Skeleton and Feeling the Form: Physical Education at the 1913 Armory Show', *Amodern*, III (2014), www.amodern.net, accessed 4 June 2016.

57 George Copland, 'Hints on Singing', *The Minim: A Musical Magazine for Everybody*, IV/43 (1897), pp. 164–5.

58 Francesco Lamperti, *The Art of Singing*, ed. and trans. J. C. Griffith (London, 1939), p. 3.

59 D. F. Lincoln, *School and Industrial Hygiene* (Philadelphia, PA, 1880), pp. 31–7. See also Tait Mackenzie, MD, 'The Influence of School Life on Curvature of the Spine', *American Physical Education Review*, III (1898), pp. 274–80; George Muller, MD, *Spinal Curvature and Awkward Deportment* (New York, 1894), pp. 3–4, 20, 24, 39.

60 Peggy Shinner, *You Feel so Mortal: Essays on the Body* (Chicago, IL, 2014), p. 39.

61 Maria Montessori, *Pedagogical Anthropology*, trans. Frederic Taber Cooper (New York, 1913).

62 Ibid., p. 119.

63 Ibid., p. 120.

64 John Dewey, *The School and Society*, 3rd edn (Chicago, IL, 1900), p. 14.

65 Montessori, *Pedagogical Anthropology*, p. 159.

66 Quoted in Allan M. Kraut, *Silent Travelers: Germs, Genes, and the 'Immigrant Menace'* (Baltimore, MD, 1994), p. 191.

67 Montessori, *Pedagogical Anthropology*, p. 166.

68 Daniel J. Kevles, *In the Name of Eugenics: Genetics and the Uses of Human Heredity* (Cambridge, MA, 1995), p. 91.

69 Montessori, *Pedagogical Anthropology*, p. 307.

70 Christine Rosen, *Preaching Eugenics: Religious Leaders and the American Eugenics Movement* (New York, 2004), p. 113.

71 Quoted in Kraut, *Silent Travelers*, p. 63.

72 Benjamin Grant Jefferis and James Lawrence Nichols, *Searchlights on Health: Light on Dark Corners: A Complete Sexual Science and a Guide to Purity and Physical Manhood: Advice to Maiden, Wife, and Mother: Love, Courtship, and Marriage* (Toronto, ON, 1894), p. 34.

73 Jessie H. Bancroft, 'New Efficiency Methods for Training the Posture of School Children', *American Physical Education Review*, XVIII (1913), pp. 309–13.

74 Robert W. Lovett, MD, 'Round Shoulders and Faulty Attitude: A Method of Observation and Record, with Conclusions as to Treatment', *American Physical Education Review*, VII/4 (1902), pp. 169–87.

75 Ethel Perrin, 'Methods of Interesting School Children in Good Postural Habits', *American Physical Education Review*, XIX (1914), pp. 503–6.

76 Ron Rosenbaum, 'The Great Ivy League Nude Posture Photo Scandal', *New York Times Magazine* (15 January 1995), pp. 26ff.

77 D. A. Sargent, 'The Physical State of the American People', in *The United States of America: A Study of the American Commonwealth, its Natural Resources, People, Industries, Manufactures, Commerce, and its Work in Literature, Science, Education and Self-government*, ed. Nathaniel Southgate Shaler (London, 1894), pp. 452–75, here 458–60.

78 Ibid., p. 472.

79 Ibid.

80 Martha H. Verbruegge, *Active Bodies: History of Women's Physical Education in Twentieth-century America* (New York, 2012), p. 69.

81 Richard T. Gray, *About Face: German Physiognomic Thought from Lavater to Auschwitz* (Detroit, MI, 2004), pp. 57–110.

82 Quoted in Anna G. Creadick, *Perfectly Average: The Pursuit of Normality in Postwar America* (Amherst, MA, 2010), p. 25.

83 William H. Sheldon, *The Varieties of Human Physique: An Introduction to Constitutional Psychology* (New York and London, 1940), p. 49.

84 Ibid., p. 5.

85 William H. Sheldon, *Varieties of Delinquent Youth: An Introduction to Constitutional Psychology* (New York, 1949), p. 15.

86 Ibid.

87 Sheldon, *The Varieties of Human Physique*, p. 145.

88 Ibid., p. 170.

89 Ibid., pp. 190–91.

90 Ibid., pp. 220–21.

91 Sheldon, *Varieties of Delinquent Youth*, p. 30.

92 Ibid., pp. 30–31, 726.

93 Sheldon, *The Varieties of Human Physique*, p. 1.

94 William H. Sheldon, *The Varieties of Temperament: A Psychology of Constitutional Differences* (New York, 1942), p. 69.

95 Ibid., p. 167.

96 Ibid., p. 199.

97 J. Knox Thompson, 'The Erect Posture', *The Lancet*, CXCIX/5150 (1922), p. 107.

98 J. Knox Thompson, 'Letter: The Erect Posture', *The Lancet*, CXCIX/5136 (1922), p. 251.

99 Wendy Dasler Johnson, 'Cultural Rhetorics of Women's Corsets', *Rhetoric Review*, XX (2001), pp. 203–33.

100 Sorge-English, *Stays and Body Image in London*, p. 126.

101 Cited in Kimberly Wahl, *Dressed as in a Painting: Women and British Aestheticism in an Age of Reform* (Boston, MA, 2013), p. 13.

102 Heather Bigg and Lætitiah Andrew-Bird, 'Civilization and the Corset', *The Lancet*, CLXXIV/4500 (1909), pp. 1630–31.

103 Cecil Fish, 'Civilization and the Corset', *The Lancet*, CLXXIV/4502 (1909), pp. 1774–5.

104 Heather Bigg, 'Civilization and the Corset', *The Lancet*, CLXXV/4507 (1910), pp. 203–5.
105 H. O. Kendall and F. P. Kendall, 'Developing and Maintaining Good Posture', *Physical Therapy*, XLVIII/4 (1968), p. 320.
106 Ibid.
107 See the turn to a social rather than a medical definition of disability and the meaning of posture in Tobin Siebers, *Disability Theory* (Ann Arbor, MI, 2008), p. 58. See also Lennard J. Davis, *Bending Over Backwards: Disability, Dismodernism and Other Difficult Positions* (New York, 2002); and Sharon L. Snyder, Brenda Brueggemann and Rosemarie Garland-Thomson, eds, *Disability Studies: Enabling the Humanities* (New York, 2002).
108 American Academy of Orthopaedic Surgeons, Posture Committee, *Posture and its Relationship to Orthopaedic Disabilities: A Report* (Chicago, IL, 1947), p. 1.
109 Laura Smith, Elizabeth L. Weiss and Don Lehmkuhl, *Brunnstrom's Clinical Kinesiology*, 5th edn (Philadelphia, PA, 1996).
110 Moshé Feldenkrais, *Body and Mature Behavior: A Study of Anxiety, Sex, Gravitation and Learning* (New York, 1949), p. 34.
111 Anson Rabinbach, *The Human Motor: Energy, Fatigue, and the Origins of Modernity* (Berkeley, CA, 1991).
112 P. Reginald Hug, 'Posture Queen Contests in Alabama', *Journal of Chiropractic Humanities*, XV (2008), p. 72. See also R.J.R. Hynes, 'The Most Beautiful Spines in America: The History of the Posture Queens', *Chiropractic History*, XXII (2002), pp. 65–71.
113 Shinner, *You Feel so Mortal*, p. 38.
114 Scott Henslcy, 'You Think Beauty Is Skin Deep? You're Not a Chiropractor', www.npr.org, 1 August 2012.
115 Les Goates, 'New Beauty Contest Places Emphasis on Proper Posture', *Deseret News* (16 June 1965), p. 16A.
116 John F. Kasson, *Rudeness and Civility: Manners in Nineteenth-century Urban America* (New York, 1991), p. 123.

SEVEN: ANTHROPOLOGY REMAKES POSTURE: LAMARCK, DARWIN AND BEYOND

1 'Aures homini tantum immobiles'. Pliny the Elder, *Natural History*, trans. H. Rackham (Cambridge, MA, 1940), vol. III, pp. 516–17.
2 Jonathan Kingdon, *Lowly Origin: Where, When, and Why our Ancestors First Stood Up* (Princeton, NJ, 2003), p. 2.
3 James Alexander Lindsay, 'The Bradshaw Lecture on Darwinism and Medicine. Delivered at the Royal College of Physicians of London on November 2, 1909', *The Lancet*, CLXXIV/4497 (1909), p. 1328.
4 C. Owen Lovejoy, 'The Natural History of Human Gait and Posture: Part 1. Spine and Pelvis', *Gait and Posture*, XXI (2005), p. 95; see C. Owen Lovejoy, 'The Natural History of Human Gait and Posture: Part 2. Hip and Thigh', *Gait and Posture*, XXI (2005), pp. 113–24; and C. Owen Lovejoy, 'The Natural History of Human Gait and Posture: Part 3. The Knee', *Gait and Posture*, XXV (2007), pp. 325–41.
5 Ann Gibbons, 'A New Kind of Ancestor: Ardipithecus Unveiled', *Science*, CCCXXVI/5949 (2009), p. 36. The entire issue was devoted to papers on the

discovery. See also the overviews by Carol V. Ward, 'Early Hominin Posture and Locomotion: Where Do We Stand?', *Yearbook of Physical Anthropology*, XLV (2002), pp. 186–215, and 'The Evolution of Human Origins', *American Anthropologist*, CV (2003), pp. 77–88.

6   Ann Gibbons, 'Habitat for Humanity', *Science*, CCCXXVI/5949 (2009), p. 40.

7   Tim D. White, Berhane Asfaw, Yonas Beyene, Yohannes Haile-Selassie, C. Owen Lovejoy, Gen Suwa and Giday WoldeGabriel, 'Ardipithecus Ramidus and the Paleobiology of Early Hominids', *Science*, CCCXXVI/5949 (2009), pp. 75–86.

8   Sir Arthur Keith, *The Construction of Man's Family Tree* (London, 1934), p. 15.

9   Jean-Baptiste de Lamarck, *Philosophie zoologique, ou exposition des considérations relatives à l'histoire naturelle des animaux* (Paris, 1809), p. 349.

10   Quoted by Gustav Muskat, 'Ist der Plattfuss eine Rasseneigentümlichket?', *Im Deutschen Reich* (1909), p. 354 (translation by the author).

11   Frederick Arthur Hornibrook, *The Culture of the Abdomen: The Cure of Obesity and Constipation* (London, 1927).

12   Robert J. Richards, *The Meaning of Evolution: The Morphological Construction and Ideological Reconstruction of Darwin's Theory* (Chicago, IL, 1993).

13   Thomas Henry Huxley, *Evidence as to Man's Place in Nature* (New York, 1863), pp. 39–40.

14   Ibid., p. 63.

15   Ibid., p. 69.

16   Robert Munro, *Prehistoric Problems, Being a Selection of Essays on the Evolution of Man and Other Controverted Problems in Anthropology and Archaeology* (Edinburgh, 1897).

17   Huxley, *Evidence*, p. 158.

18   Ibid., p. 181.

19   John Reader, *Missing Links: The Hunt for Earliest Man* (New York, 1981), p. 32.

20   W. L. Straus and A.J.E. Cave, 'Pathology and Posture of Neanderthal Man', *Quarterly Review of Biology*, XXXII (1957), pp. 348–63.

21   Stephanie Moser, *Ancestral Images: The Iconography of Human Origins* (Ithaca, NY, 1998), p. xii.

22   Quoting the report of Eugéne Dubois in Erik Trinkaus and Pat Shipman, *The Neanderthals: Changing the Image of Mankind* (New York, 1993), p. 139. The naming of this find varies over time; I have simplified it in the text using the commonly accepted designation.

23   See Constance Areson Clark, *God – or Gorilla: Images of Evolution in the Jazz Age Neanderthal* (Baltimore, MD, 2008).

24   Amédée Bouyssonie, Jean Bouyssonie and L. Bardon, 'Découverte d'un Squelette Humain Moustérien à la Bouffia de La Chapelle-aux-Saints (Corrèze)', *L'Anthropologie*, XIX (1908), pp. 513–18.

25   Marianne Sommer, 'Mirror, Mirror on the Wall: Neanderthal as Image and "Distortion" in Early 20th-century French Science and Press', *Social Studies of Science*, XXXVI (2006), p. 213.

26 Anonymous, 'The Most Important Anthropological Discovery for Fifty Years', *Illustrated London News* (27 February 1909), p. 313.

27 Sommer, 'Mirror, Mirror on the Wall', p. 226.

28 Quoted in Charles De Paolo, *Human Prehistory in Fiction* (Jefferson, NC, 2003), p. 34.

29 Graeme Donald, *They Got It Wrong: Science: All the Facts that Turned Out to be Science Fiction* (New York, 2013), p. 134.

30 Charles Darwin, *The Works of Charles Darwin*, ed. Paul H. Barrett and H. B. Freeman (London, 1992), vol. XXI, p. 56.

31 Ibid., p. 57.

32 Darwin, *The Works of Charles Darwin*, vol. XXIII, p. 283.

33 Joseph Shaw Bolton, 'The Evolution of Mind', *The Lancet*, CCXXV/5822 (1935), p. 664.

34 *The Collected Works of Karl Marx and Frederick Engels* (London and New York, 1978), vol. XXV, p. 452.

35 Ibid.

36 Ibid., p. 457.

37 Stephen J. Gould, 'Posture Maketh the Man', in *Ever Since Darwin: Reflections on Natural History* (New York, 1977), p. 208.

38 Joel E. Goldthwait, 'An Anatomic and Mechanistic Conception of Disease', *Boston Medical and Surgical Journal*, CLXXII (1915), p. 893.

39 J. Knox Thompson, 'The Erect Posture', *The Lancet*, CXCIX/5150 (1922), p. 107.

40 Albert Gresswell, 'The Application of the Theory of Evolution to Pathology', *The Lancet*, CXXXII/3390 (1888), p. 310.

41 W. H. Walshe, 'Lectures on Clinical Medicine', *The Lancet*, LIII/1332 (1849), p. 251.

42 See his contemporaries' evaluations of his social views: O. Stoessl, 'The Philosophy of Satire and the Work of T. T. Heine', *The Artist*, XXVII (1900), p. 357.

43 G. B. Shaw, *Pygmalion: A Play in Five Acts* (London, 1913), p. 58.

44 H. G. Wells, *The Island of Dr Moreau* (Garden City, NY, 1896), p. 83.

45 Ibid., p. 230.

46 Ibid., p. 233.

47 [H. G. Wells], 'The Limits of Individual Plasticity', *Saturday Review* (19 January 1895), p. 90.

48 Robert Louis Stevenson, *Strange Case of Dr Jekyll and Mr Hyde* (New York, 1903), pp. 12, 25, 37, 43, 97, 118.

49 Martha Stoddard Holmes, *Fictions of Affliction: Physical Disability in Victorian Culture* (Ann Arbor, MI, 2007), p. 199.

50 Lillian C. Drew, 'Ways and Means of Overcoming Inefficient Posture', *American Physical Education Review*, XXVIII (1923), p. 4.

51 Peter N. Stearns, *Battleground of Desire: The Struggle for Self-control in Modern America* (New York, 1999), p. 4. See also Stearns's earlier essay on posture, which was incorporated into this formidable book: David Yosifon and Peter N. Stearns, 'The Rise and Fall of American Posture', *American Historical Review*, CIII (1998), pp. 1057–95.

52 David M. Friedman, *Wilde in America: Oscar Wilde and the Invention of Modern Celebrity* (New York, 2014), p. 24.

53 Michele Mendelssohn, *Henry James, Oscar Wilde and Aesthetic Culture* (Edinburgh, 2007), p. 64.

54 Joseph John Gurney, *Thoughts on Habit and Discipline* (London, 1845), pp. 65–6.

55 George Mosse, *The Image of Man: The Creation of Modern Masculinity* (New York, 1996), pp. 191–2.

56 Quoted ibid., p. 70.

57 Sigmund Freud, 'Notes Upon a Case of Obsessional Neurosis', *The Standard Edition of the Complete Psychological Works of Sigmund Freud*, ed. James Strachey, vol. x (London, 1955), pp. 246–7.

58 Frank Sulloway, *Freud, Biologist of the Mind: Beyond the Psychoanalytic Legend* (New York, 1979), p. 377. See also the discussion of Freud and posture in Gould, 'Posture Maketh the Man', p. 209.

59 Jeffrey Moussaieff Masson, ed., *The Complete Letters of Sigmund Freud to Wilhelm Fliess, 1887–1904* (Cambridge, MA, 1985), p. 278.

60 Ibid., p. 280.

61 Sulloway, *Freud, Biologist of the Mind*, appendix D, pp. 516–18.

62 Quoting from G.W.F. Hegel, *Aesthetics*, vol. II, in Jacques Derrida, *Margins of Philosophy*, trans. Alan Bass (Chicago, IL, 1982), p. 93.

63 See Robert Jütte, *The History of the Senses: From Antiquity to Cyberspace*, trans. James Lynn (Cambridge, 2005), pp. 54–72, on Freud pp. 72ff.

64 Sigmund Freud, *Civilization and its Discontents*, in Strachey, *The Standard Edition of the Complete Psychological Works of Sigmund Freud*, vol. XXI (London, 1961), p. 104.

65 Emil du Bois-Reymond, *Über die Übung: Reden, gehalten zur Feier des Stiftungstages der militarärtzlichen Bildungs-Anstalten am 2. August 1881* (Berlin, 1881), pp. 6–7.

66 Joseph Krauskopf, *Evolution and Judaism* (Kansas City, MO, 1887), p. 128.

67 Erwin W. Straus, 'The Upright Posture', *Psychiatric Quarterly*, XXVI (1952), pp. 529–61. See also Thomas Abrams, 'Is Everyone Upright? Erwin Straus' "The Upright Posture" and Disabled Phenomenology', *Human Affairs*, XXIV (2014), pp. 564–73.

68 Straus, 'The Upright Posture', p. 536.

69 Ibid., p. 559.

70 Ibid., p. 558.

71 Ibid., p. 534.

72 Ibid., p. 541.

73 Ibid., p. 545.

74 G. H. Estabrooks, *Man: The Mechanical Misfit* (New York, 1941), p. 96.

75 Mitchell Ash, 'Wissenschaft und Politik als Ressourcen fur einander', in *Wissenschaften und Wissenschaftspolitik: Bestandsaufnahme und Perspektiven der Forschung*, ed. Rudiger vom Buch and Brigitte Kaderas (Stuttgart, 2002).

76 Klaus Theweleit, *Männerphantasien* (Frankfurt am Main, 2002), vol. II, p. 62.

77 Michael Hau, *The Cult of Health and Beauty in Germany: A Social History, 1890–1930* (Chicago, IL, 2003), p. 157.

78 Peter Sloterdijk, *Weltfremdheit* (Frankfurt am Main, 1993), p. 235 (translation by the author).

79 C. O. Lovejoy, 'The Origin of Man', *Science*, CCXI (23 January 1981),
    pp. 341–50, here p. 345.
80 C. O. Lovejoy, 'Evolution of Human Walking', *Scientific American*, CCLIX/5
    (1988), p. 120.
81 Ibid.
82 Angela Willey, 'From Pair-bonding to Polyamory: A Feminist Critique of
    Naturalizing Discourses on Monogamy and Non-monogamy', PhD thesis,
    Emory University, 2009. Expanded as *Undoing Monogamy: The Politics of
    Science and the Possibilities of Biology* (Durham, NC, 2016).

EIGHT: 'NATURAL POSTURE': POSTURE AND RACE

1 See Gordon W. Hewes, 'World Distribution of Certain Postural Habits',
    American Anthropologist, LVII (1955), p. 231.
2 More than twenty years ago it was suggested that 'the meaning of race is
    defined and contested in both collective action and personal practice.'
    Michael Omi and Howard Winant, *Racial Formation in the United States
    from the 1960s to the 1980s* (New York, 1986), p. 61. Science was and is one
    of the spaces for collective action in regard to race, for good and for ill.
3 On the history of the term and concept, see Dirk Rupnow, Veronika
    Lipphardt, Jens Thiel and Christina Wessely, eds, *Pseudowissenschaft:
    Konzeptionen von Nichtwissenschaftlichkeit in der Wissenschaftsgeschichte*
    (Frankfurt am Main, 2008).
4 William F. Bynum, 'The Great Chain of Being after Forty Years: An
    Appraisal', *History of Science*, XIII (1975), pp. 1–28.
5 See Irene Tucker, *The Moment of Racial Sight: A History* (Chicago, IL,
    2012).
6 Elizabeth Gitter, *The Imprisoned Guest: Samuel Howe and Laura
    Bridgman, the Original Deaf-blind Girl* (New York, 2001), p. 198.
7 See Robert A. Yelle, 'The Rhetoric of Gesture in Cross-cultural
    Perspective', *Gesture*, VI (2006), pp. 223–40; Mary Baine Campbell,
    'Anthropometamorphosis: John Bulwer's Monsters of Cosmetology and
    the Science of Culture', in *Monster Theory: Reading Culture*, ed. Jeffrey
    Jerome Cohen (Minneapolis, MN, 1996), pp. 202–22.
8 From the second, expanded edition of John Bulwer,
    Anthropometamorphosis: Man Transform'd (London, 1653), p. 5. See
    Stephen Greenblatt, 'Toward a Universal Language of Motion: Reflections
    on a Seventeenth-century Muscle Man', in *Choreographing History*, ed.
    Susan Leigh Foster (Bloomington, IN, 1995), pp. 25–31.
9 Bulwer, *Anthropometamorphosis*, p. 431.
10 Lynda Boose, quoted in Mary Floyd-Wilson, *English Ethnicity and Race in
    Early Modern Drama* (Cambridge, 2003), p. 45. For evidence that such
    images are well within contemporary theories of race, see Peter Erickson
    and Kim F. Hall, '"A New Scholarly Song": Rereading Early Modern Race',
    Shakespeare Quarterly, LXVII (2016), pp. 1–13.
11 Gerard Boate and Thomas Molyneux, *A Natural History of Ireland in
    Three Parts* (Dublin, 1726), p. 100. See Anne MacLellan and Alice Mauger,
    eds, *Growing Pains: Childhood Illness in Ireland 1750–1950* (Dublin, 2013).
    MacLellan's own essay on rickets covers only the early twentieth century.

12 Frank McCourt, *Angela's Ashes: A Memoir* (New York, 1996), p. 27.

13 John S. Haller, Jr, *Outcasts from Evolution: Scientific Attitudes of Racial Inferiority, 1859–1900* (Carbondale, IL, 1971), p. 49.

14 On Blackness and disability, see *Blackness and Disability: Cultural Examinations and Cultural Interventions*, ed. Christopher M. Bell (East Lansing, MI, 2011); Josh Lukin, 'Disability and Blackness', in *The Disability Studies Reader*, ed. Lennard J. Davis, 4th edn (New York, 2013), pp. 308–15; Ato Quayson, *Aesthetic Nervousness: Disability and the Crisis of Representation* (New York, 2007); Nirmala Erevelles, *Disability and Difference in Global Contexts: Enabling a Transformative Body Politic* (New York, 2011); Rosemarie Garland-Thomson, *Extraordinary Bodies: Figuring Physical Disability in American Culture and Literature* (New York, 1997), pp. 103–34.

15 Bernard Williams, 'Necessary Identities', in *Subjugation and Bondage: Critical Essays on Slavery and Social Philosophy*, ed. Tommy Lee Lott (Lanham, MD, 1998), p. 10.

16 Paul Cartledge, *The Greeks: A Portrait of Self and Others* (Oxford, 1993), p. 125.

17 Aristotle, *Minor Works*, trans. W. S. Hett (Cambridge, MA, 1936), p. 99.

18 Ingomar Weiler, 'Inverted Kalokagathia', in *Representing the Body of the Slave*, ed. Jane Gardner and Thomas Wiedemann (New York, 2013), pp. 11–28.

19 Aristotle, *The Politics*, trans. H. Rackham (Cambridge, MA, 1932), pp. 23, 25. See also Naomi Zack, *The Ethics and Mores of Race: Equality after the History of Philosophy* (Lanham, MD, 2011), pp. 78–9.

20 Johannes Fabian, *Time and the Other: How Anthropology Makes its Object* (New York, 1983).

21 John H. Van Evrie, *Negroes and Negro 'Slavery': The First an Inferior Race; The Latter its Normal Condition* (New York, 1861), p. 93.

22 Ibid., p. 96.

23 Ibid., p. 44.

24 Mrs A. C. Carmichael, *Domestic Manners and Social Conditions of the White, Coloured and Negro Populations of the West Indies* (London, 1833), vol. I, p. 322.

25 Thomas Dixon, *The Clansman: A Historical Romance of the Klu Klux Klan* (New York, 1907), p. 216.

26 Haller, *Outcasts from Evolution*, p. 16.

27 Roberto Romani, *National Character and Public Spirit in Britain and France, 1750–1914* (Cambridge, 2004), pp. 165ff.

28 Charles Carroll, *The Negro a Beast; or, In the Image of God* (St Louis, MO, 1900), p. 128.

29 Ibid., p. 219.

30 William Gallio Schell, *Is the Negro a Beast? A Reply to Chas. Carroll's Book Entitled 'The Negro a Beast'* (Moundsville, WV, 1901), p. 67.

31 R. J. Terry, 'Robert Bennett Bean, 1874–1944', *American Anthropologist*, XLVIII (1946), p. 70.

32 Robert Bennett Bean, 'Notes on the Body Form of Man', *Scientific Papers of the Second International Congress of Eugenics, September 22–28, 1921* (Baltimore, MD, 1923), vol. II, pp. 16–17. See Gregory Michael Dorr,

Segregation's Science: Eugenics and Society in Virginia (Charlottesville, VA, 2008), p. 82.

33 Erving Goffman, 'Picture Frames', in *Gender Advertisements* (New York, 1979), p. 13.

34 See the photographs taken in 1850 of seven South Carolina slaves by the naturalist Louis Agassiz that were intended to provide evidence of the supposed biological inferiority of the slave. See Molly Rogers, *Delia's Tears: Race, Science, and Photography in Nineteenth-century America* (New Haven, CT, 2010).

35 Kirk Savage, *Standing Soldiers, Kneeling Slaves: Race, War, and Monument in Nineteenth-century America* (Princeton, NJ, 1997), p. 98.

36 Erving Goffman, *Stigma: Notes on the Management of Spoiled Identity* (Englewood Cliffs, NJ, 1963), p. 3.

37 'A Citizen of New-York', 'Slavery – A Narrative', *National Anti-slavery Standard* (17 September 1840), p. 59.

38 John Warner Barber, ed., *A History of the Amistad Captives* (New Haven, CT, 1840), p. 19.

39 Thomas Clarkson, *The History of the Rise, Progress, and Accomplishment of the Abolition of the African Slave-trade by the British Parliament* (London, 1808), vol. II, pp. 191–2.

40 William Lloyd Garrison, 'The Kneeling Slave', *The Liberator* (22 February 1834).

41 Charles A. Jarvis, 'Admission to Abolition: The Case of John Greenleaf Whittier', *Journal of the Early Republic*, IV/2 (1984), pp. 161–76.

42 Marcus Wood, *Horrible Gift of Freedom: Atlantic Slavery and the Representation of Emancipation* (Athens, GA, 2010), p. 19.

43 Quoted in Benjamin Quarles, *Frederick Douglass* (New York, 1968), p. 184. See also Constance McLaughlin Green, *The Secret City: A History of Race Relations in the Nation's Capital* (Princeton, NJ, 1967).

44 Freeman Henry Morris Murray, *Emancipation and the Freed in American Sculpture: A Study in the Interpretation* (Washington, DC, 1916), p. 28. See also Benjamin Quarles, *Lincoln and the Negro* (New York, 1962), p. 12.

45 Savage, *Standing Soldiers*, p. 119.

46 Roland C. White, Jr, *American Ulysses: A Life of Ulysses S. Grant* (New York, 2016), p. 573.

47 Savage, *Standing Soldiers*, p. 78.

48 Frantz Fanon, *Black Skin, White Masks*, trans. Richard Philcox (New York, 1967), p. 119. See the discussion in Aviva Briefel, *The Racial Hand in the Victorian Imagination* (Cambridge, 2015), p. 151.

49 Fanon, *Black Skin*, pp. 152–3. We should note that subsequent generations of scholars have expanded where and how Fanon locates the root of, and identification with, the aggressor. One of the most fascinating revisions is in the emergent field of critical affect studies, where the links between Fanon's described *perception* of difference and the felt or lived corporeal effects of this perception of difference work in tandem to produce a *lived experience* of racialization. In her essay 'A Phenomenology of Hesitation', the philosopher Alia Al-Saji recalls Fanon's use of 'affective ankylosis' (Fanon, *Black Skin*, p. 121) to describe the condition of the colonizer, but turns it around to describe the 'rigidity, immobility, and numbing that

characterize racializing affects' in the 'epidermalized' bodies of racial Others. See Alia Al-Saji, 'A Phenomenology of Hesitation: Interrupting Racializing Habits of Seeing', in *Living Alterities: Phenomenology, Embodiment and Race*, ed. Emily S. Lee (Albany, 2014), pp. 137, 140–41.

50 Malcolm X, 'Afro-American History', *International Socialist Review*, 28 (1967), p. 14.

51 Michael Eric Dyson, *I May Not Get There with You: The True Martin Luther King Jr* (New York, 2000), p. 109.

52 Martin Luther King, Jr, 'The Rising Tide of Racial Consciousness', in *The Papers of Martin Luther King Jr*, ed. Clayborne Carson, vol. v: *The Threshold of a New Decade, January 1959–December 1960* (Berkeley, CA, and Los Angeles, CA, 2005), pp. 505–6.

53 Ibid.

54 Garnett S. Huguley, *Growing up African American: Struggling through the Legacy of Slavery and Jim Crow Segregation* (New York, 2003), p. 51.

55 Robert Burton, *The Anatomy of Melancholy: What It Is, with All the Kinds, Causes, Symptomes, Prognostickes and Severall Cures of It* [1621] (New York, 1977), pp. 211–12.

56 Johann Jakob Schudt, *Jüdische Merkwürdigkeiten* (Frankfurt am Main, 1718), vol. II, p. 368.

57 See Leah Hochman, *The Ugliness of Moses Mendelssohn: Aesthetics, Religion and Morality in the Eighteenth Century* (New York, 2014), p. 6.

58 Joseph Rohrer, *Versuch über die jüdischen Bewohner der österreichischen Monarchie* (Vienna, 1804), pp. 25–6 (translation by the author).

59 Balduin Groller, 'Die körperliche Minderwertigkeit der Juden', *Die Welt*, XVI (19 April 1901), p. 4 (translation by the author).

60 Ibid.

61 Joseph Pennell, *The Jew at Home: Impressions of a Summer and Autumn Spent with Him* (New York, 1891), pp. 77–8.

62 Jack London, *The People of the Abyss* (New York, 1904), p. 220.

63 Eva Brinkschulte, Muniz de Faria and Yara Lemke, 'Patienten im Atelier: die fotografische Sammlung des Arztes Heimann Wolff Berend 1858 bis 1865', *Fotogeschichte*, LXXX (2001), pp. 17–27.

64 Max Nordau, *Degeneration* (New York, 1895), p. 11.

65 Franz Rosenzweig, *Briefe und Tagebücher*, ed. Rachel Rosenzweig and Edith Rosenzweig-Scheinmann (The Hague, 1979), vol. I, p. 392.

66 Ulrich Dunker, *Der Reichsbund jüdischer Frontsoldaten, 1918–1938* (Düsseldorf, 1977), p. 541.

67 Athena S. Leoussi and David Aberbach, 'Hellenism and Jewish Nationalism: Ambivalence and its Ancient Roots', *Ethnic and Racial Studies*, XXV (2002), p. 755.

68 Quoted in Todd Samuel Presner, '"Clear Heads, Solid Stomachs, and Hard Muscles": Max Nordau and the Aesthetics of Jewish Regeneration', *Modernism/modernity*, X/2 (2003), p. 296.

69 Quoted in Paul R. Mendes-Flohr and Jehuda Reinharz, eds, *The Jew in the Modern World: A Documentary History* (New York, 2011), p. 547.

70 Quoted in Max Simon Nordau and Gustav Gottheil, *Zionism and Anti-Semitism* (New York, 1905), p. 45.

71 Quoted ibid., p. 176.

72 In Mann's untitled contribution to Julius Moses, ed., *Die Lösung der Judenfrage: Eine Rundfrage* (Berlin, 1907), pp. 242–8. We are citing from the original edition, since it presents the text in its original context. Reprinted in Thomas Mann, 'Zur jüdischen Frage', in *Gesammelte Werke in 13 Bänden* (Frankfurt am Main, 1974), vol. VII, pp. 466–75. All translations are by the author.

73 Todd Kontje, *Thomas Mann's World: Empire, Race, and the Jewish Question* (Ann Arbor, MI, 2011), pp. 19–24.

74 Mann in Moses, *Die Lösung*, pp. 244–5.

75 Thomas Mann, *Tonio Kröger and other Stories*, trans. David Luke (New York, 1970), p. 5.

76 Alex Bein, *Theodor Herzl: Biographie* (Vienna, 1974), p. 173.

77 Paul Higate, *Military Masculinities: Identity and the State* (Westport, CT, 2003), p. 189.

78 Sharon Gillerman, 'Samson in Vienna: The Theatrics of Jewish Masculinity', *Jewish Social Studies*, IX/2 (2003), p. 85.

79 Breitbart often performed in the United States, and his work had a presence there. Siegmund Breitbart, *Muscular Power* (New York, 1924).

80 Elias Auerbach, 'Die Militärtauglichkeit der Juden', *Jüdische Rundschau*, L (1908), pp. 491–2.

81 Max Zirker, 'Vom Basler Schauturnen', *Die jüdische Turnzeitung*, IX (1903), pp. 164–9.

82 Anatole Leroy-Beaulieu and Frances Hellman, *Israel Among the Nations: A Study of the Jews and Antisemitism* (New York and London, 1895), p. 198.

83 Oskar Panizza, 'The Operated Jew', trans. Jack Zipes, *New German Critique*, XXI (1980), p. 64.

84 Ibid., p. 68.

85 Alexander Granach, *There Goes an Actor* (Garden City, NY, 1945), p. 189. See Arnold Zweig, *Juden auf der deutsche Bühne* (Berlin, 1928), pp. 149–56.

86 Ibid., p. 189.

87 Ibid., p. 172.

88 Quotations taken from Douglas C. Baynton, 'Disability and the Justification for Inequality in American History', in Davis, ed., *The Disability Studies Reader*, p. 28.

89 Quoted in Allan M. Kraut, *Silent Travelers: Germs, Genes, and the 'Immigrant Menace'* (Baltimore, MD, 1994), p. 208.

90 James Truslow Adams, *The Epic of America* (Boston, MA, 1931), pp. 404–5.

91 Keith A. Livers, *Constructing the Stalinist Body: Fictional Representations of Corporeality in the Stalinist 1930s* (Lanham, MD, 2004), p. 204.

92 George L. Mosse, *Nationalism and Sexuality: Respectability and Abnormal Sexuality in Modern Europe* (New York, 1985), pp. 134–6.

93 Jan Robert Bloch, 'How Can We Understand the Bends in the Upright Gait?', trans. Capers Rubin, *New German Critique*, XLV (1988), pp. 9–39. With reference to Ernst Bloch, *Natural Law and Human Dignity*, trans. D. J. Schmidt (Cambridge, MA, 1986).

94 Rainer Traub, Harald Wiesner and Otto Klemperer, eds, *Gespräche mit Ernst Bloch* (Frankfurt am Main, 1975), pp. 123ff.

95 Ernst Bloch, *The Principle of Hope*, trans. Neville Plaice, Stephen Plaice and Paul Knight (Cambridge, MA, 1995), vol. II, p. 453.

96 Ibid., p. 467.

97 Ibid., p. 472.

98 Miriam Rürup, 'Capitalism and the Jews Revisited: A Comment', *Bulletin of the German Historical Institute Washington*, LVIII (2016), p. 27.

99 Ibid., p. 472.

100 Gary Shteyngart, *The Russian Debutante's Handbook* (New York, 2002), p. 44. See also Natalie Friedman, 'Nostalgia, Nationhood, and the New Immigrant Narrative: Gary Shteyngart's "The Russian Debutante's Handbook" and the Post-Soviet Experience', *Iowa Journal of Cultural Studies*, V (2004), pp. 77–87.

101 Shteyngart, *The Russian Debutante's Handbook*, p. 46.

102 Michael Chabon, *Moonglow: A Novel* (New York, 2016), p. 158.

NINE: 'POLITICAL POSTURING': POSTURE DEFINES THE GOOD CITIZEN

1 Benedict Anderson, *Imagined Communities: Reflections on the Origin and Spread of Nationalism* (London, 1983), p. 19.

2 Ibid., pp. 6–7.

3 Ibid., p. 147.

4 Ernest Gellner, 'Do Nations Have Navels?', *Nations and Nationalism*, II (1996), pp. 366–70.

5 Ernest Gellner, *Nations and Nationalism* (Ithaca, NY, 1983), p. 85.

6 Anderson, *Imagined Communities*, p. 89.

7 William Bloom, *Personal Identity, National Identity and International Relations* (Cambridge, 1990), p. 52.

8 Ibid., p. 74.

9 Ibid., p. 31.

10 Charles Taylor, 'Self-interpreting Animals', in *Philosophical Papers* (Cambridge, 1985), vol. I, pp. 45–76.

11 Jürgen Habermas, *The Future of Human Nature*, trans. Hella Beister, Max Pensky and William Rehg (Cambridge, 2003).

12 Johann Gottfried Herder, *Outlines of a Philosophy of the History of Man*, trans. T. Churchill (New York, 1966), p. 468.

13 Ibid., p. 658.

14 Quoted in Heikki Lempa, *Beyond the Gymnasium: Educating the Middle-class Bodies in Classical Germany* (Lanham, MD, 2007), p. 4.

15 Ibid., p. 8.

16 Benjamin Braude, 'How Racism Arose in Europe and Why It Did Not in the Near East', in *Racism in the Modern World: Historical Perspectives on Cultural Transfer and Adaptation*, ed. Manfred Berg and Simon Wendt (New York, 2011), p. 54.

17 George Mosse, *The Image of Man: The Creation of Modern Masculinity* (New York, 1996), p. 41.

18 Johann Christoph Friedrich Guts Muths, *Gymnastics for Youth, Or, A Practical Guide to Healthful and Amusing Exercises* (Philadelphia, PA, 1803), pp. 332–3.

19 Jonathan Black, *Making the American Body* (Lincoln, NE, 2013), p. 3.

20 Ibid., p. 67.

21 Quoted ibid., p. 90.

22 Friedrich Jahn, *A Treatise on Gymnastiks*, trans. Charles Beck (Northampton, MA, 1828), p. 1.

23 Friedrich Jahn, *Deutsches Volksthum* (Lübeck, 1810), pp. 14–15. Jakob and Wilhelm Grimm, in *Wörterbuch*, vol. XXVIII, col. 1571, give this citation for *weltflüchtig* with the translation 'durch die welt fliehend, nomadisierend, unstet', www.woerterbuchnetz.de, accessed 30 June 2016.

24 Jahn, *Deutsches Volksthum*, p. 15.

25 Thus the note under *Gesund*: 'Auch das antike *sanum corpus et sana mens* taucht in der humanistisch beeinfluszten sprüchwörterlitteratur auf (Lehmann 302) und erhält mit dem neu erwachenden sinne für leibesübungen und körperpflege seine neue prägung *mens sana in corpore sano*: wir wünschen einen gesunden geist in einem gesunden körper. Göthe (farbenlehre) 53, 130.' In Grimm, *Wörterbuch*, vol. V, col. 4292.

26 Robert Knight Barney, 'Forty-eighters and the Rise of the Turnverein Movement in America', in *Ethnicity and Sport in North American History and Culture*, ed. George Eisen and David K. Wiggins (Westport, CT, 1995), p. 28.

27 Karl-Heinz Schodrok, *Preußische Turnpolitik: Preußische Turnpolitik mit Blick auf Westfalen* (Berlin, 2013), p. 301.

28 Quoted in David J. Rothman, Steven Marcus and Stephanie A. Kiceluk, eds, *Medicine and Western Civilization* (New Brunswick, NJ, 1995), p. 96.

29 *Marriage: Sex Facts and Conduct: For Girls and Matured Women* (n.p., 1925), p. 4.

30 Quoted in W. Grant Hague, *The Eugenic Marriage: A Personal Guide to the New Science of Better Living and Better Babies* (New York, 1914), p. 25.

31 Havelock Ellis, *The Philosophy of Conflict and Other Essays in War-time: Second Series* (London, 1919), p. 183.

32 Heinrich von Treitschke, *The Organization of the Army*, trans. Adam L. Gowans (London, 1914), p. 10.

33 Quoted in Richard S. Levy, ed., *Antisemitism in the Modern World: An Anthology of Texts* (Lexington, MA, and Toronto, ON, 1991), pp. 69–73.

34 Heinrich von Treitschke, *History of Germany in the Nineteenth Century*, trans., Eden and Cedar Paul (New York, 1917), vol. III, p. 46.

35 Hajo Bernett, 'Das Jahn-Bild in der Nationalsozialistischen Weltanschauung', *Stadion*, IV (1978), pp. 225–47.

36 Treitschke, *History of Germany*, vol. III, p. 7.

37 Ibid., p. 229.

38 Ibid., p. 230.

39 Ibid., p. 233.

40 Thomas Weber, *Hitler's First War: Adolf Hitler, the Men of the List Regiment, and the First World War* (Oxford, 2010), p. 119.

41 Tara Magdalinski, 'Beyond Hitler: Alfred Baeumler, Ideology and Physical Education in the Third Reich', *Sporting Traditions*, XII (1995), pp. 61–79.

42 Alfred Baeumler, 'Die weltanschaulichen Grundlagen der deutschen Leibesübungen', in *Sport und Staat* (Berlin, 1934), vol. I, pp. 31–2 (translation by the author).

43 Quoted by Bernett, 'Das Jahn-Bild', p. 240 (translation by the author).

44 Hajo Bernett, ed., *Nationalsozialistische Leibeserziehung* (Schorndorf bei Stuttgart, 1966), p. 20 (translation by the author).

45 'United States Holocaust Memorial Museum', www.ushmm.org, accessed 23 September 2016.

46 M. Kohn, *The Race Gallery: The Return of Racial Science* (London, 1995), p. 36.

47 Michael Hau, *The Cult of Health and Beauty in Germany: A Social History, 1890–1930* (Chicago, IL, 2003), p. 157.

48 Peter Longreich, *Heinrich Himmler: A Life* (Oxford, 2013), pp. 600–601.

49 Susan Brownell, *Training the Body for China: Sports in the Moral Order of the People's Republic* (Chicago, IL, 1995), p. 10.

50 Larissa N. Heinrich, *The Afterlife of Images: Translating the Pathological Body between China and the West* (Durham, NC, 2008), pp. 41–2, for the discussion of representations of pathological Chinese posture.

51 David E. Mungello, *Curious Land: Jesuit Accommodation and the Origins of Sinology* (Honolulu, HI, 1989), pp. 300–328.

52 Christopher Frayling, *The Yellow Peril: Dr Fu Manchu and the Rise of Chinaphobia* (London, 2014), p. 252.

53 Karl Friedrich A. Gützlaff, *A Sketch of Chinese History, Ancient and Modern: Comprising a Retrospect of the Foreign Intercourse and Trade with China* (London, 1834), p. 54.

54 William Hamilton Jeffreys and James L. Maxwell, *The Diseases of China: Including Formosa and Korea* (Philadelphia, PA, 1911), pp. 305–6.

55 Jing Tsu, *Failure, Nationalism, and Literature: The Making of Modern Chinese Identity, 1895–1937* (Redwood City, CA, 2005).

56 Lu Xun, quoted in James Reeve Pusey, *China and Charles Darwin* (Cambridge, 1983), p. 16.

57 Luo Shimin, *The History of Sport in China* (Beijing, 2008), vol. II, p. 204.

58 Francis Graham Crookshank, *The Mongol in our Midst: A Study of Man and his Three Faces* (London, 1924), p. 15.

59 L. A. Rocha, 'Sex, Eugenics, Aesthetics, Utopia in the Life and Work of Zhang Jingsheng (1888–1970)', PhD thesis, University of Cambridge, 2010.

60 Madalina Yuk-Ling Lee, 'The Intellectual Origins of Lin Yutang's Cultural Internationalism, 1928–1938', PhD thesis, University of Maryland, 2009, pp. 116–18.

61 See Benjamin I. Schwartz, *In Search of Wealth and Power: Yen Fu and the West* (Cambridge, MA, 1964); and James Reeve Pusey, *China and Charles Darwin* (Cambridge, MA, 1983).

62 Chen Duxiu, 'Jinride Jiaoyo Fanghen' (The Objectives of a Modern Education), *Xin Qingnian*, I/2 (1915, repr. 1962), p. 118.

63 Frank Dikötter, *Sex, Culture and Modernity in China: Medical Science and the Construction of Sexual Identities in the Early Republican Period* (Honolulu, HI, 1995), p. 175.

64 A complete French translation of Mao's essay, along with explanatory notes and an introduction, was published as Stuart Schram, ed. and trans., *Mao Zedong: Une Étude de l'Éducation Physique* (Paris and The Hague, 1962).

65 All quotations from this text are from the partial English translation available as Mao Tse-tung, 'A Study of Physical Education', www.marxists. org, accessed 8 November 2013. This has been compared to the more complete French translation.

66 Quoted in Edgar Snow, *Red Star over China*, revd edn (Harmondsworth, 1972), p. 174.
67 Quoted ibid., pp. 172–3.
68 Mao, 'A Study of Physical Education'.
69 Ibid.
70 Ibid.
71 Amos Elon, *Herzl* (New York, 1975), p. 63.
72 Konrad Hugo Jarausch, *Students, Society, and Politics in Imperial Germany: The Rise of Academic Illiberalism* (Princeton, NJ, 1982), p. 350.
73 Ibid., p. 272.
74 Oz Almog, *The Sabra: The Creation of the New Jew*, trans. Haim Watzman (Berkeley, CA, 2000), p. 134.
75 Stuart Schram, ed., *Mao's Road to Power: Revolutionary Writings, 1912–49* (Florence, 1992), vol. I. Schramm transliterates the Chinese characters as 'Sonntag', but this is an error, since Mao is transcribing the Japanese transliteration of Sandow's name into Chinese characters. I am grateful to Zhou Xun for correcting this error. Sandow was first translated into Chinese in Fubao Ding, *Shi yan que bing fa* (Shanghai, 1915).
76 Theodore Roosevelt, 'To the Holy Name Society at Oyster Bay, NY, August 16, 1903', in *The Works of Theodore Roosevelt: Presidential Address and State Papers* (New York, 1905), vol. XIV, p. 460.
77 Eugen Sandow, *Strength and How to Obtain It* (London, 1897), p. 10.
78 David Waller, *The Perfect Man: The Muscular Life and Times of Eugen Sandow, Victorian Strongman* (Brighton, 2011), p. 146.
79 All quotations are from Arthur Conan Doyle's foreword to Eugen Sandow, *The Construction and Reconstruction of the Human Body: A Manual of the Therapeutics of Exercise* (London, 1907), p. x.
80 Mark Singleton, *Yoga Body: The Origin of Modern Posture Practice* (Oxford, 2010), p. 89.
81 Waller, *The Perfect Man*, p. 184.
82 Ibid., p. 145.
83 See Zhou Xun, *Chinese Perceptions of the 'Jews' and Judaism: A History of the Youtai* (New York, 2000), pp. 11–14.
84 Carey A. Watt, 'Physical Culture as "Natural Cure" – Eugen Sandow's Global Campaign against the Diseases and Vices of Civilization c. 1890–1920', in *Global Anti-vice Activism, 1890–1950*, ed. Jessica Pliley, Robert Kramm and Harald Fischer-Tiné (Cambridge, 2016), pp. 74–100.
85 Sandow, *Construction and Reconstruction*, p. 29.
86 Ibid.
87 Eugen Sandow, 'Talk XIII: Exercise versus Medicine', in *The Gospel of Strength According to Sandow* (Melbourne, 1902), p. 134.
88 Mao, 'A Study of Physical Education'.
89 Quoted in Lu Zhouxiang and Fan Hong, 'From Celestial Empire to Nation State: Sport and the Origins of Chinese Nationalism (1840–1927)', *International Journal of the History of Sport*, XXVII (2010), p. 493.
90 Mao Dun, *My Life* (Beijing, 1997), p. 72.
91 Anonymous, 'Foot-binding', *Medical News*, XLI (22 August 1882), p. 242.
92 Andrew D. Morris, *Marrow of the Nation: A History of Sport and Physical Culture in Republican China* (Berkeley, CA, 2004).

93 Lu Zhouxiang and Fan Hong, *Sport and Nationalism in China* (New York, 2014), p. 111.

94 Vivienne Lo, ed., *Perfect Bodies: Sports, Medicine and Immortality* (London, 2012), p. 82.

95 Ibid., p. 12.

96 Ibid., p. 5.

TEN: CONTEMPORARY POSTURE AND DISABILITY STUDIES

1 Georges Canguilhem, *Ideology and Rationality in the History of the Life Sciences*, trans. Arthur Goldhammer (Cambridge, MA, 1989), p. 246.

2 Nikolas Rose, *Inventing our Selves: Psychology, Power, and Personhood* (Cambridge, 1998), p. 157.

3 Nicholas Mirzoef, *Silent Poetry: Deafness, Sign, and Visual Culture in Modern France* (Princeton, NJ, 1995). See also Lennard J. Davis, *Enforcing Normalcy: Disability, Deafness, and the Body* (London, 1995), pp. 26–9; and Jennifer L. Nelson and Bradley Berens, 'Spoken Daggers, Deaf Ears, and Silent Mouths: Fantasies of Deafness in Early Modern England', in *The Disability Studies Reader*, 1st edn, ed. Lennard J. Davis (New York, 1997), pp. 52–74.

4 Sander L. Gilman, 'What is the Color of the Gonorrhea Ribbon? Stigma, Sexual Diseases and Popular Culture in George Bush's World', *Cultural Politics*, II (2007), pp. 175–202.

5 Lennard J. Davis, *Bending Over Backwards: Disability, Dismodernism and Other Difficult Positions* (New York, 2002), p. 105.

6 Thomas Abrams, 'Is Everyone Upright? Erwin Straus' "The Upright Posture" and Disabled Phenomenology', *Human Affairs*, XXIV (2014), p. 571.

7 Rosemarie Garland-Thomson, 'The Case for Conserving Disability', *Journal of Bioethical Inquiry*, IX (2012), p. 341.

8 Ibid., p. 342.

9 Ibid.

10 Rosemarie Garland-Thomson, *Extraordinary Bodies: Figuring Physical Disability in American Culture and Literature* (New York, 1996), p. 8. Garland-Thomson coined the term 'normate' to indicate the non-stigmatized figure – a body that is 'normal' that serves as the unspoken standard against which society measures difference. The 'normate' is a dynamic concept and changes over time.

11 Elizabeth Barnes, *The Minority Body: A Theory of Disability* (Oxford, 2016), p. 2.

12 Erving Goffman, *Stigma: Notes on the Management of a Spoiled Identity* (Harmondsworth, 1968), p. 4.

13 Ibid., p. 110.

14 Ibid., p. 11.

15 Ibid., p. 16, citing L. Baker, *Out on a Limb* (New York, 1946), p. 73.

16 Rosemarie Garland-Thomson, *Staring: How We Look* (New York, 2009).

17 Aimi Hamraie, 'Designing Collective Access: A Feminist Disability Theory of Universal Design', *Disability Studies Quarterly*, XXXIII (2013), www.dsq-sds.or, accessed 15 January 2016.

18 Isabel Dyck, 'Geographies of Disability: Reflecting on New Body Knowledges', in *Toward Enabling Geographies: 'Disabled' Bodies and Minds*

in Society and Space, ed. Vera Chouinard, Edward Hall and Robert Wilton (Burlington, VT, 2010), p. 254.

19 The debate about metaphor in Disability Studies looks at the inherent physicality of metaphor and the ability or inability to transcend such limiting cases. Here I am engaging with what is not seen as a metaphor, being upright as a moral category, but which has deep metaphoric roots in shaping both our notion of the body and our sense of moral rectitude. This leads to what Ato Quayson in *Aesthetic Nervousness: Disability and the Crisis of Representation* (New York, 2007) calls 'aesthetic nervousness', a critical reassessment of David Mitchell and Sharon Snyder's *Narrative Prosthesis: Disability and the Dependencies of Discourse* (Ann Arbor, MI, 2001), pp. 7–9, claims about the literary representation of disability as a form of 'narrative prosthesis'. This Quayson views as too narrow in scope. Aesthetic nervousness identifies that the 'prostheticizing function [of narrative] is bound to fail, not because of the difficulties in erasing the effects of disability in the real world, but because the aesthetic domain itself is short-circuited upon the encounter with disability'. For this debate, see Amy Vidali, 'Seeing What We Know: Disability and Theories of Metaphor', *Journal of Literary and Cultural Disability Studies*, IV (2010), pp. 33–54.

20 Robert Murphy, *The Body Silent: The Different World of the Disabled* (New York, 1987), p. 93.

21 Barnes, *The Minority Body*, pp. 76–7.

22 Tobin Siebers, 'My Withered Limb', *Disability, Art, and Culture (Part One)*, XXXVII/2 (1998).

23 Ibid.

24 There seem to be only two photographs of Roosevelt in his wheelchair. In 1992, then President Bill Clinton urged that an additional statue of Roosevelt in a wheelchair be added to the new FDR memorial in Washington, DC, in response to calls from 'advocates for the disabled, who had threatened to protest at the memorial's dedication'. He wrote: 'I'm pleased to offer this legislation so that generations of Americans will know that this great President was great with his disability.' See David Stout, 'Clinton Calls for Sculpture of Roosevelt in Wheelchair', *New York Times* (24 April 1997).

25 David Citino, 'New Roosevelt Sculpture Includes Wheelchair', *Southern Review*, XXXVIII (2002), pp. 7–8.

26 Lothar Scharf, '*Schutzabzeichen für Schwerhörige*', '*Taubstummen-Armbinde*' oder '*Blindenabzeichen*'? *Die Geschichte der gelben Armbind mit den drei schwarzen Punkten* (Berlin, 2013).

27 Quoted in Carol Poore, *Disability in Twentieth-century German Culture* (Ann Arbor, MI, 2007), p. 16.

28 See Eleoma Joshua and Michael Schillmeier, eds, *Edinburgh German Yearbook* (Edinburgh, 2004), vol. IV; and Elsbeth Bösl, Anne Klein and Anne Waldschmidt, eds, *Disability History: Konstruktionen von Behinderung in der Geschichte: Eine Einführung* (Bielefeld, 2010).

29 Poore, *Disability in Twentieth-century German Culture*, pp. 26–32.

30 Ibid., p. 30.

31 Reinhold Heller, *Art in Germany: 1901–1936: From Expressionism to Resistance. The Marvin and Janet Fishman Collection* (Munich, 1990), p. 162.

32 This becomes the litmus test and is, of course, extended to exclude Jews. See Paul Wehner, 'Arbeit der blinden Hitlerjugend' (1937), reprinted in Sven Degenhardt and Waldraut Rath, eds, *Blinden- und Sehbehinderenpädagogik* (Weinheim, 2009), pp. 125–32.

33 Sieglind Ellger-Rüttgardt, 'Blinde Menschen im Dritten Reich', in *200 Jahre Blindenbildung in Deutschland (1806–2006)*, ed. Wolfgang Drave and Hartmut Mehls (Würzburg, 2006), pp. 161–71.

34 Poore, *Disability in Twentieth-century German Culture*, pp. 126–30.

35 Anson Rabinbach and Sander L. Gilman, eds, *The Third Reich Sourcebook* (Berkeley, CA, 2013), p. 333.

36 Malin Büttner, *Nicht Minderwertig, Sondern Mindersinnig . . . : Der Bann G für Gehörgeschadigte in der Hitler-Jugend* (Frankfurt am Main, 2005).

37 Brenda Ralph Lewis, *Illustrierte Geschichte der Hitlerjugend: 1922–1945 – Die verlorene Kindheit* (Vienna, 2001), p. 55.

38 Werner Brill, *Pädagogik der Abgrenzung: Die Implementierung der Rassenhygiene im Nationalsozialismus durch die Sonderpädagogik* (Bad Heilbrunn, 2011), p. 175 n. 406.

39 Horst Biesold, *Crying Hands: Eugenics and Deaf People in Nazi Germany* (Washington, DC, 1999), p. 97.

40 Quoted by Gabriel Richter, 'Blind Jews in the Third Reich', trans. Gail Snider, *Braille Monitor*, www.nfb.org, accessed 9 October 2016. See also Gabriel Richter, *Blindheit und Eugenik (1918–1945)* (Freiburg, 1986).

41 Richter, 'Blind Jews'.

42 Brill, *Pädagogik der Abgenzung*, p. 14.

43 Michael Buddrus, *Totale Erziehung für den totalen Krieg: Hitlerjugend und nationalsozialistische Jugendpolitik* (Munich, 2003), vol. II, pp. 929–31.

44 Quoted in Richter, 'Blind Jews'.

45 See Rabinbach and Gilman, eds, *The Third Reich Sourcebook*, pp. 68–71.

46 Kevin McSorley, *War and the Body: Militarisation, Practice, and Experience* (New York, 2013).

47 Poore, *Disability in Twentieth-century German Culture*, pp. 129–30.

48 Jacques Lusseyran, *And Then There Was Light: The Extraordinary Memoir of a Blind Hero of the French Resistance in World War II*, trans. Elizabeth R. Cameron (Novato, CA, 1963), p. 265.

49 Richter, 'Blind Jews'.

50 Kay Boyle, *Generation without Farewell* (New York, 1960), pp. 134–5.

51 Ingeborg Bachmann, *Eine Ort für Zufälle* (Berlin, 1965). See Christian Däufel, *Ingeborg Bachmanns 'Ein Ort für Zufälle'* (Berlin, 2013), pp. 276–7.

52 Olaf Berwald, 'The Ends of Blindness in Max Frisch's *Mein Name Sei Gantenbein*', in *A Companion to the Works of Max Frisch*, ed. Olaf Berwald (Rochester, NY, 2013), pp. 156–71.

53 Max Frisch, *A Wilderness of Mirrors*, trans. Michael Bullock (New York, 1966), pp. 40, 45.

54 Moshé Feldenkrais, *Body and Mature Behavior: A Study of Anxiety, Sex, Gravitation and Learning* (Berkeley, CA, 2005).

55 Ibid., p. 139.

56 Rod Michalko, *The Mystery of the Eye and the Shadow of Blindness* (Toronto, ON, 1998), p. 93.

57 Feldenkrais, *Body and Mature Behavior*, p. 69.

58 Michalko, *The Mystery of the Eye*, p. 19.
59 Alexander and Margarete Mitscherlich, *Die Unfähigkeit zu trauern: Grundlagen kollektiven Verhaltens* (Munich, 1967); Alexander and Margarete Mitscherlich, *The Inability to Mourn: Principles of Collective Behavior*, trans. Eric Mosbachs (New York, 1974). See Tobias Freimüller, ed., *Psychoanalyse und Protest – Alexander Mitscherlich und die 'Achtundsechziger'* (Göttingen, 2008).
60 Aimi Hamraie, 'Historical Epistemology as Disability Studies Methodology: From the Models Framework to Foucault's Archaeology of Cure', *Foucault Studies*, XIX (2015), pp. 108–34.
61 Georges Canguilhem, *The Normal and the Pathological*, trans. Carolyn R. Fawcett (New York, 1978), p. 159. See especially in this context Jan Branson and Don Miller, *Damned for their Difference: The Cultural Construction of Deaf People as Disabled* (Washington, DC, 2002), p. 37.
62 Canguilhem, *The Normal and the Pathological*, p. 69.
63 Elizabeth Guffey, 'The Scandinavian Roots of the International Symbol of Access', *Design and Culture*, VII/3 (2015), pp. 357–76. See also Paul Arthur and Romedi Passini, *Wayfinding: People, Signs and Architecture* (New York, 1992).
64 Nora Ellen Groce, *From Charity to Disability Rights: Global Initiatives of Rehabilitation International, 1922–2002* (New York, 2002), p. 52.
65 Victor Papanek, *Design for the Real World: Human Ecology and Social Change* (Chicago, IL, 1985), pp. 106–7, 332.
66 Ibid., p. 129.
67 Selwyn Goldsmith, *A Symbol for Disabled People: The Report of a Research Study* (London, 1969), p. 10.
68 'No Stigma', *The Times* (9 September 1967), p. 10.
69 Jenny Morris, 'Impairment and Disability: Constructing an Ethics of Care that Promotes Human Rights', *Hypatia*, XVI (2001), p. 9.
70 Liat Ben-Moshe and Justin J. W. Powell, 'Sign of our Times? Revis(it)ing the International Symbol of Access', *Disability and Society*, XXII (2007), p. 498.
71 D. Courvant, 'Coming Out Disabled: A Transsexual Woman Considers Queer Contributions to Living with a Disability', *International Journal of Sexuality and Gender Studies*, IV (1999), p. 105.
72 See the detailed account in Brian Glenney, 'Emergent Learning in Independent Studies: The Story of the Accessible Icon Project', in *Experiential Learning in Philosophy*, ed. Julinna Oxley and Ramona Illea (New York, 2016), p. 126. See also 'The "Accessible Icon" Project', www.accessibleicon.org.
73 Ankur Paliwal, 'Why Are Wheelchairs More Stigmatized than Glasses?', *NAUTILUS* (17 March 2016), www.nautil.us, accessed 17 November 2016.
74 Ibid.
75 Indra Kagis McEwen, *Vitruvius: Writing the Body of Architecture* (Cambridge, MA, 2002), p. 2.
76 Toby Lester, *Da Vinci's Ghost: The Untold Story of the World's Most Famous Drawing* (London, 2011), pp. 222–3.
77 Vitruvius, *On Architecture*, trans. Frank Granger (Cambridge, MA, 1962), p. 79.
78 McEwen, *Vitruvius*, p. 230.
79 Dennis Cosgrove, 'Ptolemy and Vitruvius: Spatial Representation in the Sixteenth-century Texts and Commentaries', in *Architecture and the*

Sciences: Exchanging Metaphors, ed. Antoine Picon and Alesandra Ponte (Princeton, NJ, 2003), pp. 22–4.

80 Andreas Vesalius, *On the Fabric of the Human Body*, trans. William Frank Richardson and John Burd Carman (Novato, CA, 2007), vol. V, p. 59.

81 Roger Griffin, *Modernism and Fascism: The Sense of a Beginning under Mussolini and Hitler* (New York, 2007), p. 337.

82 Selwyn Goldsmith, *Designing for the Disabled* (London, 1963) and still in print. See Louis-Pierre Grosbois, 'The Evolution of Design for All in Public Buildings and Transportation in France', in *Universal Design Handbook*, ed. Wolfgang F. E. Preiser and Elaine Ostroff (New York, 2001), p. 27.4.

83 Selwyn Goldsmith, *Designing for the Disabled: The New Paradigm* (Oxford, 1997), p. 7.

84 Ibid., p. 12.

85 Ibid., p. 15.

86 Ibid., p. 30.

87 'No Stigma', p. 10.

88 Ibid.

89 These were published as specially numbered sections of the *Architects' Journal*, CXLVII/3 for 13, 20 and 27 March 1968. The anthropometric section compiled by Goldsmith was in 13 March 1968, pp. 32–6. The special issues were then collected in the first edition of the *AJ Metric Handbook* (London, 1968) that same year. The quotation here is from the *AJ Metric Handbook*, 2nd edn (London, 1969), p. ii.

90 *AJ Metric Handbook*, p. 45.

91 Jim Sandhu, 'An Integrated Approach to Universal Design: Toward the Inclusion of All Ages, Cultures, and Diversity', in *Universal Design Handbook* (New York, 2001), pp. 3.3–3.14.

92 Grosbois, 'The Evolution of Design for All', p. 27.4. I am indebted to the dissertation by Aimi Hamraie, 'What Can Universal Design Know?: Bodies as Evidence in Disability-accessible Design', PhD thesis, Emory University, 2013. A revised version of this has been published as Aimi Hamraie, *Building Access: Universal Design and the Politics of Disability* (Minneapolis, MN, 2017).

93 Mitra Kanaani and Dak Kopec, eds, *The Routledge Companion for Architecture Design and Practice* (New York, 2016), p. 258.

94 Friedrich Nietzsche, *Human, All too Human*, trans. R. J. Hollingdale (Cambridge, 1996), p. 293.

95 Hans-Georg Gadamer, *The Enigma of Health*, trans., Jason Gaiger and Nicolas Walker (London, 1996), p. 113.

96 Giorgio Colli und Mazzino Montinari, eds, *Nietzsche: Sämtliche Werke: Kritische Studienausgabe* (Berlin, 1980), vol. III, p. 57 (translation by the author).

97 Davis, *Bending Over Backwards*, p. 117.

98 Lennard Davis, *Enforcing Normalcy: Disability, Deafness, and the Body* (London, 1995), p. 5.

99 See Gary Gutting, *Michel Foucault's Archaeology of Scientific Reason* (Cambridge, 1989), p. 82; also Sander L. Gilman, 'The Mad as Artist: Medicine, History and Degenerate Art', *Journal of Contemporary History*, XX (1985), pp. 575–97.

100 Ronald Mace, 'Universal Design: Barrier-free Environments for Everyone', *Designers West*, XXXIII/1 (1985), pp. 147–52.
101 Ibid., p. 147.
102 Nancy Mairs, *Waist-high in the World: A Life Among the Nondisabled* (Boston, MA, 1997), p. 68.
103 Ibid., p. 32.
104 Ibid., p. 56.
105 Jay Dolmage, 'Between the Valley and the Field: Metaphor and Disability', *Prose Studies*, XXVII (2005), p. 116.
106 Tobin Siebers, *Disability Theory* (Ann Arbor, MI, 2008).
107 Ibid., p. 57.
108 Ibid., p. 58.
109 Ibid.
110 David Mitchell and Sharon Snyder, *Narrative Prosthesis* (Ann Arbor, MI, 2003), p. 47.
111 Ibid., p. 49.

CONCLUSION: MAPS OF MORAL POSTURE

1 Clifford Geertz, *The Interpretation of Cultures* (New York, 1973), p. 381.
2 Pierre Bourdieu, *Distinction: A Social Critique of the Judgment of Taste*, trans. Richard Nice (Cambridge, MA, 1987), p. 84.
3 Pierre Bourdieu, *Masculine Domination*, trans. Richard Nice (Stanford, CA, 2001), pp. 22–3.
4 Ibid., p. 238.
5 Ibid., p. 215.
6 Oswald Spengler, *Der Untergang des Abendlandes: Umrisse einer Morphologie der Weltgeschichte* (Munich, 1963), p. 136 (translation by the author).
7 Ibid.
8 Henry Head and Gordon Holmes, 'Sensory Disturbances in Cerebral Lesions', *Brain,* XXXIV (1911), p. 188. For an excellent overview of these debates, see the collected papers of John M. Krois, *Bildkörper and Körperschema: Schriften zur Verkörperungstheorie ikonischer Formen*, ed. Horst Bredekamp and Marion Lauschke (Berlin, 2011).
9 Sir Henry Head, *Studies in Neurology* (London, 1920), vol. II, p. 608.
10 Ibid.
11 Katja Guenther, *Localization and its Discontents: A Genealogy of Psychoanalysis and the Neuro Disciplines* (Chicago, IL, 2015), pp. 39–152, on Wernicke, Schilder and Freud.
12 Paul Schilder, *The Image and Appearance of the Human Body* (Oxford, 1935), p. 273.
13 See the discussion of Maurice Merleau-Ponty and Schilder in Gail Weiss, *Body Images: Embodiment as Intercorporeality* (New York, 1999), pp. 7–28.
14 Isadore Ziferstein, 'Psychoanalysis and Psychiatry: Paul Ferdinand Schilder 1886–1940', in *Psychoanalytic Pioneers*, ed. Franz Alexander, Samuel Eisenstein and Martin Grotjahn (London and New York, 1966), p. 458.
15 Erwin Straus, *Phenomenal Psychology* (New York, 1966), p. 139.
16 Aron Gurwitsch, *Marginal Consciousness* (Athens, OH, 1985), p. 31.

17 Maurice Merleau-Ponty, *Phenomenology of Perception*, trans. Colin Smith (New York, 1962), pp. 470–71.
18 Schilder, *The Image and Appearance of the Human Body*, p. 270.
19 Elias Canetti, *Crowds and Power*, trans. Carol Stewart (New York, 1962), p. 387.
20 'Whether the memory of the first time one stood alone as a child contributes to this, or the sense of our superiority to animals, hardly any of whom by nature stand unsupported on two legs, the fact remains that a man who is standing feels confident and self-sufficient.' Ibid., pp. 387–8.
21 Ibid., p. 387.
22 John A. Schumacher, *Human Posture: The Nature of Inquiry* (Albany, NY, 1989), pp. 18ff.
23 Gordon W. Hewes, 'World Distribution of Certain Postural Habits', *American Anthropologist*, LVII (1955), p. 242.
24 Karen Barad, *Meeting the Universe Halfway: Quantum Physics and the Entanglement of Matter and Meaning* (Durham, NC, 2002), p. 390.
25 Ibid., p. 389.
26 Peggy Shinner, *You Feel so Mortal: Essays on the Body* (Chicago, IL, 2014), p. 40.
27 Donna J. Haraway, *Modest_Witness@Second_Millennium.FemaleMan_Meets_OncoMouse: Feminism and Technoscience* (New York, 1997), p. 142.
28 Judith Butler, *Bodies that Matter: On the Discursive Limits of 'Sex'* (New York, 1993), p. ix.
29 Elizabeth Cashdan, 'Smiles, Speech, and Body Posture: How Women and Men Display Sociometric Status and Power', *Journal of Nonverbal Behavior*, XXII (1998), pp. 209–28.
30 Gayle Salamon, *Assuming a Body: Transgender and Rhetorics of Materiality* (New York, 2010), esp. pp. 29ff.
31 Simon Williams, 'Medical Sociology, Chronic Illness and the Body: A Rejoinder to Michael Kelly and David Field', *Sociology of Health and Illness*, XVIII (1996), p. 702.
32 Robert S. Williams, Jr, 'Ability, Dis-ability and Rehabilitation: A Phenomenological Description', *Journal of Medicine and Philosophy*, IX (1984), p. 93.
33 Nishitani Osamu, 'Anthropos and Humanitas: Two Western Concepts of "Human Being"', in *Translation, Biopolitics, Colonial Difference*, ed. Naoki Sakai and Jon Solomon, trans. Trent Maxey (Hong Kong, 2006), p. 265.
34 'The Marquis was a tall, upstanding man of spare figure', *Strand Magazine*, VIII (1894), p. 156, from www.oed.com, accessed 24 January 2013.
35 'A white-headed clergyman was called upon to say prayers, which he did upstanding', *Illustrated London News* (1 June 1861), p. 505, col. 1, from www.oed.com, accessed 24 January 2013.
36 'A lot of game upstanding chaps, that acted like men', Rolf Boldrewood, *Robbery Under Arms: A Story of Life and Adventure in the Bush and in the Goldfields of Australia* (London, 1888), from www.oed.com.
37 Susan Wendell uses the term 'rejected' to refer to bodily appearances and experiences that are ostracized or rejected from society and cultural inclusion in her *The Rejected Body: Feminist Philosophical Reflections on Disability* (New York, 1996), p. 85.

ACKNOWLEDGEMENTS

I am grateful to Ben Hayes at Reaktion Books, who guided the manuscript from my computer to you. I have taught classes on postural studies at Emory University at graduate and undergraduate level. The graduate seminar produced a collection of essays dedicated to this topic in volume VI of *Jahrbuch für Medizin und Literatur*. I want to thank the editor, Florian Steger, for his support in this endeavour. My thanks also go to Lindsey Grubb and Jennifer van der Grinten, who aided in the production of the manuscript and clearing of the permissions for the images, as well as to Marie Hansen of the Woodruff Library at Emory, for her aid in producing useable images for the book.

PHOTO
ACKNOWLEDGEMENTS

The author and publishers wish to express their thanks to the below sources of illustrative material and/or permission to reproduce it. Some locations of artworks are also given below, in the interests of brevity. While every effort has been made to identify and credit copyright holders, we would like to apologize to anyone who has not been formally acknowledged.

From Bernard Siegfried Albinus, *Tabulae sceleti et musculorum corporis humani* (Leiden, 1747): p. 109; from *Amazing Stories*, I/8 (November 1926): p. 234; from Nicolas Andry de Bois-Regard, *Orthopedia or the Art of Correcting and Preventing Deformities in Children*, vol. I (London, 1743): p. 176; from Domenico Angelo, *The School of Fencing, with a General Explanation of the Principal Attitudes and Positions Peculiar to the Art – by Mr. [Domenico] Angelo* (London, 1765): p. 76; from *The Architects' Journal*, CXLVII/3 (13 March 1968): pp. 342, 343; from John Warner Barber, ed., *A History of the Amistad Captives: Being a Circumstantial Account of the Capture of the Spanish Schooner Amistad, by the Africans on Board; Their Voyage, and Capture Near Long Island, New York; with Biographical Sketches of Each of the Surviving Africans* . . . (New Haven, CT, 1840): p. 257 (photo Emory University, Atlanta, GA – Pitt Theological Library, Rare Book Room); from Johann Bernhard Basedow, *Des Elementarwerks* (Dessau and Leipzig, 1774): pp. 187, 188 (photos Beinecke Library, Yale University, New Haven, CT); from Govert Bidloo, *Anatomia Humani Corporis centum & quinque tabulis* . . . *illustrata* (Amsterdam, 1685): p. 105; from Friedrich Eduard Bilz, *The Natural Method of Healing: A New and Complete Guide to Health* (Leipzig and New York, 1898): p. 124; from Pierre Boaistuau, *Histoires Prodigieuses les plus memorables qui ayent esté obseruées, depuis la natiuité de Iesus Christ, iusques à nostre siecle* . . . (1560): p. 66; from Hans Brandenburg, *Der moderne Tanz* (Munich, 1921); p. 171; from Christian Wilhelm Braune and Otto Fischer, *Über den Schwerpunkt des menschlichen Körpers mit Rücksicht auf die Ausrüstung des deutschen Infanteristen* (Leipzig, 1889): p. 88; from John Bulwer, *Anthropometamorphosis: Man Transform'd* (London, 1653): p. 249 (photo Dartmouth College Library, Hanover, NH); from J. M. Charcot et al., *Nouvelle Iconographie de la Salpêtrière: clinique des maladies du systeme nerveux*, vol. XIV (Paris, 1901): p. 118; from *La Culture Physique: Revue Binensuelle Illustrée*, 23 (1905): p. 214; from Calvin Cutter, *A Treatise on Anatomy, Physiology, and Hygiene Designed for Colleges, Academies, and Families* (Philadelphia, PA, 1849): p. 194; from Jacques Mathieu Delpech, *De l'orthomorphie, par rapport a L'espèce humaine*... (Paris, 1828): p. 18; Deutsches Historisches Museum, Berlin: pp. 69, 292 (I. Desnica), 318 (I. Desnica); Deutsches Hygiene-Museum, Dresden: pp. 139, 140; from Charles Dickens, *A Christmas Carol in Prose* (Boston, MA, 1869): p. 11; from Charles Dickens, *David Copperfield*, household edition (London, 1871–9): p. 27; from Paul Diday, *A Treatise on Syphilis in New-born Children and Infants at the Breast* (New York, 1883): p. 53; Dilbert © 2016 Scott Adams – used by permission of UNIVERSAL CLICK – all rights reserved: pp. 10, 26; from Galen, *Opera ex nona Juntarum editione* ... (Venice, 1625): p. 100 (photo courtesy of The New York Academy of Medicine); Galleria dell'Accademia, Venice: p. 336; from Jacob de Gheÿn, *Wapenhandelinghe Van Roers, Mvsqvetten, Ende Spiessen: Achtervolgende de ordre van Sÿn Excellentie Maurits, Prince van Orangie* ... ('sGraven Hage, 1607): pp. 72, 73, 75; from Ann Gibbons, 'Ardipithecus ramidus', in *Science*, CCCXXVI/5960 (2009): p. 222 (with permission of Jay Matternes); from John William Gibson, *Golden Thoughts on Chastity and Procreation* (Toronto, ON, and Naperville, IL, [1903]): p. 215; from Hans Günther, *Rassenkunde des jüdischen Volkes* (Munich, 1930): p. 293; from Ernest Haeckel, *Anthropogenie, oder, Entwickelungsgeschichte des menschen Keimes- und Stammesgeschichte* (Leipzig, 1874): p. 252; from J. G. Heck, *Iconographic Encyclopedia of Science, Literature, and Art*, vol. II (New York, 1851): p. 58; from Heinrich Hoffmann and Baldur von Schirach, ed., *Hitler wie Ihn keiner kennt* (Berlin, [1940]): p. 290; from F. A. Hornibrook, *The Cultures of the Abdomen* (London, 1927): p. 224; from Thomas Henry Huxley, *Man's Place in Nature* (London, 1863): p. 226; from *The Illustrated London News* (27 February 1909): p. 228; J. Paul Getty Museum, Los Angeles: pp. 23, 70; from William Jardine, *The Naturalist's Library: Mammalia*, vol. I: *Monkeys* (Edinburgh, 1844): p. 231; from *Kikeriki*, XXXIX (23 April 1899): p. 271; from Emil Kraepelin, *Psychiatrie: Ein Lehrbuch für Studierende und Ärtze* (Leipzig, 1896): p. 130; from A. F. Thomas Levacher de la Feutrie, *Traité du rakitis, ou l'art de redresser les enfants contrefaits* (Paris, 1772): p. 114; Library of Congress, Washington, DC: p. 192 (Lessing J. Rosenwald Collection); photos Library of Congress, Washington, DC (Prints and Photographs Division): pp. 30 (Frank G. Carpenter Collection), 82, 116 (photo Lewis Wickes Hine – National Child Labor Committee Collection), 144, 200, 203, 215, 235 (Theatrical Poster Collection), 261, 285, 314; from Carl Linnaeus, *Amoenitates academicæ: seu dissertationes variæ physicæ, medicæ, botanicæ antehac seorsim editæ* . . ., vol. VI ([1763] Stockholm, 1749–90): p. 40; Logan University Archive, Chesterfield, MO (Posture Queen Collection): p. 219; photo Los Angeles County Museum of Art, Los Angeles: p. 33; from Robert W. Lovett, MD, 'Round Shoulders and Faulty Attitude: A Method of Observation and Record, with Conclusions as to Treatment', in *American Physical Education Review*, VII/4 (1902): p. 205; from [Christian von Mechel], *Soldaten- und Plotons-Schule für die Infanterie, aus dem französischen Reglement vom 1. August 1791, übersetzt. Herausgegeben mit 13 meist neu gezeichneten Kupfer-Tafeln von Christian von Mechel* (Basel, 1799): p. 79; from Bess M. Mesendieck, *Körperkultur des Weibes: Praktisch Hygienische und Praktisch*

Ästhetische Winke (Munich, 1906): p. 96 (photo Boston Athenæum Library); from Eadweard J. Muybridge, *Animal Locomotion: An Electro-photographic Investigation of Consecutive Phases of Animal Movements* . . . (Philadelphia, PA, 1887): pp. 91, 92 (photos George Eastman Museum, Rochester, NY); from Franz Carl Naegele, *Das weibliche Becken: betrachtet in Beziehung auf seine Stellung und die Richtung seiner Höhle: nebst Beyträgen zur Geschichte der Lehre von den Beckenaxen* (Karlsruhe, 1825): p. 86; National Gallery, Washington, DC: p. 162; photo National Gallery, Washington, DC (Rosenwald Collection): p. 176; photos National Library of Medicine, Bethesda, Maryland: pp. 85, 194, 276, 350, 355; from *La Nature*, XI/2 (1883): p. 95; from Cesare Negri, *Nuove Inventioni di Balli opera Vaghissima nella quale si danno i giusti modi del ben portar la vita, et di accommodarsi con ogni leggiadria di movimento alle Creanze et Gratie d'Amore* . . . (Milan, 1604): p. 144; photo Niedersächsische Staats- und Universitätsbibliothek Göttingen: p. 79; from Joseph Pennell, *The Jew at Home: Impressions of a Summer and Autumn Spent with Him* (New York, 1891): p. 267; private collections: pp. 173, 275, 316, 319; from *Das Programm, Artistisches Fachblatt*, no. 1187 (4 January 1925): p. 272 (courtesy of Sharon Gillerman); from *Punch* (30 October 1880), p. 238; from Qian Xiuchang, *Shangke buyao* (*no loc.*, 1818): p. 102; photos Rijksmuseum, Amsterdam (Rijksprentenkabinet): pp. 72, 73, 74, 75, 225; from [Jean-Jacques Rousseau], *Collection complète des oeuvres de J. J. Rousseau*, vol. III ('London' [=Brussels], 1774): p. 185; from Eugen Sandow, *Life Is Movement: The Physical Reconstruction and Regeneration of the People (A Diseaseless World)* (London, [192?]): p. 302; from Lewis A. Sayre, *Spinal Disease and Spinal Curvature: Their Treatment by Suspension and the Use of the Plaster of Paris Bandage* (London, 1877): p. 115; from Daniel Gottlieb Moritz Schreber, *Die schadlichen Körperhaltungen und Gewohnheiten der Kinder: nebst Angabe der Mittel dagegen* (Leipzig, 1853): pp. 121, 122; from *Scientific Papers of the Second International Congress of Eugenics, September 22–28, 1921*, vol. II (Baltimore, MD, 1923): p. 255; from Nathaniel Southgate Shaler, *The United States of America: A Study of the American Commonwealth, its Natural Resources, People, Industries, Manufactures, Commerce, and its Work in Literature, Science, Education and Self-government* (London, 1894): p. 208; from W. H. Sheldon, *The Varieties of Human Physique: An Introduction to Constitutional Psychology* (New York and London, 1940): p. 211; from *Simplicissimus*, I/14 (1896): p. 232; Sistine Chapel, Vatican City, Rome: p. 37; Staatlichen Museen zu Berlin, Berlin (Preussischer Kulturbesitz): p. 141 (photo Johannes Laurentius); from John Thomson, *Illustrations of China and its People*, IV (London, 1873–4): p. 295; photo Jörg Bittner Unna: p. 37; from Andreas Vesalius, *De humani corporis fabrica libri septem* (Basel, 1543): p. 106; Victoria and Albert Museum, London: pp. 25 (Guy Little Collection), 195, 199, 258; from *M. Vitruvius per Iocundum solito castigatior factus cum figuris et tabula ut iam legi et intelligi possit* [*De Architectura*] (Venice, 1511): p. 335; from Charles White, *An Account of the Regular Gradation in Man, and in Different Animals and Vegetables; and from the Former to the Latter* . . . (London, 1799): p. 60; from Wilhelm and Eduard Weber, *Mechanik der menschlichen Gehwerkzeuge: eine anatomisch – physiologische Untersuchung* (Göttingen, 1836): p. 85; Wellcome Library, London (Archives and Manuscripts): p. 66 (WMS 136); photos Wellcome Images: pp. 18, 40, 50, 66, 86, 102, 105, 106, 107, 108, 114, 115, 118, 127, 128, 149, 156, 159, 176, 214, 224, 252, 295, 297, 302, 335, 361; photo courtesy Yale Centre for

British Art, New Haven, CT: p. 152; photos courtesy Yale University, New Haven, CT (Harvey Cushing/John Hay Whitney Medical Library): pp. 157, 305.

INDEX